Self-Care in the Elderly

Fatemeh Bahramnezhad
Editor

Self-Care in the Elderly

Springer

Editor
Fatemeh Bahramnezhad
Tehran University of Medical Sciences
Tehran, Iran

ISBN 978-981-96-9020-6 ISBN 978-981-96-9021-3 (eBook)
https://doi.org/10.1007/978-981-96-9021-3

This Springer imprint is published by the registered company Springer Nature Singapore Pte Ltd.
The registered company address is: 152 Beach Road, #21-01/04 Gateway East, Singapore 189721, Singapore

The health of older adults is a priceless asset that must be protected with love, respect, and care

Preface

Aging is an inevitable part of life, bringing its own set of challenges and opportunities. As the global population of older adults continues to grow, the importance of self-care within this group is becoming more evident than ever. Maintaining independence, managing chronic conditions, and promoting overall health depend largely on awareness and the effective implementation of self-care strategies.

This book, *Self-Care in Older Adults*, offers a comprehensive exploration of the physical, psychological, spiritual, and social dimensions of self-care for older adults. Topics covered include nutrition, exercise, mental health, medication management, and preventive care. Drawing on scientific research and real-life examples, this book serves as an invaluable resource for older adults, caregivers, and healthcare professionals alike.

One of the key objectives of this book is to empower older adults by providing them with the knowledge and skills necessary to actively engage in their own health maintenance. Self-care is not just about treating illnesses; it encompasses a holistic approach to well-being, including emotional resilience, social interaction, and lifestyle changes. This book also highlights the importance of family, community, and healthcare systems in supporting self-care practices.

Given the complexities of the aging process, it is crucial to view self-care as a dynamic and personalized journey. Each chapter offers practical, evidence-based strategies to help older adults enhance their quality of life and sustain their independence for as long as possible.

I hope this book will serve as a valuable guide, an inspiring resource, and a source of motivation for all those dedicated to improving the lives of older adults. By fostering a culture of self-care, we can contribute to a more fulfilling and enriching aging experience for individuals and society as a whole.

Tehran, Iran Fatemeh Bahramnezhad

Contents

An Overview of Self-Care

1

Fatemeh Bahramnezhad and Zahra Asadi

In the end, the learner should be able to:

- Understand the importance of self-care for health and well-being
- Identify key components of self-care: physical, emotional, mental, and social aspects
- Recognize how self-care affects resilience, stress management, and quality of life
- Develop personalized self-care strategies that suit individual needs and preferences
- Evaluate self-care practices' effectiveness and adjust for a balanced lifestyle
- Advocate for self-care in healthcare settings to promote well-being and resilience among professionals

1.1 Introduction

Since humans first appeared, they've come up with ways to fight sickness and stay safe. People of early cultures had rituals, ate certain foods for health, and passed down knowledge to keep themselves well. Self-care has deep roots in many cultures and ways of thinking throughout time. Thinkers from old societies like Greece, Rome, and China stressed how crucial it is to take care of yourself and know yourself. Greek philosophy, for instance, linked self-care with loving yourself (philautic) and growing as a person. Big names like Socrates, Plato, and Aristotle talked about how vital it is to think about yourself, control yourself, and not go overboard to have a good life. In Eastern traditions, things like yoga, meditation, and Ayurveda from ancient India focused on self-care to make your body, mind, and spirit healthy. These methods help you know yourself better, pay attention to the present, and look at health as a whole to grow and heal yourself. Many religious and spiritual beliefs also include ways to take care of yourself as part of becoming more spiritual and reaching enlightenment. For instance, Buddhism, Christianity, Islam, and other faiths often teach about being kind to yourself, accepting who you are, and taking care of yourself. They see this as a way to help others better and live a life with more meaning. The idea of self-care we know today has its roots in past movements. The self-help and wellness trends of the 1800s and 1900s played a big part. These movements pushed people to take charge of their own health and well-being. They said that looking after yourself could make you stronger and help you reach your full potential. Even with this knowledge, people didn't have a clear picture of what self-care meant until the late 1900s. As more people started getting long-term illnesses, experts began to see how important it was for people to take care of themselves.

F. Bahramnezhad (✉) · Z. Asadi
Tehran University of Medical Sciences, Tehran, Iran
e-mail: bahramnezhad@tums.ac.ir

F. Bahramnezhad (ed.), *Self-Care in the Elderly*, https://doi.org/10.1007/978-981-96-9021-3_1

1.1.1 Definition of Self-Care

Self-care involves intentional, learned, and deliberate actions that a person takes to survive and boost their own or their family's health. It forms a part of daily life and covers taking care of kids, family, friends, neighbors, and local communities. In essence, self-care encompasses a broad range of actions and activities that people can do to nurture their physical, emotional, mental, and spiritual well-being. It calls for putting your needs first and taking specific steps to ensure balance, toughness, and overall health when facing challenges and stress. Self-care plays a key role in maintaining overall health and preventing burnout, stress, and sickness. It gives people the power to look after themselves, focus on their needs, and build self-awareness and self-kindness. Self-care habits can differ a lot from person to person based on what they like and need and their situation, but the main aim is to create a sense of balance, adaptability, and overall wellness.

Self-care got its start in the nursing field way back when nurses like Henderson and Hall talked about it in their nursing models, but Dorothea Orem was the one who really nailed it down in the 1950s. She called self-care those smart, good-for-you things folks do to keep themselves healthy and grow as people. Her idea of self-care was about three things: getting folks to take charge of their own health, paying attention to what sick people need, and figuring out how to live with sickness. Come 1971, Orem developed a whole nursing theory about this concept. There's the self-care theory, which spells out what self-care is; a self-care deficit theory, which shows where nurses come in when people can't do their self-care solo; and the nursing systems theory, which is all about how nurses connect with each other. These ideas gave nurses a plan for what to do and tied the whole self-care shebang right back to nursing itself.

Back in 1979, Levine was a trailblazer in sociology, coming up with a way to talk about self-care. He said it's all about people taking charge of their own health game, like staying healthy, preventing sickness before it starts, and handling treatment. Then, in 1983, Idler was like, "Yeah, that's right," and spelled out self-care as all the stuff we do to keep in shape, get back on our feet, prevent illness, and put a cap on it.

In 1984, the big guns at the World Health Organization (WHO) chimed in and dropped their take: "Self-care in health means all the things folks, their families, and their communities pull off to stay healthy, dodge illness, keep it under wraps, and bounce back. It's all about what you learn from both expert and street-smart experiences. Regular people get down to this business on their own or team up with pros."

Fast forward to 1998, the WHO hit us with another definition in their piece on pharmacists getting in on the self-care action. They pretty much laid it down that self-care is what you do for yourself to build and keep health, ward off sickness, and duke it out with disease. It's this huge idea that takes in your well-being, what you chow down on, how you live it up where you're planted, who you hang with, the cash in your pocket, and your cultural vibe. Oh, and yes, taking care of your own medical needs too.

Back in 2013, on World Health Day, the WHO took the concept of self-care up a notch. It's not just something a person does on their own. No, it's also the power people, their families, and whole neighborhoods have to keep themselves healthy, prevent sickness before it starts, and handle illness and disability even if they don't have medical pros backing them up. They summed it up by saying "self-care is the ability of individuals, families, and communities to promote health, prevent disease, and maintain health and cope with disease and disability with or without the support of a healthcare provider."

Taking care of yourself is a daily thing. It's about looking after your health as well as taking care of your kids, family, buddies, and people around your area. It's made up of stuff everyone does to keep in shape and have solid mental and physical health. It's not just about staying fit; it's also about satisfying social and emotional needs. Plus, it's about preventing sickness or mishaps from happening, dealing with small sicknesses and ongoing health problems, and staying well after you get over a serious sickness or come back home from the hospital. All these definitions focus on healthy people, zeroing in on preventing sickness as a big aim for taking care of oneself. It's like most healthcare setups are built to handle illnesses only when they show up. The things you do to stay healthy or keep yourself from getting sick, like what you eat, working out, and steering clear of risky stuff, are all up to you, no matter how much doctors try to steer you right. Tons of definitions also give the idea that patients and doctors have to work together. If you think about it, anything that isn't happening in the doc's office counts as your own health gig. When you talk about working together, it means that you're supposed to be all hands-on with your health stuff, not just sitting back and letting the treatment happen to you.

These definitions also include the behavior of individuals as self-care, but several extend this to families and communities. That suggests that caregivers essentially do self-care vicariously and also that some elements of self-care (e.g., the prevention of accidents and provision of facilities to encourage exercise) cannot be attained unless people act in concert. The terms self-care, self-management, and self-reliance are very important to be differentiated.

Self-care refers to people's responsibility for their own health by adopting a healthy lifestyle, planning to prevent accidents and diseases, maintaining good physical and mental health, using over-the-counter drugs for minor diseases, and opting for optimal care of chronic diseases.

Self-management: Self-management means the responsibility and participation of people with chronic diseases in informed clinical decisions, cooperation with people who are responsible for their healthcare, minimizing the impact of the disease on functional status, emotions, and interpersonal communication, as well as monitoring and management of signs and symptoms. Illness is meant to minimize the frequency and consequences of exacerbation of the disease.

Self-reliance: Self-reliance may be understood as the potential and belief of an individual in being independent with regard to performing activities of daily living and life goals themselves without depending on others.

1.1.2 The Difference Between Self-Care and Self-Treatment

Sometimes, the concept of self-care is misunderstood and mixed with self-treatment. Self-treatment is the concept of taking treatment without having enough information about symptoms and diseases or making arbitrary and non-standard treatment decisions. Among the behaviors of arbitrariness that do not comply with the standards of self-care is the wrong use of medicine; not only does it not cure the disease, but it also causes long-term side effects.

Self-care: The active process of looking after one's health, well-being, and happiness, in particular during periods of stress. It involves those activities and actions that one does and recommends for the maintenance of physical, mental, and emotional health.

1.1.3 Definitions of Some Self-Care Concepts

Self-care activities: These involve specific actions or actions that people take in looking after their physical, emotional, and psychological needs, for example, exercising, eating healthily, relaxing, spending time with friends, and seeking emotional support.

Self-care plan: A personal strategy or set of guidelines developed by an individual to prioritize self-care needs and integrate self-care practices into their daily routine. It generally includes goals, strategies, and activities that support overall well-being.

Self-care assessment includes the process of checking on the current physical, emotional, and mental status of a person; pointing out aspects to be watched or improved; and describing appropriate self-care strategies.

Self-care maintenance: The regular process and commitment to engage in the practice of self-care to maintain long-term health and promote well-being. This includes consistency and purposefulness in self-care practices.

Self-care deficit: The inability of a person to care for himself or herself properly because of some physical limitations, emotional stress, lack of knowledge, or possibly external factors. Nursing interventions might be required to assist with such self-care deficits.

These definitions give a broader meaning to the essential concepts and principles of self-care in health and wellness.

1.1.4 The Progress of Self-Care

Self-care has gone through an evolutionary process through cultures, social influences, and history to become the varied practices and approaches we have today. The roots of self-care can be traced back to ancient civilizations such as Egypt, Mesopotamia, Greece, Rome, India, and China. In these cultures, people learned the value of keeping the physical, mental, and spiritual body healthy through bathing, massage, herbal medicine, meditation, and spiritual ceremonies. These ancient civilizations realized the connection between mind, body, and spirit and developed holistic health approaches that placed self-care as an integral part of daily life. It also drew upon the rich philosophical traditions around the world, including Greek, Roman, Hindu, Buddhist, and Taoist philosophies. Aristotle, Confucius, and Lao Tzu were among the many philosophers who taught the ways of self-awareness, moderation, and self-discipline on the path to excellence and harmony of the person. Many of these philosophies advocated practices that cultivate the self, inner peace, and overall well-being. The custom of self-care in the religious and medical traditions continued through the Middle Ages and into the Renaissance. Monastic communities promoted self-discipline, prayer, and meditation as ways of caring for oneself. Physicians prescribed treatments that would maintain health and prevent disease: herbal remedies, diet, and exercise. In the twentieth century, health movements developed centered on holistic well-being, self-improvement, and integrating the mind, body, and spirit. The modern concept of self-care gained momentum in the twentieth century with the rise of self-help movements, wellness trends, and the integration of psychology and holistic health practices. Figures such as Carl Rogers, Abraham Maslow, and Carl Jung emphasized the importance of self-actualization, self-compassion, and self-exploration as pathways to personal growth and fulfillment. The self-care movement has expanded to encompass a wide range of practices and approaches, from mindfulness and meditation to fitness, nutrition, and self-improvement. Over time, multiple and often imprecise definitions of self-care have led to different descriptions in several disciplines. The elusive and complex phenomenon of self-care reflects confusion about the integration of terms such as symptom management, self-efficacy, self-management, and self-monitoring. The concept of selfhood is also linked with wider concepts of autonomy, responsibility, and self-direction. In some circumstances, individuals depend solely on self-care because of a lack of healthcare services. Even though there was a belief in the notion that self-care is an inherently human entity, the use of the same received less attention during the scientific era. This can be said to be in relation to the expansion of nursing and medical schools, where people sought care, mainly in acute conditions. As technological advances increased the knowledge and discretion of health professionals, self-care further declined until the latter half of the twentieth century, when a dramatic shift in disease patterns from acute to chronic illnesses facilitated the spread and need for self-care. Self-care intervention was also considered in view of the increased emphasis on enhancing the inherent capacity of older people to manage their chronic diseases. Autonomy was welcomed by the community and thus marked the beginning of support groups and motivation for involvement in healthcare. Acceptance of a new dimension of healthcare continued to gain more speed as the population was rising along with chronic diseases.

During recent years, self-care has been considered more of a mainstream movement or a mainstream concept regarding the holistic promotion of well-being, management of stress, and development of resilience toward the challenges in daily living today. These are seen in social media and wellness trends that show that there is a surge in various industries and sectors that underscore mental health and self-care practices. Today, individuals are increasingly being encouraged to take active responsibility for themselves with self-care to maintain balance and flexibility in a rapidly changing world. Generally, the evolution of self-care reflects the exploration and adjustment of practices and philosophies supportive of personal well-being, empowerment, and growth amid changes in social norms and values. Self-care is now recognized as a necessary aspect of overall health and wellness, promoting self-awareness, self-compassion, and self-empowerment in individuals who are trying to thrive in a complex and demanding world.

Two major developments justify the revival of the study of care in twenty-first-century society and, in particular, within the scientific field of the psychology of aging. On one hand, population aging is about to become one of the most important social developments of this century. The unstoppable aging trend in most countries should be an opportunity to exchange the concept of older people as passive recipients of care with a preventive model of aging that guarantees shared responsibility for care. On the other hand, the COVID-19 experience has identified the need for a paradigm shift regarding the understanding of care as a right but also a duty. The concept of self-care reached its apogee in the modern COVID-19 pandemic. The COVID-19 pandemic has widely affected healthcare systems in general and, particularly, primary care across the world. In many countries, healthcare services have been overloaded, while nonurgent services have considerably shrunk. This deep transformation of care delivery underlines the key role of patient self-care behaviors in maintaining contagion risk as low as possible and keeping themselves healthy.

1.1.5 Self-Care in Nursing

The term self-care was first used in the nursing literature in the 1950s to describe the learned, positive, and practical activities of individuals in their own time frame to maintain their health and well-being while continuing their personal growth. Although much information is available on self-care, there are still differences in how self-care is conceptualized in the elderly and chronically ill population across disciplines. The findings of the conceptual analysis revealed common features of the self-care process that contribute to long-term individual benefits and the maintenance of general well-being. These features include knowledge and education (health literacy), self-monitoring or self-control, which involve the ability and self-confidence to perform certain activities, and relationships that act as joint ventures. Additionally, action skills related to health needs, goals, and problems are important. The process also involves various self-care activities, including physical, mental, social, and spiritual care. Furthermore, informed decision-making, positive attitudes, active participation in changes, role management, effective use of resources, and adherence to the self-care plan are essential components. Three types of antecedents relevant to the client's self-care were identified: those associated with healthcare providers, those linked to the positive outcomes mentioned, and those related to the systems responsible for maintaining health and well-being. These include increasing knowledge and awareness, increasing adaptation to the disease, reducing symptoms, increasing self-esteem, increasing active participation, reducing the use of healthcare resources, reducing the risk of disease complications, improving the ability to achieve autonomy, improving treatment adherence, improving health status, improving health outcomes, increasing functional ability, improving self-efficacy, increasing patient satisfaction, and improving the quality of life through education, social support, functional skill development, and lifestyle modification. The negative consequences described include poor functional ability, loss of strength capabilities, increased dependence, decreased self-esteem and confidence, decreased well-being, decreased health outcomes, increased risk of disease complications, more healthcare visits, and physical and mental states that are negative. Some psychological factors were found to have negative effects. Seven concepts related to self-care included coping, adherence, empowerment, active participation, self-management, self-monitoring, and self-efficacy.

1.1.6 Different Areas of Self-Care

Physical Self-Care

It includes attention to the body by ways of adequate restful sleep, being physically active, eating the right amount of a balanced diet, being hydrated, and keeping oneself clean. Regular physical exercise contributes not only to physical health but also to mental health by dissipating stress and stimulating the release of endorphins, which are the body's natural mood elevators.

Emotional Self-Care

It focuses on the acceptance and processing of one's emotions in a healthy manner. This may include acts such as journaling, talking to a trusted friend or counselor, practicing mindfulness or meditation, engaging in hobbies or activities that bring happiness, and setting boundaries in relationships for emotional protection.

Mental Self-Care

It involves the stimulation and nourishment of the mind through activities such as reading, learning new things, engaging in creative endeavors, solving puzzles or playing brain games, and seeking opportunities for personal growth and development. It also involves taking breaks, being in the moment, and dealing with stress.

Spiritual Self-Care

It involves the things that one feels nurture their sense of purpose, meaning, and a connectedness to something bigger than one's self. Examples might include prayer, meditation, spending time in nature, celebration and rituals, and developing an attitude of gratitude and compassion. Spiritual self-care can establish a feeling of grounding, calmness, and congruence of one's values and beliefs.

Overall, the general understanding of self-care is that it is an active and deliberate process of listening to one's needs, setting boundaries, seeking balance, and paying attention to self-nurturing practices. People can develop resilience by incorporating self-care into their daily routine and, in turn, decreasing levels of stress while enhancing the overall quality of life.

Recently, self-care has been theorized as an umbrella concept in nursing, which consists of three main functions: maintenance of self-care, monitoring of self-care, and management of self-care.

Maintaining Self-Care

Self-care refers to those behaviors performed to enhance well-being, maintain health, or stabilize physiological and psychological functioning. Among the healthy, self-care emphasizes self-improvement. Among those with chronic illnesses, many self-care behaviors often reflect advice received from their providers, for instance, lifestyle-related or those concerned with medical regimen; the former includes quitting smoking, healthy eating, and stress management; examples of the latter would include following a medication regimen. These activities can be imposed by others—for example, healthcare professionals or family members—and then agreed to by the patient or selected by a patient in an effort to reach his or her goals.

Self-care is maintained through reflection on the utility of the behavior, vigilance regarding the performance of the behavior, and ongoing evaluation regarding the activities' effectiveness. Adaptation is often needed to adjust to changed conditions.

Adherence is a major component of self-care. Adherence to treatments that are evidence-based has the best outcomes. Healthcare providers strive to work with patients to adopt as many evidence-based behaviors as the patient can tolerate and accept.

Self-Care Surveillance

Self-care monitoring involves the habitual and conscious awareness of one's body, often termed "listening to the body." This instinctive behavior is common among humans; for instance, many individuals regularly weigh themselves to track weight fluctuations. Many visit the dentist to check their success in avoiding cavities. In chronic disease self-care, regular and routine monitoring yields the best results. For individuals with asthma, consistent peak flow monitoring and symptom assessment are key components of following their asthma action plan, which helps them respond proactively to changes in their condition. Similarly, other chronic conditions, like diabetes and heart failure, benefit from regular monitoring activities—such as checking blood sugar levels and daily weight checks—contributing to better management and healthier outcomes. Additionally, monitoring emotional well-being is crucial for individuals with mental illness, as it aids in achieving overall physical and emotional stability. These practices promote a comprehensive approach to health management, enabling patients to take informed actions toward improving their quality of life.

Three criteria are needed to effectively monitor self-care. First, clinically significant changes in conditions must be possible over time. Second, there must be a way to reliably detect these changes. Finally, a reasonable action must be possible in response.

The purpose of self-care monitoring is to detect change. This change may or may not be related to a chronic disease, but the self-care process discussed here is a change that occurs due to chronic disease. Detection of a physical change is facilitated by somatic awareness, which is defined as sensitivity to physical sensations and bodily activities. Recognizing emotional change is aided by personal insight and interpersonal awareness. For people with chronic illness, symptoms or signs are diagnosed.

It highlights that when patients can identify and understand their health status, they can take proactive steps before issues worsen. Additionally, it underscores the role of self-care monitoring, where patients track their health and communicate effectively with healthcare providers. This collaboration enhances the care provided and ensures better management of health conditions, making self-care monitoring a crucial element in the self-care maintenance and management continuum.

Self-Care Management

Self-care management requires monitoring changes in physical and emotional symptoms to determine if action is required, which may be due to disease, treatment, or environmental causes. Those with self-care expertise recognize the meaning of such changes, can mentally rehearse alternative actions, and choose an appropriate response. If action is indicated, effective self-care requires action implementation and treatment evaluation concerning specific chronic disease symptoms. For example, asthma-related dyspnea may require the use of a bronchodilator, whereas dyspnea due to heart failure would require an added diuretic. Also, treatment changes may involve consulting health providers based on recommendations about patient self-determination regarding changes in treatments. Finally, self-care management includes evaluating a treatment to decide whether the strategy is to be used again sometime in the future. Situational awareness enhances treatment evaluation through an understanding of events and their significance, the prediction of outcomes that includes awareness of bodily sensations, and the ability to make accurate assessments of changes in response to treatment.

1.1.7 Basic Processes of Self-Care

Decision-Making

The complexity of self-care involves complex decision-making. Successful symptom management requires cognitive judgments based on multiple signs and symptoms, as classical decision theory postulates a deliberate and analytical approach to the evidence before reaching a conclusion. However, our observations showed that this theoretical approach is not the practice in reality for patients.

That is, they do not typically generate and evaluate options systematically. Naturalistic decision-making is a far better description of the process patients use in self-care. The term "naturalistic decision-making" refers to the automatic, impulsive, and contextual choices people make within complex real-world situations. Real-world situations are commonly ambiguous, options are often ambiguous, and decisions must be made quickly. Real-world decisions involve dynamically changing conditions, uncertainty, ambiguity, missing information, time stress, and high stakes. These decisions may have ill-defined, changing, or competing goals. Sometimes several people are involved in the decision-making. For example, patients presenting acute symptoms face a high-stakes decision. That situation is sure to change, and the evolution may be fast. The full decision analysis is not reasonable, given these conditions of expectation.

Reflection

Reflection has its relation to the acquisition of knowledge, both of which are necessary for self-care. Self-care may be adequate or insufficient, purposeful or unintentional, rational or reflective, or automatic or invisible. This duality of process is based on Orem's statement that "self-care is purposeful actions taken in sequence and pattern."

Patients who have poor self-care knowledge tend to carry out fewer self-care behaviors of lower quality. Oddly enough, some patients do practice self-care, however, in ways considered unusual or invisible. For example, many have been known to take their medicines without even knowing why, and others learn to monitor but do not know how to interpret findings. It is reasonable to assume that those with little knowledge might participate in specific education and increase their self-care activity. However, the lack of sufficient reflection is a contribution in its own right. Possibly, these patients will benefit from situational discussions that encourage reflection. Other patients are reflective; however, they do not actively engage in their care. They may understand and know what must be done as self-care for a condition yet rationally decide not to do as recommended. In the literature, this is called reasoned decision-making, intelligent non-adherence, or self-regulation behavior.

1.1.8 Factors Affecting Self-Care

Below are the key factors that serve as barriers and facilitators to self-care:

Experience and Skill

Experience is the foundation of self-care skills. It helps identify patterns and allows suggestions of likely outcomes and reasonable goals and actions that are appropriate in a given situation. For situations that have not previously been experienced, options must be explored by mental simulation.

Self-care skills are crucial; patients should be able to plan, set goals, and make decisions. The development of skills is also facilitated through experience, although some patients can have a particular disease for many years and never develop the skill. Healthcare professionals have to confront the challenge of recognizing the learned experiences of patients, confirming their knowledge, and promoting the development of self-care skills that are necessary.

Motivation

Motivation can be defined as the force that drives people to achieve their goals. Motivation is called internal or external. Intrinsic motivation originates from the desire to absorb and learn and includes the aspects of pleasure and interest. Intrinsic motivation is driven by an internal desire to do a particular task because that task is enjoyable. Conversely, extrinsic motivation refers to changing behavior because it leads to a specific predetermined outcome that is desirable for some reason (e.g., to improve health or please others). Many self-care behaviors are motivated and directed, at least initially, by external stimuli. That is, a person may not have an internal motivation to perform a behavior, but the perception of others about the importance of performing the behavior may motivate self-care.

Cultural Beliefs and Values

While self-care may be important in countries and cultures that prize independence, in some cultures, self-care is not important. In these situations, showing love and concern through care and attention is even more critical when a family member is ill.

Sometimes, self-care recommendations conflict with one's cultural beliefs, as is the case with the encouragement of rest versus activity in patients with chronic heart failure.

Self-Confidence
These aspects of attitudes and beliefs—very important for self-care, especially the belief in self-efficacy—are described as the belief in being able to act and continue through difficulties. Confidence to take appropriate actions at each of these stages of self-care is crucial.

Habits
Daily habits greatly impact self-care. Some patients turn self-care into a habit, while to others, it is a chore. The most successful individuals with self-care may be those who are willing to become compulsive about performing certain behaviors until, over time, the behaviors become a habit.

Functional and Cognitive Abilities
Self-care requires the ability to display necessary behaviors (e.g., balancing a scale). Problems with hearing and vision, impaired manual ability, and limited energy hinder self-care. Moreover, an increasing number of scientific reports indicate that most chronic medical conditions are accompanied by decrements in cognition, including the cognitive aspects of mood disorders, further complicating self-care.

Supporting Others
Although self-care is, by definition, performed by individuals, it would be naive to suggest that self-care is always done alone. Instead, most people with chronic illness acknowledge the necessary communication, decision-making, and reciprocity by family and friends—a process called shared care when it involves two competent adults.

Access to Care
While chronic disease self-care is many times partly influenced by providers after accessing the healthcare system to receive care, one must also recognize that, due to various reasons, such as economic and locational reasons, a considerable proportion of chronic disease sufferers do not have access to the providers of the organized healthcare system. It is to the community workers, parents, neighbors, and friends that they look to guide them. Without exposure to trained healthcare providers, though, chronic disease outcomes remain poor most of the time.

1.1.9 The Importance of Self-Care

Self-care is the linchpin for the management of chronic diseases and plays a basic role in all health aspects and levels of care. Due to the growth in the global market for drugs, diagnostics, and devices, added to the rapid development of digital technologies, new configurations of self-care are becoming possible. Bearing in mind the rise in the number of new interventions, the importance of communication with care, and the supportive role that may be played by the health system, there is an urgent need for a clearer conceptualization of self-care to support health policy. With the rise of chronic diseases, self-care turns out to be the major source of care. It is important that people are forced to take greater responsibility in providing care. Self-care interventions allow individuals to be in a position to make informed choices about their health by having more available, accessible, and affordable care options. Finally, the driving force for shared decision-making, coproduction, and competent self-management reflects self-care practices reinforced in patient education and instructions. They take care of themselves rather than spending time with their providers. Validating this knowledge as a legitimate component of medical care in the context of chronic disease strengthens the rationale for spreading this information to both professional and lay communities. Self-care is an intentional choice-making process through which individuals can take an active part in their care. Self-care encompasses everything from a set of activities to a set of capacities. It contributes to personal agency and independence, accessing and using social and family resources, which, in turn, determine health outcomes. Hence, self-care is about care and relational context, finding ways to create self-care, and avoiding the social and cultural harms of self-medication. From this point of view, the capacity to fulfill physical, physiological, psychological, and self-actualization needs is important.

Self-care is critical to overall well-being and maintaining a healthy balance between work and life. The practice of self-care through regular exercise, proper nutrition, adequate sleep, and annual medical checkups can prevent diseases. Self-care in mental health can positively influence well-being by mitigating stress, anxiety, and depression. Mindfulness, meditation, journaling, and therapy or counseling can all help manage emotions, improve mood, and increase mental well-being. Self-care enables a person to deal with his or her emotions, have self-compassion, and spend much time in growth and self-awareness. This helps an individual become more emotionally resilient, build stronger relationships, and develop emotional well-being. The most common goal of self-care is the prevention of stress and burnout. Lower levels of stress, a better capacity for coping with daily demands, and personal fulfillment might be facilitated through participation in relaxation-enhancing leisure activities, time spent outdoors, and/or other relaxation techniques.

Also, self-care is important in increasing productivity and efficiency. Taking breaks, setting boundaries, and prioritizing self-care activities can reenergize people, increase focus, and increase motivation to get things done effectively. Generally, self-care is necessary in maintaining physical, mental, and emotional health, dealing with stress, enhancing productivity, strengthening relationships, and avoiding burnout. People can develop a healthy and fulfilling life by incorporating self-care into their daily routine, which allows them to spend time on activities that help maintain health and happiness.

1.1.10 Consequences of Self-Care

These common outcomes related to improved abilities include maintaining health and well-being, increasing knowledge and awareness, enhancing adjustment to illness, alleviating symptoms, boosting self-esteem, encouraging active participation, reducing healthcare resource use, lowering the risk of disease complications, achieving autonomy, and improving treatment adherence. Such benefits enable patients to reach a higher level of competence in self-care. The consequences of an independent attitude toward the care process include improved health status, improved health outcomes, increased functional ability, improved self-efficacy, increased patient satisfaction, and improved quality of life through education, social support, development of action skills, and lifestyle changes. Self-care is positive.

1.1.11 Theories and Models Related to Self-Care

Theories of self-care in nursing encompass various frameworks and conceptual models that focus on the active role of individuals in ensuring health and well-being. These theories emphasize the idea that patients have the ability and responsibility to engage in activities that support their physical, emotional, and mental health so as to maintain or improve their overall quality of life. Self-care theories provide a guide to healthcare professionals in a way that the latter may work with patients in the analysis of needs, establishment of priorities, establishment of goals, and the implementation of strategies toward the desired health outcomes. With self-care theories incorporated into nursing practice, caregivers can assist patients to develop the necessary knowledge, skills, and confidence in effectively managing their health. This leads to increased independence, better self-management, and better health-related outcomes.

1.1.11.1 Orem's Self-Care Theory

The Self-Care Theory by Dorothea Orem is a nursing theory that emphasizes self-care activities as the main strategy for maintaining health and wellness. This theory, introduced by Dorothea Orem, a renowned nurse theorist in the 1950s and 1960s, focuses on the role of individuals in assuming responsibility for their health and on the need for nurses to support and facilitate self-care behaviors in situations where individuals cannot meet their own self-care needs. At the core of Orem's theory is the emphasis on self-care or the action of individuals for their own selves to maintain their health and prevent diseases or manage disorders. Self-care includes a collection of activities such as eating and preparing nutritious foods, exercising routinely, managing stress, taking medication as prescribed, and seeking appropriate healthcare as needed. This theory is based on the belief that people are capable of self-care and that they must be encouraged and empowered in terms of their participation in the activities of self-care in promoting health and well-being. This theory also acknowledges that individuals may experience self-care deficits due to various factors, such as illness, injury, lack of knowledge or resources, or environmental barriers, and that nurses play a key role in helping individuals with these deficits. Orem's self-care theory emphasizes the need for the person to take part in maintaining his or her health and well-being while, at the same time, recognizing the professional and valuable role of a nurse in helping people with deficits in self-care. It shows how individuals and care providers work together in terms of health promotion and an enhanced quality of life.

Orem's theory details the concepts of self-care, self-care agency, self-care deficiency, and the nursing system to outline how people, self-care, and nursing care are interrelated. This theory leads nurses to assess patients for their potential for self-care, recognize self-care deficits, plan care, and implement specific nursing interventions to support and promote self-care practices.

Key Concepts of Orem's Self-Care Theory

Nursing self-care theory consists of three related theories:

1. Self-care theory
2. Self-care deficit theory
3. The theory of nursing systems, which are classified as fully compensatory, partially compensatory, and supportive-educational

Self-Care

At the core of this theory is the concept known as self-care, defined by activities that individuals perform for themselves to either maintain or restore their health or both. These activities also include some basic activities of daily living, such as eating and dressing, and more complex ones, such as managing medications or seeking medical care when such needs arise. In this theory, the nurses believe that patients are not passive and only receive health services. Instead, the patients are considered to be strong, reliable, responsible, and capable of making decisions for their health properly.

According to Orem's theory, nursing is defined as "the act of assisting others in providing and managing self-care to maintain or improve human functioning at the level of home effectiveness." The theory specifically focuses on an individual's capability for self-care, which has been defined as "the performance of activities that individuals initiate and carry out on their behalf to maintain life, health, and well-being."

Self-Care Deficit

Orem proposed that individuals might develop self-care deficits if they could not meet their own self-care needs. The defect in self-care arises due to factors such as illness, injury, or limitation of the physical or cognitive ability of a person. In this case, a person requires the help of a healthcare professional or a caregiver to meet their self-care needs. Self-care deficit is an important concept used to describe a state or condition where an individual fails to meet their self-care needs. Understanding self-care deficits involves the identification of specific self-care activities that a person is struggling with and the assessment of the reasons for an inability to meet these needs. For instance, a chronic illness may hinder one from managing his or her medications appropriately, leading to a lack of self-care in medication management. Similarly, personal hygiene may be compromised, as one with a physical disability may struggle with activities of daily living, such as bathing or dressing.

Nurses are very instrumental in the identification and solution of self-care deficits among people. They assess the patient's ability to care for themselves, train them to enhance their self-care skills, and develop a care plan that meets their needs and preferences. In such a way, nurses contribute to returning patients to independence, improving health outcomes, and enhancing their quality of life by meeting the self-care deficits.

The concept of deficits in self-care underscores the prominence of individual factors in self-care within Orem's self-care theory, taking into consideration that one might need external support and assistance in cases where the self-care abilities are compromised. The health professional thus provides personalized interventions and support to address these self-care deficits and, in turn, enable the individual to achieve optimal health and well-being despite the limitations.

In other words, this theory identifies when an adult (or in the case of a dependent, the parent or guardian) is unable or has limited capacity to provide continuous, effective self-care and nursing is needed by identifying and doing the following:

- Acting for others and doing for others
- Guiding others
- Supporting another
- Providing an environment to promote personal development in meeting future demands
- Teaching another

"The condition which confirms the need for nursing in adults is the inability to maintain continuously that amount and quality of self-care necessary to preserve life and health, to recover from illness or injury, or to counteract their effects in the case of children, this state of parental incapacity (or the guardian) is in maintaining the continuity of the amount and quality of care for the child, that is therapeutic."

Assumptions of Self-Care Deficit Theory

The assumptions of Dorothea Orem's self-care theory are as follows:

1. In order to survive and be efficient, humans are in constant communication and connection between themselves and their environment.
2. The power of deliberate action is exercised to identify needs and make necessary judgments.
3. Adult humans may experience deficits in self-care and other activities essential for sustaining life and regulating performance.
4. Human agency is applied in discovering, developing, and communicating to others the ways and means of identifying needs and creating inputs for self and others.
5. Groups of humans with structured relationships cluster tasks and assign responsibilities to group members for providing care.

Main Concepts of Self-Care Deficit Theory

The basic concepts of Orem's self-care deficiency theory are defined in this section:

Nursing can be defined as the art, and a nurse provides specialized help and assistance to persons with disabilities who require ordinary assistance for maintaining their self-care needs and intelligently participates in obtaining medical care that the person receives from the doctor.

People: People are defined as "men, women, and children cared for singly or as social units" and are the "material objects" of nurses and others who provide direct care.

Environment: The environment has physical, chemical, and biological characteristics. It includes family, culture, and society.

Health: Health is "being structurally and functionally complete or sound." Also, health is a state that includes both the health of individuals and groups, and human health is the ability to reflect on oneself, symbolize experience, and communicate with others.

Nursing System

In Dorothea Orem's theory of self-care, the nursing system is an important component that defines the role of nurses and other healthcare providers in helping people with self-care deficits. This theory describes the role of the nursing system in helping people with self-care deficits. The nursing system includes formal healthcare providers and informal caregivers who provide support, education, and resources to help people meet their self-care needs. Nurses assess a person's abilities and limitations, develop care plans, and provide interventions to promote self-care and independence.

Compensatory nursing system: This is indicated by a condition in which the individual cannot "participate in those self-care activities that require self-directed and controlled movement and manipulative movement or medical prescription to refrain from such activity." People with these limitations are socially dependent on others for their survival and well-being.

An example would be caring for a newborn or caring for a client recovering from surgery in a postanesthesia care unit.

Partial compensatory nursing system: This applies when both the nurse and the patient share major roles in performing care actions or other activities involving manipulation or movement.

Example: A nurse can assist a postoperative client to ambulate, or a nurse can bring a tray of food to a client who can feed himself or herself. Educational support system: This system is also referred to as a developmental support system. A person "can do, or can and must learn to do, external or internal therapeutic self-care, but cannot do it without help."

The key aspects of the nursing system in Orem's theory are as follows:

Evaluation: Nurses evaluate the patient's ability to care for himself or herself, identify any self-care deficits, and determine the extent of assistance and resources required to achieve optimal health and well-being. This helps the nurse formulate an individualized care plan that will address the specific self-care needs of each individual.

Planning: Nurses, through assessment findings, collaborate with the individual to formulate a care plan that identifies priorities of self-care activities, establishes goals for improving the person's self-care, and determines interventions to promote and support the person's self-care abilities. Care plans are individualized to reflect the person's specific needs, preferences, and abilities.

Implementation: Nurses implement the care plan by providing education, support, guidance, and encouragement to help individuals effectively perform self-care activities. This may include teaching self-care skills, helping with tasks when needed, and empowering people to take an active role in managing their health.

Evaluation: Nurses evaluate the effectiveness of the care plan by assessing the individual's progress in achieving self-care goals, identifying any barriers to self-care, and modifying interventions necessary to promote positive health outcomes. Assessment helps determine the impact of nursing interventions on a person's self-care abilities and overall well-being.

Application of Orem's self-care theory: Orem's self-care theory has been widely used in different healthcare settings, guiding nursing practice, education, and research. As guides, nurses assess patients' self-care abilities, develop care plans, teach self-care skills, and promote independence. By focusing on enhancing self-care agency and supporting individuals in meeting their self-care needs, health professionals can improve outcomes and empower individuals to take an active role in their health.

Limitations

Orem's theory is considered, in general, as one unit, and Orem defines a system as a unit. Orem's theory is simple yet complicated. The use of the word self-care in a number of terms, such as self-care agency, self-care demand, self-care deficit, self-care needs, and universal self-care, is a bit confusing for the reader. Orem limits health to three stable states, which she describes as a "concrete nursing system" that implies rigidity. The individual's emotional needs are recognized minimally throughout her work. Health can often be conceptualized as dynamic and changing.

Result

It advocates for all patients who intend and desire to take their own care. Patients recover and will do better if they manage on their own as long as it is possible or could take care of themselves. This theory mainly assists rehabilitation and primary care that help the patient perform some activities independently.

Apart from Dorothea Orem's nursing theory of self-care deficits, there are a number of nursing theories on self-care. Some of the most recognized nursing theories that also focus on self-care include the following:

1.1.11.2 Neuman Systems Model

The Neuman systems model, developed by Betty Neuman, is a comprehensive nursing theory directed at assisting individuals to maintain optimal health and wellness through a holistic approach. Based on the concept of stress and the reaction of a person to stressful factors, this model emphasizes the importance of balance and stability to achieve well-being. The key components of the Neuman systems model include the following:

Basic structure: This model has a central core, representing the basic structure or characteristics of the individual, and shows three concentric circles around the core: lines of resistance, lines of conventional defense, and lines of flexible defense.

Stressors and reactions: The stressors, which may be internal or external, are considered disturbances to the stability of a person. This model focuses on how individuals respond to the stressful factors through lines of defense and resistance mechanisms.

Prevention: Neuman's model focuses on prevention as a means of maintaining stability and preventing stressors from causing damage. The nurse is in a prime position to identify potential stressors, strengthening defense mechanisms by the promotion of self-care activities to enhance resilience.

Holistic view: In the model, a holistic view is taken by considering all aspects of the person, including physical, psychological, social, and spiritual aspects. Assessment and interventions are made at various levels to address the comprehensive needs of the person.

Open system: Neuman views individuals as open systems in which there is interaction between the individual and his or her environment and constant energy and information exchange. Such a perspective reinforces the dynamic nature of health and the importance of adaptation to change.

Prevention consists of three components: primary prevention, which consists of the prevention of stressors; secondary prevention, which decreases the impact of the stressor; and tertiary prevention, which consists of promotion and rehabilitation of an individual's well-being. Nurses at all these levels work for health and wellness promotions.

Application to nursing practice: In the Neuman systems model, nurses assess stability and stressors, plan care promoting adaptive responses, and validate intervention effectiveness. This helps in guiding the nurse for holistic care regarding the physical, emotional, social, and spiritual needs of the person.

The Neuman systems model provides an all-inclusive framework for nursing practice through which the resilience of people can be heightened, self-care behaviors enhanced, and optimum health and well-being promoted through stressors and challenges.

1.1.11.3 Levine's Conservation Model

The Levine's conservation model, developed by Myra Levine, is a nursing theory that has focused on promoting adaptation and maintaining holistic health by the maintenance of a person's energy and integrity. This model views humans as holistic beings with interconnected systems striving to maintain balance and well-being. Here are the key components and concepts of Levine's conservation model:

Protection principles: This model is based on four protection principles:

- *Energy conservation*: People need to conserve their energy to maintain their balance and overall well-being.
- *Maintaining structural integrity*: Physical and physiological structures must be maintained to support health.
- *Maintaining individual integrity:* To promote mental health, psychological and emotional integrity must be maintained.
- *Maintaining social cohesion:* Social relationships and interactions must be maintained to support social well-being.

Adaptation: Levine's model emphasizes the importance of adaptation as individuals strive to maintain stability and balance in response to internal and external stressors. Adaptive responses help people conserve energy and maintain health.

Environmental stimuli: This model considers environmental stimuli that can affect an individual's protection principles. Nurses assess these triggers and work with individuals to promote adaptive responses and enhance protection.

Holistic approach: Levine's model has a holistic approach and recognizes the interrelationship of physical, psychological, social, and environmental factors in maintaining health and well-being. Nurses address individual needs at various levels to support adaptive and protective strategies.

Protective nursing theory: Protective nursing is a key concept in Levine's model that focuses on promoting health by helping people maintain energy and integrity. Nurses have a vital role in assessing protection needs, implementing interventions to support adaptation, and evaluating outcomes.

Conservation of resources: To maintain health, people must effectively manage and preserve their resources, including physical, emotional, and social resources. Nurses help people identify and use resources to promote well-being.

Application in nursing practice: Using Levine's protective model, nurses assess the individual's protective needs, develop care plans to support adaptation and maintain energy and integrity, and evaluate the effectiveness of interventions. This model guides nurses in promoting comprehensive health and wellness through the principles of protection.

Overall, Levine's conservation model provides a framework for nursing practice that focuses on promoting adaptation, maintaining energy and integrity, and maintaining overall health and well-being. By addressing the interconnected nature of person protection principles, nurses can support people in achieving optimal health outcomes.

1.1.11.4 Roy Adaptation Model

The Roy Adaptation Model, developed by Sister Calista Roy, is a nursing theory in which individuals and groups continually interact with their environment through an adaptation process. In such a model, people represent adaptive systems through which balanced human development can be gained by continuously making necessary changes in maintaining a balance to meet one's needs. Components of the Adaptation Model the key concepts and components are listed as follows:

Adaptation model: The main concept of the adaptation model is adaptation itself. Adaptation refers to the process of responding to environmental stimuli through a process of maintaining internal equilibrium. Adaptation involves coping with stressors and making adjustments to promote health and well-being.

The model identifies two types of stimuli, namely internal and external. The internal stimuli come from within the individual and might include physiological processes or feelings, while the external ones come from the environment and thus can be physical or social in nature. Responses are behaviors and actions taken up by the individual to adapt themselves to such stimuli.

Adaptive modes: Roy categorizes adaptive responses into four modes:

Physiological state: It involves the physical ways in which the body responds, such as with an increase or reduction in heart rate and hormone secretion.

Self-concept: It concerns the person's view of himself or herself and his or her abilities to deal with problems.

Role performance model: It concerns the social functions and responsibilities of a person in relation to others.

Interdependence model: It deals with the interactions and relationships of people with others within their environment.

Adaptive processes: The model describes three important adaptive processes:

- Regulation: This is the way the body maintains balance through mechanisms that restore balance following a stimulus.
- Coping mechanisms: These are the ways in which individuals manage stressors to maintain adaptation.
- Integration: It refers to the process of incorporating new experiences and learning into one's adaptive responses.

Focal and contextual stimuli: Zinc differentiates between focal and contextual stimuli. Focal triggers are immediate stressors that directly impinge on individuals' adjustment, whereas contextual triggers are broad environmental factors that affect adjustment over time.

Nursing process: Roy Adaptation Model guides nursing practice by assessing people's adaptation levels, identifying their adaptive states, intervening to promote adaptation, and evaluating the effectiveness of nursing interventions in supporting people's adaptation processes.

Application in nursing practice: The adaptation model has been used by nurses to assess individual adaptive responses, identify stressors and stimuli that influence adaptation, and plan interventions to promote adaptation and health and the outcomes of nursing care to promote the processes. They assess the compatibility of people.

The adaptation model provides a framework for nursing practice in which people's adaptive responses to environmental stimuli are highlighted, the promotion of adaptation is important for health and well-being, and the role of nurses is crucial in supporting people's adaptation processes. In such a way, nurses, while addressing people's adaptive states and processes, help people reach optimal adaptation and well-being.

1.1.11.5 Watson's Theory of Human Care

Jean Watson's theory of human care, also called Human Caring Theory, is a nursing theory that centers on the importance of human connection, empathy, and a holistic approach toward care. This theory, by nursing theorist Jean Watson, focuses on the promotion of healing and wholeness through caring relationships between nurses and patients.

The following are the major components and concepts of Watson's theory of human care:

The phenomenon of care: At the heart of Watson's theory lies the concept of care as the essence and moral ideal of nursing. Caring is seen as a unique human-to-human interaction that involves deep communication, empathy, and mutual understanding between nurses and patients.

Transpersonal care relationship: Watson emphasized the importance of developing a transpersonal care relationship between nurses and patients—a relationship that transcends the physical and emotional aspects of caring to the spiritual and existential dimensions and leads to growth and maturation.

Curative factors: Watson proposed a set of ten curative factors that guide nursing practice and augment the care environment. These include developing a helping–trusting relationship, promoting and cultivating the feelings of faith and hope, being sensitive to self and others, and creating a healing presence.

The approach within Watson's theory is holistic; in general, it considers that humans are multidimensional beings interpenetrated by physical, emotional, social, and spiritual aspects, and nurses should approach care focusing on the whole person to support all dimensions of a patient's being.

Moment of care: Watson emphasizes the importance of "moments of care," which are opportunities for authentic and meaningful connections between nurses and patients. These moments are seen as transformative encounters that have the potential to promote healing, comfort, and understanding.

Science of care: The theory developed by Watson is based on the science of care, wherein empirical knowledge, personal wisdom, and ethical principles are integrated into nursing. Science of care emphasizes the importance of attention, compassion, and reciprocity in caring for people.

Application to nursing practice: The nurses, when applying Watson's theory of human care, show concern and empathy and try to establish a therapeutic relationship with the patient. They also include factors that cause disruptions in their practice, prioritize care holistically, and facilitate healing and well-being through proper care environments.

In summary, Watson's theory of human care underlines the importance of caring relationships in nursing, the transformational power of compassion and empathy, and a holistic approach to the promotion of healing and wellness. It is by embracing the principles of human-centered care that nurses will be able to enhance the quality of care they provide and support patients in their journey toward healing.

1.1.11.6 Bandura's Social Cognitive Theory

Albert Bandura's social cognitive theory, also known as social learning theory, puts great emphasis on the cognitive processes, social interactions, and observational learning that shape human behavior. This theory is based on the idea that people learn not only through direct reinforcement and punishment but also by observing others and modeling their behaviors.

Key Concepts and Components of Bandura's Social Cognitive Theory

Triple mutual determinism: Bandura proposed the concept of triple mutual determinism, wherein behavior is said to be influenced by continuous interactions between personal factors (like beliefs and emotions), environmental factors (such as social influences and situational cues), and behavioral factors, for example, actions and responses. These factors dynamically and mutually influence one another.

Observational learning is one of the key components of Bandura's theory. People learn behaviors and actions by observation and imitation of others. This learning can occur by a process known as observational learning, involving the stages of attention, retention, reproduction, and motivation.

Self-efficacy: Bandura proposed the concept of self-efficacy, defined as an individual's belief in his or her capability to successfully execute a certain action or behavior. Self-efficacy beliefs determine the level of motivation and persistence in achieving performance outcomes. Individuals with high self-efficacy are more likely to set challenging goals, strive, and persevere in the face of obstacles.

Outcome expectations: According to Bandura's theory, individuals have outcome expectations. The theory asserts that people weigh consequences and make decisions according to their expectations of certain outcomes. Positive outcomes increase the chances of repeating a behavior, while negative ones may discourage it.

Vicarious reinforcement and punishment: According to social cognitive theory, individuals can learn from others through vicarious reinforcement and punishment. One will be more or less likely to engage in certain behaviors if they see others receive rewards or punishments for that behavior.

Reciprocal determinism shows that Bandura's theory is a dynamic interaction, where people are interacting and being influenced by their surroundings, social interactions, and personal experiences. This interaction goes on continuously to shape behavior and cognitive processes.

Application to behavior change: Bandura's social cognitive theory finds wide application in the fields of education, psychology, health promotion, and organizational behavior. Understanding the role of cognitive processes, social influences, and observational learning provides a basis for interventions on behavior change, skill development, and personal growth.

In summary, Bandura's social cognition theory encompasses the complex interactions between cognitive processes, social influences, and behaviors within a broad framework. The knowledge of the importance of observational learning, self-efficacy beliefs, and environmental factors enables individuals and professionals to apply this theory in enhancing learning, motivation, and personal growth.

These provide good examples of nursing theories that have addressed the concept of self-care in different ways. Each of these offers a distinct perspective on self-care and provides nurses with valuable frameworks for understanding and promoting self-care practices among those in their care.

1.1.12 Importance of Self-Care in Old Age

Self-care is an integral part of human life and is essential in every stage of life, but it is more important in old age due to specific physical, emotional, and social challenges that older adults may go through. Aging is a global issue that has turned into one of the serious social challenges these days. This unstoppable trend of aging societies in most countries is an opportunity to exchange the concept of older people as passive recipients of care with a preventive model of aging that guarantees shared responsibility for care. Currently, older people—those 60 years and above—have the highest population growth rate in the world compared to other age groups. This is due to the advancement of medical science and the improvement in the quality of nutrition and the prevention of many diseases along with it. In the next couple of decades, the percentage of the world's older population is expected to rise from about 12.3% in 2015 to about 21.5% in 2050, according to United Nations projections. The number of people over 65 years in industrialized countries has been growing consistently, adding to a greater challenge for social welfare, healthcare systems, and informal caregivers. Successful aging is not only a question of the right genes but also a matter of how it depends on how people manage their aging process themselves. Two trends underline the role of active self-management and empowerment in old age. First, the growth of an older population and the threat of an overburdened healthcare and welfare system make it increasingly important that older people can take care of themselves for as long as possible. Second, the increasing number of healthy years encourages older people to "find their way" because these added years have a relatively lower stable social structure and fewer meaningful roles. Here, successful aging is understood to be the capability for self-care and orienting oneself with increasing age. This does not happen to be an equal competence for everybody, and once we have found out what exactly is necessary for such an ability to be enhanced, then we shall also be in a position to help overcome both of the problems referred to. Therefore, there is a need for guidelines or interventions aimed at self-management of health in old age, not only to support older people who have suffered certain injuries but also to help prevent and delay age-related problems and help them create (actively) and maintain their well-being. Most needed may be those self-management interventions that provide individuals with a coherent set of cognitive and behavioral capabilities to deal with the various and interrelated difficulties associated with aging while building on their strengths to achieve well-being. Most programs in healthcare are focused on keeping older adults in their homes for as long as possible and preserving their identity, independence, and quality of life. Many factors affect the ability of older people to live in their own homes, such as health status, functional capacity, availability of healthcare services, and self-care abilities. Therefore, autonomy and self-care are key factors for maintaining the functional capacity of older people and achieving maximum lifespan and quality of life.

This becomes obvious since the incidence of chronic diseases increases with age, and increasingly, older people live with a number of comorbid chronic diseases. The cumulative effects of chronic diseases are highly individualized and mostly increase with age. Given the continued growth in the number of people worldwide who live with chronic conditions, there is an increased understanding needed for our care response to living with chronic conditions at individual, societal, and systemic levels. Although healthcare providers and formal healthcare services play a central role in the treatment of chronic diseases, it has been noted that "most of the burden of chronic disease management rests with patients and their families." In particular, chronic disease management requires monitoring symptoms; adhering to prescribed treatments and medication regimens; coping with physical limitations and the emotional consequences of illness; regulating diet, exercise, and other lifestyle modifications; and seeking a specialist's advice and intervention only if necessary. In this context, self-care has become a vital and growing necessity for many older people living in society with multiple complications.

One clear reason why older persons especially need assistance in maintaining and developing such a constellation of skills and behaviors is that more often than not, the aging process is characterized by the depletion of reserve capacities and resources in more than one area, with interactions commonly amplifying losses. For instance, the loss of social roles might affect one's mood negatively, which, in turn, may undermine one's energy to care for one's health and physical condition. The latter may subsequently lead to further loss of social activities and resources. Therefore, a small loss in one area may lead to a downward spiral of resource loss in several areas. With diminished reserve capacity to fully compensate for losses of selected resources, older persons may be especially vulnerable or frail and thus more susceptible than younger persons to diminished well-being. It may, therefore, be particularly relevant for older adults to have a set of self-management skills in place that can interrupt potential downward spirals in multiple important domains of well-being. Simultaneously, this set should contain abilities to enhance one's strengths and build and stabilize important resources to maintain well-being. Therefore, older adults may benefit mostly from self-management interventions that do not focus only on a specific problem but cover all fundamental aspects of well-being, including those that help them actively maintain well-being.

Among the older population, added complexity includes living with chronic health conditions and related functional limitations. Self-care is described as an individual's capacity, tendency, or practice in managing chronic conditions while living, serving as a modifier of health outcomes and symptoms.

However, successful aging requires maintaining not only physical health but also social and psychological well-being. It is, therefore, also important to identify self-management behaviors in the social and psychological domains and examine how to learn or improve them. At the individual level, there are changes in health status that affect a person's ability and capacity to take care of themselves. Disease manifestations at an individual level are believed to be major barriers to self-care; these include functional changes in the form of altered cognition, psychological changes, and physiological changes. Any impairment due to a disturbed mental and physical function can lead to disability and weakness, as it may be related to the formation of chronic diseases. While disability is described as a barrier, the outcome of well-controlled chronic conditions has the positive effect of delaying the progression of chronic conditions, leading to controlled symptoms and positive reinforcement for self-care practices. Perception affects the ability to care for oneself at the individual level. Self-care is influenced positively by factors like self-care self-efficacy, perceived self-care agency, belief in the efficiency of self-care, and optimism since these factors provide the means for producing reinforcing behaviors across the lifespan. Illness perceptions represent a precursor to self-care, suggesting that an older person's perception about the benefit of self-care relates to their preconceived beliefs regarding illness and health. The perceived benefit of health attention for specific symptoms has a strong influence in self-care action.

An active, participatory, and engaged response versus a passive attitude to health at the individual level influences self-care among older people. An active role provides the decision-making capacity needed to determine the course of action in response to symptoms and fluctuating states of health and well-being.

During the past two decades, many studies on self-care have been conducted in the older population. Most of the research on self-care has been carried out with a focus on chronic diseases, such as heart failure, arthritis, or diabetes. Few studies have addressed self-care in the context of health promotion for older people living in the community. However, the study of self-care is important in health promotion, in that it contributes to healthy aging or serves to prevent or delay the onset of chronic diseases, or at least reduces their consequences. In addition, health-promoting self-care activities are important to both healthy older adults and those who are chronically ill.

Understanding the older adult's perspective about health-promoting self-care can help health professionals who can promote self-care behaviors, prevent self-care deficits, and plan educational interventions to keep older adults in their homes as long as possible. It's very important. The meaning that the older people attribute to self-care, the self-care activities experienced, and the attitude toward self-care have been investigated mainly through qualitative studies.

The concept of successful aging, developed through the compensatory selection optimization model developed by Baltes, provides a comprehensive framework for understanding how individuals can navigate the challenges of aging while striving for continued growth, productivity, and fulfillment in later life. The life of this model is based on the recognition that aging is a complex and dynamic process that involves both gains and losses and that successful adaptation requires a strategic approach to managing these changes.

Choice, the first component of the Selection, Optimization, and Compensation (SOC) model, is a process of conscious selection and prioritization of goals, activities, and commitments, in accordance with values, interests, and capabilities. People manage to reduce complexity by devoting energy and resources only to those pursuits that are truly important and realistic for them.

Compensation, the second component of the model, involves the development of adaptive strategies to overcome limitations, challenges, or losses that might occur as a result of aging. Examples include finding alternative ways of reaching goals, reallocating resources to areas of strength, or finding creative solutions to maintain performance and independence in the face of obstacles.

The third component of the SOC model, optimization, involves maximizing potentials, strengths, and resources to realize valued outcomes and promote further development of overall well-being. Through active investment in personal development, skill acquisition, resilience enhancement, and the development of a positive attitude, people can optimize their adaptive capacities and sustain a sense of purpose and vitality in later life.

Empirical support from the biological and social sciences testifies to the principles underlying the SOC model and presents evidence of the efficiency of these adaptive processes in successful aging and improving the quality of life for older adults. By incorporating self-care practices that reflect the guiding principles of selection, compensation, and optimization, the potential of individuals to cope with the challenges of aging, maintain independence and self-efficacy, and strive for personal growth and fulfillment is enhanced. At the end of life, the exploration of new avenues of research may provide deeper insights into the interplay between selection, compensation, and optimization as related to aging in order to better understand how people adapt effectively, grow, and flourish as they age. By embracing the principles of the SOC model and self-care strategies to support successful adaptation, the individual is able to promote resilience, a sense of purpose, and a fulfilling life throughout the course of aging.

Here's a look at the importance of self-care in old age:

Physical health: The maintenance of physical health in old age is crucial for the prevention of disease, injury, and functional decline. Regular exercise, proper nutrition, adequate sleep, and proper hygiene are the essential components of physical self-care in the older people. By prioritizing physical self-care, seniors can increase their overall quality of life, mobility, and independence.

Mental health and emotional well-being: The practice of self-care, including relaxation techniques, mindfulness, social engagement, and mental stimulation, is vital in the promotion of mental health and emotional well-being during older age.

Loneliness, depression, anxiety, and cognitive decline are some of the common issues that are seen in this age group and can be eased with the help of self-care activities promoting emotional resilience and psychological well-being.

Social communication and support: The maintenance of social contacts is a very important aspect of self-care in older adults. Engaging in social activities, spending time with loved ones, joining social groups, and seeking professional support when needed can help seniors fight off feelings of isolation and loneliness and develop a sense of belonging and connection.

Preventive healthcare and medical management: Most adults develop complex healthcare needs over time that necessitate rigorous self-care practices through regular checkups, medication management, chronic disease management, and preventive healthcare practices. In addition, seniors may actually take responsibility for their health and well-being by actively managing their healthcare, advocating for healthcare needs, and adhering to medical advice.

Quality of life and independence: The quality of life in old age and independence can well be promoted when the activities that support physical, mental, and emotional well-being are cared for. In this regard, it will be possible for seniors to increase their functional ability and maintain independence in life for a fulfilling and meaningful existence.

Basically, the role of self-care at old age is priceless. Seniors can increase health, happiness, and their overall quality of life simply by adapting to self-care activities in physical, mental, emotional, and social respects, which will really allow them to grow old gracefully and with dignity. Supporting older people to place significance on self-care is therefore necessary for healthy aging and well-being in later years.

1.1.13 Recommendations Are Also Given for Family Caregivers and Older People

Family caregivers need to first search for educational resources and programs on caregiving, management of chronic conditions, and self-care promotion among older people. These may equip them with the necessary knowledge and competencies for proper support. It is also important to identify and join support groups or networks of caregivers for older adults, as these will help in sharing experiences, seeking advice, and gaining emotional support from others in similar caregiving roles. Such groups strengthen self-care by increasing knowledge and skills while reducing feelings of helplessness and isolation in older people.

Family caregivers must focus on building resilience and other coping strategies to deal with the challenges and stresses related to caregiving. Mindfulness, self-care practices, and seeking professional support can help caregivers maintain their well-being.

Advance care planning is best, and older adults and their family caregivers should participate in advance care planning discussions to clarify priorities for medical care, end-of-life decisions, and future healthcare choices. Having these conversations early can ensure that the older person's wishes are honored and respected. Family caregivers can also be enabled to consider the use of technological tools such as mobile health apps, wearable devices, and telehealth services for remote monitoring of the status of older adults' health, medication, and other vital signs. These help the caregiver stay in close contact with the care receiver. It is also important that family caregivers consider the financial implications of caregiving and seek advice on planning for long-term care costs, financial management, and access to available benefits and resources. Financial planning can help reduce stress and ensure long-term care support.

One of the most important things that needs consideration and observation is the issue of caregivers taking care of themselves to provide better-quality care. Family caregivers are encouraged to practice self-care by maintaining healthy lifestyle habits, regularly seeking rest and respite care, setting boundaries, and seeking emotional support when necessary. The well-being of caregivers is crucial in sustaining long-term caregiving responsibilities. Care by both family caregivers and older adults should be person-centered, respecting the individual's preferences, values, and autonomy in decision-making. This involves collaboration on care plans and solutions that reflect the individual's goals and needs in promoting well-being. Also, the holistic approach to health, having an integrated perspective, and promoting self-care in all dimensions of health—physical, emotional, social, and spiritual—endorsing all aspects of well-being may lead to comprehensive and sustainable self-care practices. Family caregivers and older adults should regularly assess self-care routines, assess progress toward health goals, and make adjustments as needed. Openness in communication and flexibility in the care plan significantly improve health outcomes.

By expanding on these recommendations, family caregivers and older adults can work together to establish a supportive and enabling caregiving relationship that focuses on self-care, well-being, and quality of life for all parties involved.

1.1.14 Advice for Family Caregivers and Older Adults on Self-Care

- *Establish a routine:* Encourage the older person to develop a daily schedule that includes time for self-care activities, such as personal hygiene, physical activity, medication management, and relaxation.
- *Communication:* Establish open and honest communication between family caregivers and seniors to discuss self-care needs, preferences, and challenges. Encourage older people to express their feelings and concerns about their health and well-being.
- *Support independence*: Empower older people to participate in their care and decision-making process. Encourage independence and self-efficacy by involving them in setting goals and making choices about their health.
- *Promote healthy habits:* Encourage older adults to get regular physical activity, eat a balanced diet, get enough sleep, and stay hydrated. Provide guidance on managing chronic conditions and adhering to treatment plans.
- *Seek professional help*: Encourage older adults to see their doctor regularly for check-ups, medication management, and preventive care. Encourage them to seek help from professionals such as nurses, therapists, or social workers if needed.
- *Social participation:* Encourage social interaction and participation in social activities, hobbies, and events. Combat isolation and loneliness by connecting with friends, family, or support groups.
- *Mental health support:* Look after the emotional health of older people and provide support to manage stress, anxiety, or depression. Encourage activities that increase relaxation, mindfulness, and emotional flexibility.
- *Respite care:* Ensure that family caregivers have opportunities for rest and self-care to prevent burnout and maintain well-being. Enlist the help of other family members, friends, or caregiving services to give caregivers a chance to rest and rejuvenate.
- *Safety measures:* Ensure that the home environment is safe and accessible for older adults to prevent falls, accidents, or injuries. Install grab bars, eliminate trip hazards, and provide assistive devices as needed.
- *Celebrate successes:* Appreciate and celebrate seniors' efforts and accomplishments in self-care. Offer praise, encouragement, and rewards to encourage them to continue their self-care routine.

Self-care is essential for the well-being of nursing home residents, who often encounter various physical, cognitive, and emotional challenges that impact their daily functioning and quality of life.

Effective self-care practices in nursing home environments help ensure that residents maintain their independence, dignity, and sense of agency in making decisions about their personal care routines.

Physical health: Self-care in the nursing institution may refer to personal hygiene, cleaning, nutrition, mobility, medication management, and the like. Encouraging them toward this practice of self-care may enhance physical health and prevent pressure ulcers, infection, malnutrition, and medication errors.

Mental well-being: It also enhances the mental health of residents as well as their emotional well-being through involvement in self-care activities. Self-concepts of independence and being able to handle their daily activities give them self-confidence and self-respect, thus creating in themselves a sense of self-worth.

Social participation might also be facilitated by self-care practices in nursing homes and help residents communicate and create a feeling of community and belonging to the place. Group activities, shared meals, and recreational programs regarding self-care will help build a supportive, inclusive living environment.

The level of quality of life could also be increased for the nursing home residents when they become empowered to perform self-care activities in line with their desires and unique needs. In fact, such usual activities could bring about personal identities and a sense of continuity and independence, thus giving the residents satisfying and meaningful lives.

Person-centered care: Emphasizing self-care in nursing homes supports a person-centered care model that respects the independence of residents, their choices, and preferences about daily routines and personal care needs. It is important to involve healthcare providers in care planning and decision-making processes that reflect the values and goals of the residents regarding the practice of self-care.

Prevention and rehabilitation: Such preventive and rehabilitative self-care practices also take place in nursing homes, developing the physical and cognitive abilities of the residents to the fullest possible extent. Participation in activities that maintain or improve functional capacity can therefore be associated with better outcomes in terms of mobility and independence and overall health.

Training and supporting staff: Staff contribute a lot to the encouragement of self-care practices among residents. Comprehensive training for staff, resources, and continuous encouragement will go a long way in ensuring individualized care that is compassionate to meet the needs and self-care preferences of the resident.

Quality assurance and compliance: Implementation of self-care assessments and goals within nursing home care plans enhances the quality assurance and facility compliance measures. By monitoring residents for their self-care outcomes and then making necessary adjustments in interventions, nursing homes are assured that needs are met effectively and efficiently.

Generally speaking, acknowledging and promoting self-care in nursing facilities will increase the physical, mental, and emotional well-being of residents and foster a culture of empowerment, dignity, and person-centered care in these settings. With self-care practices a priority, nursing homes have an opportunity to create supportive, enriching living environments that support residents' rights, independence, and overall quality of life.

1.2 Summary of the Chapter

Self-care is derived from nursing and has been expanded in the literature to include numerous activities that promote health, well-being, and self-preservation. The concept of self-care was first popularized through nursing theorist Dorothea Orem as the theory of self-care deficits. According to Orem, the activities one performs to maintain healthy functioning are referred to as self-care, including hygiene, nutrition, rest, and activity. This theory emphasizes the importance of people taking responsibility for their own care and well-being, while nurses support them in the performance of self-care activities.

Self-care is, therefore, important in nursing because the patient can then be an active participant in the care with the ability for autonomy and independence. Assisting and encouraging patients through self-care practices will help build the competency and confidence required to carry out their tasks of management of health conditions and treatment regimens and informed decision-making about their care. The reason self-care is an important part of nursing practice is because it improves patient outcomes and also enhances the quality-of-care delivery in general.

In the context of the older population, with advancing age, self-care becomes more important and may be challenged by physical and cognitive decline, chronic health conditions, and social isolation. The promotion of self-care practices among older adults is essential for maintaining independence, dignity, and quality of life. Healthcare providers should encourage self-care activities that are pertinent to the needs and abilities of each individual to help seniors maintain health, activity, and social involvement in their daily lives.

A number of theories and models, such as the health promotion model, self-efficacy theory, and transtheoretical model of change, have been developed that can guide the delivery of self-care interventions within nursing practice. These theories delineate the role of individual factors, social influences, and environmental factors in affecting self-care behaviors and their outcomes. The integration of such theoretical input will, therefore, enable nurses to devise appropriate self-care interventions, which not only result in positive health behaviors but also empower the patients to take responsibility for their health.

1.3 Summary of Research Studies

Research studies on self-care cover a wide range of topics and methodologies that aim at understanding, promoting, and enhancing people's ability for self-care of their health and well-being. The following are some studies and findings related to self-care among older people:

In the year 2021, a study entitled "The effect of self-care self-efficacy program on life satisfaction of the Iranian elderly" was conducted by Shafiei et al., who noted that having a self-care self-efficacy program improves the life satisfaction of older people. It follows then that this self-care self-efficacy program is an apt approach toward ensuring that life satisfaction is improved among older people, and it is one that nurses could use to assist older people in reaching an ideal state of old age with much satisfaction in life.

In 2014, a study by Min Hui et al., "A correlational study of illness knowledge, self-care behaviors, and quality of life in elderly patients with heart failure," was designed to explore the relationship between disease knowledge, self-care behaviors, and quality of life in older people suffering from heart failure in Taiwan. They conducted descriptive studies, analyzed data, and drew a conclusion that younger-aged participants with higher self-care behavior and better knowledge of the disease have a greater quality of life. Moreover, there has been a marked difference in physical performance and independence while managing daily life. In such care, the educational aspect for heart failure symptoms should be provided to these heart failure patients, particularly older people. It is very important to improve the patient's quality of life by helping older people and heart failure patients improve and maintain physical functions to perform the activities of daily living independently.

In 2019, Qing Wang et al. conducted a study, "Effectiveness of a community-based self-care promoting program for community-dwelling older adults: a randomized controlled trial," to establish whether this self-care program can enhance self-efficacy, quality of life, essential and instrumental life activities of daily living, and medication adherence, as well as reduce health service use for community-dwelling older adults, and established that this program can help raise community-dwelling older adults' self-efficacy for self-care. The slow pace allows them to maintain well-being while staying in the community.

In this context, Qing Wang et al., in the year 2020, attempted to find the effectiveness of a preventive mobile health application, together with community social healthcare team support, for older adults living in the community, by proposing a study titled, "A Proactive Mobile Health Application Program for Promoting Self-Care Health Management among Older Adults in the Community: Study Protocol of a Three-Arm Randomized Controlled Trial." The result of this study was that mHealth programs, effective in providing accessible health content and facilitating communication between older people and healthcare professionals, are invaluable. Through the interactive functions of the apps, seniors can also stay in touch with their healthcare providers across time and geographic boundaries.

In all, self-care research studies contribute valuable insights into the factors that influence people's self-care behavior, the effectiveness of interventions and strategies promoting self-care, and the use of technology to support self-care practices. By advancing our understanding of self-care and its impact on health and well-being, research in this area is contributing significantly to shaping healthcare practices, policies, and interventions toward helping people lead healthier lives.

1.4 Critical Thinking (Scenario-Based)

Scenario Case: 1

Anna is a 75-year-old female who has lost her husband several years ago and lives alone in a rural area. In the past few years, she experienced several chronic diseases, including diabetes and high blood pressure. He also faces challenges but has tried to follow self-care routines such as monitoring his blood sugar levels, taking medication on time, and maintaining an average nutritional intake. However, he often feels tired and withdrawn, which ultimately increases his anxiety and depression. She often gets tired and withdrawn that ultimately increases anxiety and depression in her.

Critical Thinking Questions

1. How would the healthcare provider assess Anna's current self-care practices and then identify factors that may need more support?
2. What barriers might prevent Anna from managing her chronic illness effectively and practicing self-care? And how can those barriers be overcome to achieve better health outcomes?
3. What resources and social support services are available to help Anna improve her self-care routines and overall well-being? How can these resources be accessed and integrated into her care plan?
4. How can communication and collaboration between Anna's healthcare providers and her family members be improved to ensure a comprehensive, patient-centered approach to her self-care needs?
5. What can be done to make Anna an active participant in her self-care and ensure the development of self-efficacy in managing her chronic diseases independently?
6. How would you make a suitable self-care plan for Anna, considering her personal needs, preferences, and competencies, with regard to age, life situation, and supporting networks?

Scenario Case: 2

Mrs. Smith is an 80-year-old lady who lives in a small apartment alone. Her limited mobility is contributed to by arthritis, and she is mostly tormented by loneliness and isolation. The grown children residing in other states visit infrequently. Mrs. Smith is lax in self-care—she mostly forgoes eating properly and forgets when and which medicines to take on prescription. She hardly goes outside the apartment and also misses occasions that may be both socially engaging and physically enhancing.

Critical Thinking Questions

1. What are the potential consequences of Mrs. Smith's lack of self-care on her physical health, psychological well-being, and overall quality of life?
2. How can social factors, such as limited access to healthcare services or social support, affect an older person's ability to perform self-care?
3. What role do family members, caregivers, and community support services play in promoting self-care among the older population?
4. How might technology be utilized to support the self-care of older adults, such as Mrs. Smith, and maintain her connectedness with others?
5. What are the ethical concerns in addressing self-care issues among older people, especially in instances where independence and autonomy may be compromised?
6. How can health professionals and policymakers collaborate to devise viable solutions that would support self-care and overall well-being of older adults?
7. What are some barriers to or challenges in implementing interventions aimed at the improvement of self-care practices among older adults, and how can such barriers be successfully resolved?
8. How could the attitude toward aging be changed to ensure that, societally, self-care

practice prioritizes the well-being and dignity of older people?
9. What role can educational and awareness campaigns play in empowering older persons and their caregivers toward strengthened self-care practices for healthy aging?
10. How does the holistic, person-centered approach in providing appropriate self-care strategies help the older adults continue being independent with dignity and in good health?

Scenario Case: 3

Mr. Johnson is a 75-year-old retiree living in a nursing home because of advanced Alzheimer's disease. In spite of very attentive care by the nursing home staff, Mr. Johnson often resists efforts at self-care activities, such as personal grooming, eating nutritious meals, and participating in social activities. His family visits regularly and tries to encourage him to participate in self-care programs.

Critical Thinking Questions

1. How does a cognitive impairment, like Alzheimer's disease, impact the ability of older adults to engage in self-care activities, and what interventions may be helpful to support a person such as Mr. Johnson to maintain his personal health and nutrition?
2. What are the implications concerning autonomy and decision-making capacity if an older individual refuses to engage in self-care activities, and how can this resistance be surmounted while supporting the person's dignity and well-being?
3. How does interdisciplinary collaboration among healthcare professionals, caregivers, and mental health experts establish individualized care plans that address the specific self-care needs of older adults with cognitive impairment?
4. What are the ethical concerns in the care of older adults with cognitive impairment, particularly with regard to the balance between beneficence, autonomy, and respect for persons?
5. How might assistive technologies and environmental modifications be used to support older adults with cognitive impairment in maintaining their independence and dignity in performing self-care activities?
6. In what ways might caregiver education and training programs be enhanced to better equip families and healthcare providers with the skills and knowledge to effectively support older adults with cognitive impairments in their self-care routines?
7. How do cultural factors, coupled with individual preferences, influence the approach to the promotion of self-care among older people with cognitive impairment, and how will the principles of person-centered care be incorporated into the care plan to respect each resident's unique identity and values?
8. What is the role of advocacy and policy initiatives in ensuring that high-quality, respectful care of rights, preferences, and dignity in self-care practices is accorded to older adults with cognitive impairment?
9. In what ways do ongoing communication and collaboration between healthcare providers, families, and community resources support the holistic well-being of older adults with cognitive impairment in the areas of physical, emotional, and social needs related to self-care?
10. How might a strengths-based approach be utilized to help older adults with cognitive impairments take an active role in their self-care routines, recognizing their capabilities, preferences, and goals, in order to feel a sense of purpose and satisfaction in daily life?

Bibliography

Alavijeh MS, Zandiyeh Z, Moeini M. The effect of self-care self-efficacy program on life satisfaction of the Iranian older people. J Educ Health Promot. 2021;10(1):167.

Alqahtani J, Alqahtani I. Self-care in the older adult population with chronic disease: concept analysis. Heliyon. 2022;8(7):e09991.

Baltes MM, Carstensen LL. The process of successful ageing. Ageing Soc. 1996;16(4):397–422. https://doi.org/10.1017/S0144686X00003603.

Bandura A. Social foundations of thought and action. Englewood Cliffs, NJ. 1986;1986(23–28):2.

Bandura A. Social cognitive theory: an agentic perspective. Annu Rev Psychol. 2001;52(1):1–26.
Bandura A. Social cognitive theory of moral thought and action. In: Handbook of moral behavior and development. Psychology press; 2014. p. 45–103.
Biggs A. Orem's self-care deficit nursing theory: update on the state of the art and science. Nurs Sci Q. 2008;21(3):200–6.
Clarke LH, Bennett EV. Constructing the moral body: self-care among older adults with multiple chronic conditions. Health. 2013;17(3):211–28.
Dean K. Self-care components of lifestyles: the importance of gender, attitudes and the social situation. Soc Sci Med. 1989;29(2):137–52.
Haug MR, Wykle ML, Namazi KH. Self-care among older adults. Soc Sci Med. 1989;29(2):171–83.
LeBlanc RG, Jacelon CS. Self-care among older people living with chronic conditions. Int J Older People Nursing. 2018;13(3):e12191.
Levine ME. The four conservation principles of nursing. Nursing Forum. 1967;6(1):45–59. Oxford, UK: Blackwell Publishing Ltd.
Levine ME. The conservation principles: a model for health. In: Levine's conservation model: a framework for nursing practice. Philadelphia: FA Davis; 1991. p. 1.
Lommi M, Matarese M, Alvaro R, Piredda M, De Marinis MG. The experiences of self-care in community-dwelling older people: a meta-synthesis. Int J Nurs Stud. 2015;52(12):1854–67.
Martínez N, Connelly CD, Pérez A, Calero P. Self-care: a concept analysis. Int J Nurs Sci. 2021;8(4):418–25. https://doi.org/10.1016/j.ijnss.2021.08.007. PMID: 34631992; PMCID: PMC8488814.
Matarese M, Lommi M, De Marinis MG, Riegel B. A systematic review and integration of concept analyses of self-care and related concepts. J Nurs Scholarsh. 2018;50(3):296–305.
McEwan M, Wills EM. Theoretical basis for nursing. Lippincott Williams & Wilkins; 2021.
Meleis AI. Theoretical nursing: development and progress. Lippincott Williams & Wilkins; 2011.
Narasimhan M, Allotey P, Hardon A. Self care interventions to advance health and wellbeing: a conceptual framework to inform normative guidance. BMJ. 2019;365:l688.
Neuman BM, Fawcett J. The Neuman systems model. Boston: Pearson; 2011.
Ong-Artborirak P, Seangpraw K. Association between self-care behaviors and quality of life among older people minority groups on the border of Thailand. J Multidiscip Healthc. 2019;12:1049–59.
Orem, Dorothea E. Self-care deficit theory of nursing. Nursing theorists and their work, edited by Ann Marriner-Tomey, 2nd ed., Mosby, 1989,
Polit DF, Beck CT. Nursing research: generating and assessing evidence for nursing practice. Lippincott Williams & Wilkins; 2008.
Riegel B, Jaarsma T, Strömberg A. A middle-range theory of self-care of chronic illness. Adv Nurs Sci. 2012;35(3):194–204.
Roy C, Whetsell MV, Frederickson K. The Roy adaptation model and research. Nurs Sci Q. 2009;22(3):209–11. https://doi.org/10.1177/0894318409338692. PMID: 19694080.
Roy C, Andrews H. The Roy adaptation model. Stamford: Appleton & Lange; 1999.
Sabo K, Chin E. Self-care needs and practices for the older adult caregiver: an integrative review. Geriatr Nurs. 2021;42(2):570–81.
Sitzman K, Watson J. Caring science, mindful practice: implementing Watson's human caring theory. Springer Publishing Company; 2018.
Toljamo M, Hentinen M. Adherence to self-care and social support. J Clin Nurs. 2001;10(5):618–27.
Truscott A, Hayes D, Bardsley T, Choksi D, Edbrooke-Childs J. Defining young people's mental health self-care: a systematic review and co-development approach. Eur Child Adolesc Psychiatry. 2023:1–21.
Watson J. Nursing: human science and human care: a theory of nursing. Jones & Bartlett Learning; 1999.
Watson J. Nursing: the philosophy and science of caring, revised edition. In: Caring in nursing classics: an essential resource; 2013. p. 243–64.
Webber D, Guo Z, Mann S. Self-care in health: we can define it, but should we also measure it? Selfcare J. 2015.
Wei H, Wei TL. The power of self-care: an ENERGY model to combat clinician burnout. Am Nurse J. 2020;15(10):28–31.
Wong AK, Wong FK, Chang K. Effectiveness of a community-based self-care promoting program for community-dwelling older adults: a randomized con trolled trial. Age Ageing. 2019;48(6):852–8.
Wong AK, Wong FK, Chang KK. A proactive mobile health application program for promoting self-care health management among older adults in the community: study protocol of a three-arm randomized controlled trial. Gerontology. 2020;66(5):506–13.
Yip JY. Theory-based advanced nursing practice: a practice update on the application of Orem's self-care deficit nursing theory. SAGE Open Nursing. 2021;7:23779608211011993.

2 Physical Self-Care

Zahra Asadi

In the end, the learner should be able to:

- Describe physiological changes due to aging on mobility, balance, strength, and overall health.
- Learn how to develop appropriate and safe exercise programs tailored for the needs, preferences, and abilities of older adults.
- Understand the dietary needs of older adults and their role in maintaining proper nutrition and hydration.
- Learn to identify risks for falls and how to prevent them, including modifications to the environment and assistive devices.
- Focus on promoting autonomy, dignity, and respect in care for older adults by encouraging patients to participate in decisions about their self-care.
- Recognize the interrelationship of physical health with mental health and learn how to address specific issues such as depression and anxiety among older adults.
- Describe the implications of polypharmacy, appropriate administration of medications, and monitoring for adverse effects in older adults.
- Understand the principles of interprofessional collaboration to deliver comprehensive, holistic care addressing the multifaceted needs of older adult patients.
- Describe community resources and programs that promote physical self-care and overall wellness among older adults.
- Improve communication skills to have discourses with the older people and their families regarding proper care and self-care.

2.1 Physical Health

Aging is a slow, chronic, and unavoidable part of the human life cycle that begins at birth. We are living longer than our ancestors today, essentially because of the reduced mortality at younger ages from infectious diseases, accidents, and malnutrition. However, with longevity comes challenges. For the first time in history, we are living long enough to confront a variety of disorders. Heart diseases, stroke, cancer, diabetes, kidney disease, Alzheimer's, and Parkinson's currently represent the major causes of morbidity and mortality in modern societies, and aging represents the major risk factor for each of these conditions.

Estimates are that by the year 2050, the number of adults over age 65 will surpass 88.5 million, further taxing healthcare providers and hospital systems. According to the United Nations, between 1950 and 2000, the percentage of individuals over age 60 rose from 8% to 10% of the total population, an increase of 2%. It is also forecasted that

Z. Asadi (✉)
Tehran University of Medical Sciences, Tehran, Iran

F. Bahramnezhad (ed.), *Self-Care in the Elderly*, https://doi.org/10.1007/978-981-96-9021-3_2

the older population will increase to comprise 22% of the total population by 2050 due to increased life expectancy. A person can differ in chronological age (the elapsed time since birth), biological age (the physiological age of organ systems), psychological age (the perception of feeling of age), and social age (roles and relationships related to age). One can note that age 65 was selected as the threshold for Social Security benefits and services in 1935. However, this threshold has become more flexible over time and continues to be extended as longevity increases and careers last longer.

Aging encompasses several changes across a continuum of body systems, each with its specific care and management needs. Biologically, the process of aging or senescence represents the chronic and natural culmination of the loss of certain regenerative and protective mechanisms that occur over time in an organism. Extending this idea to humans, we can see that by default, aging implies a pre-disease state. Although aging is a major contributor to chronic diseases and these disorders are diseases of aging, it needs to be underscored that aging itself is not a disease, but a unique and natural biological process occurring in all members of all multicellular animal species after they attain reproductive maturity. However, although aging is not a disease, it increases our vulnerability to disease.

Several theories have emerged about the origins of our aging processes. Some believe that aging is a biologically "programmed" mechanism that occurs because there is little evolutionary benefit to being very old, the idea being that if organisms can age for long enough, they will be another competitor for scarce resources that are being pursued by younger generations of organisms. Further extending this idea of programmed aging to humans, aging has been proposed to be mediated by genetically preprogrammed hormones. More specifically, the growth hormone and insulin pathways, which are well associated with growth and controlled by the neuroendocrine system, may have a central role in mediating the aging process of the organism through various forms of gene expression and subsequent hormonal fluctuations. In contrast, another mechanism that might explain the development of aging is the "lifetime accumulation of damage at the cellular level." This hypothesis depends on the idea that production of reactive oxygen species and subsequent methylation changes in our DNA could be one of the basic mechanisms leading to aging. Another more plausible mechanism of aging in which this gene is linked is via the generation of reactive oxygen species leading to oxidative damage.

2.2 Cellular Level

At the cellular level, the basic mechanisms associated with aging arise when cell proliferation eventually slows to a point of complete standstill. Furthermore, increased protein production, resistance to apoptosis, and altered cellular biochemical activity, combined with the accumulation of many similar cells in this state, result in the phenotype we associate with aging. When we are young, the total amount of these senescent cells in our bodies is rather low and manageable, with the greater number of cells not having come to that point of aging functioning in accordance with the normal physiology of the body. It is when the ratio of senescent cells to young cells increases and accumulates in the cells that the onset of aging-related diseases begins. For instance, the development of osteoarthritis is characterized by the accumulation of senescent cells in damaged areas, promoting subsequent degeneration and ultimately a decline in the function of that joint and its usefulness in our mobility. Accompanying the aging of body tissues and organs is a progressive decline in their regenerative capacity. Classically, tissue homeostasis, regeneration, and repair often involve the sequential appearance and parallel incorporation of new parenchymal cells that are produced from undifferentiated precursors.

2.3 Mechanism

Aging has been thought to be caused by various factors associated with cellular aging. It is generally believed that human cells can only replicate a number of times before becoming senescent. Previous research has indicated that telomeres on the DNA strand shorten gradually with cell division. The mechanism for this may be summarized by understanding that telomeres seem to protect the chromosomes. This results in a loss of the protective quality of proteins normally at the distal end of the telomere and allow DNA repair enzymes to recognize telomeres among sites of DNA damage. Thus, as one loses telomere length, one also loses these protective proteins, exposing chromosome ends to DNA repair enzymes. This process is combined with the activation of the transcription factor p53 by the DNA repair complex, which, in association with the cyclin-dependent kinase inhibitor p21, can lead to subsequent cell senescence and, ultimately, the cessation of metabolic functions and replication. One of the major barriers to achieving increased health span, reduced morbidity, and optimal lifespan in individuals and populations is the decline in physiological function that occurs with aging. These impairments give rise to functional limitations, increased risk of chronic diseases and disability, reduced productivity/independence/quality of life, and increased risk of mortality. The impaired physiological function of aging is a threat to longevity and optimal lifespan from various perspectives.

2.4 Pathophysiology of Aging

Three distinct processes can reasonably explain the pathophysiology underlying the aging process:

2.4.1 Free Radical Generation

Free radicals are very well known in the biochemical world to be a natural by-product of healthy physiology in relatively small and regulated amounts. These molecules contain a single, unpaired valence electron. In other words, they exist in highly reactive states around the substances surrounding them because they need to gain other valence electrons from other substances to make the electron configuration balanced. Of note, free radicals can denature proteins and damage membrane lipids, nucleic acids, and some organelles such as lysosomes and proteasomes. The importance of understanding degenerative changes caused by free radicals or reactive oxygen species lies in the belief that accumulated cellular damage through these molecules over time cumulatively overwhelms the cell's damage repair mechanisms, leading to the ultimate physiological collapse of the cell and then the entire organism.

2.4.2 Glycation

Advanced glycation end products are formed when reactions take place between the aldehyde groups of reducing sugars and the amino groups of proteins. The formation of metabolic products is dependent on increased blood glucose. In the older people, the less-controlled blood glucose and changes in glucose tolerance can take wide deviations. Advanced glycosylation end-products predominantly lead to abnormalities such as vascular fibrosis, thickening of basement membranes, impairment of lipid metabolism, and loss of elasticity in collagen. Furthermore, AGEs are linked to the induction of inflammatory responses resulting in the release of substances of inflammation and reactive oxygen species, which further cause damage to tissues.

2.4.3 Reduced Regenerative Capacity

In healthy individuals, the apoptosis of one cell balances with the maturation and healthy growth of another cell, which essentially takes the place of the first cell. Mechanisms within the cell cycle control the programmed death of an old cell and also signal to other cells the need to create a new, healthy cell to fill any metabolic demands that the old cell could meet. Progression between stages in the cell cycle is controlled by regulatory proteins, whose function is markedly reduced in old cells compared to younger, healthier cells. These signaling pathways, derived from these proteins, seem to lose their ability to signal for cellular regeneration and maturation in healthy, younger cells during the aging process, while the signaling through the pro-apoptotic pathway does not, leading to a net loss of healthy, functioning cells.

2.5 Organ Systems Involved

Almost all organ systems participate in the physiological changes associated with aging. All cells undergo age-related changes, becoming larger and less able to divide and replicate. Collectively, the loss of cell turnover, decreased function of mucous membranes, cachexia, wasting of skeletal muscle mass, increased atherosclerotic reduction in vascular compliance, cerebral atrophy, and increased pigmentation ultimately all contribute to the variety of changes we see with aging. It is important to differentiate the normal aging processes from the pathologic changes seen in disease states but which are much more severe due to the loss or complete reduction of compensatory mechanisms. While aging starts at different times in different people, some physiologic systems may show declines as early as age 30, while other aging processes may not occur until much later. Also unlike adolescence, where the developmental timelines are fairly predictable, aging timelines vary from individual to individual. Signs of aging can either be easily seen externally or may be more subtle and occur internally.

2.5.1 Nervous System

Aging is considered to be a risk factor in neurological disorders. In normal aging of the brain, many changes take place which may result in neurological disorders. Generally, with increasing age, many natural changes take place in the brain and the nervous system, but this again differs from person to person. In the early years of life, the brain makes over one million new neural connections every second. In the 30s and 40s, the brain begins to shrink, at an even faster rate by age 60.

2.5.2 Neural Tissue

The aging brain loses neurons and neuroglia; the rate increases after the age of 60, but there is an average annual loss of about 0.1% of neurons from the age of 20 until age 60. By age 90, brain mass will decrease by about 11% compared with a 50-year-old, a loss of approximately 150 grams of neural tissue. Residual tissues exhibit heightened concentrations of possibly cytotoxic elements, including iron, aluminum, and free radicals. Senescent neural tissues furthermore exhibit additional pigmentation, which is mainly attributed to the accumulation of two pigments: lipofuscin, with its brown color, and neuromelanin, with its black color. Lipofuscin accumulation correlates with amyloid protein deposition and neurofibrillary tangle formation. While these features of neuropathology usually occur at a low density within aging brain tissue in the absence of pathology, their density is greatly increased in Alzheimer's disease.

2.5.3 Cerebral Cortex

The loss of neurons is most obvious in the cerebral cortex. The sulci, which demarcate the superficial convolutions of the cerebral cortex, are much more pronounced in the brains of older individuals. Initially, the frontal lobes were believed to be especially sensitive to neuronal destruction, but similar lesions occur in other regions of the cerebral cortex, for example, in the parietal lobes.

Impaired memory is linked with changes in the frontal and parietal lobes, but the majority of people in their 80s have low to moderate amyloid protein deposits and have normal memory. Generally, people with higher amyloid protein deposition have more compromised working, or short-term, memory. Nevertheless, in recent years, the role of amyloid deposits in impaired memory has been questioned and the role of tau protein deposition may prove to be more important.

2.5.4 Hippocampus

The hippocampus is the area of the brain that is responsible for memory functions as well as learning new skills. As we age, there is a progressive loss of a considerable amount of neural tissue in the hippocampus, which may partly account for the increased difficulty that people have learning new languages, for example, as they get older. Further, recent research has shown that navigating a virtual computer environment increases spatial awareness and reduces the loss of hippocampal tissue in both young and older participants. Therefore, at least in principle, virtual reality computer programs could be used to prevent atrophy (shrinkage) in this significant brain area.

2.5.5 Somatomotor Cortex

In all, about 35% of individuals over the age of 70 face challenges with walking. There are many contributing factors, including age-related changes in muscles and joints; however, the nervous system plays a role as well. The somatomotor cortex lies in the frontal lobes of the brain and is responsible for the control of muscles used during locomotion. Beginning in middle age, this part of the brain starts to atrophy neurons, which causes some loss of coordination that can interfere with walking ability and contribute to a more sedentary lifestyle among older people.

2.5.6 Brain Ventricles

Aging is characterized by the gradual enlargement of the ventricles (fluid-filled interiors) of the brain, mostly perhaps due to a slow loss of cells lining these cavities. Enlarged ventricles hold more cerebrospinal fluid and can be visualized by imaging techniques like magnetic resonance imaging. This increase in volume of the ventricular system roughly averages 2.9% yearly. Expansion thus appears to be accelerating with age: those over 70 have an average rate of expansion of about 4.25% per year. While ventricular enlargement is, therefore, a feature of aging in most older people, the impacts of this on cognition remain unknown.

2.5.7 Brainstem and Autonomic Function

The areas of the medulla oblongata and the brainstem appear to have the least neuronal loss. For this reason, the brainstem may be the most preserved area of the brain, reflecting its role in maintaining life, which results from control of breathing, peristalsis, heart rate (HR), and blood pressure. However, with increasing age, such autonomic functions of the brain become compromised, thereby diminishing the ability of the body to respond quickly to internal and external environment changes. Hence, the entire autonomic nervous system (ANS), including the parasympathetic and sympathetic branches, becomes more susceptible to the adverse effects of aging.

These functional changes can lead to undesirable consequences in the aged individual. Diminished baroreceptor responsiveness leads to increased postural hypotension. Standing after prolonged sitting may precipitate a fall and, with it, injury. Another adverse change is involuntary loss of bladder control. Adequate urination requires contraction of the bladder and relaxation of the urinary sphincter, with signals to the brain depending on sensory stretch receptors engaged along with involuntary input from the ANS. Together, these other systems send conscious messages of bladder fullness from exposed regions of the cerebral cortex. With age, all these components become less functional; therefore, these age changes, further compounded by changes in other body systems, including an enlarged prostate in men and weakening of the pelvic floor muscles in women, may ultimately lead to reduced bladder sensitivity and control mechanisms, with the possible sequelae of urinary control problems.

Cerebral blood flow and blood–brain barrier flow density drop by 0.38 % per year, leading to a 27 % reduction over a 70-year lifespan. It should be noted that these changes are induced directly by aging changes in the heart and arteries, and possibly exacerbated in patients with atherosclerotic occlusion of the carotid arteries. The tight junctions between endothelial cells form the major constituents of the blood-brain barrier (BBB) separating adjacent blood vessels in the brain. Neuroglial cells called astrocytes surround brain vessels and provide additional protection to the blood-brain barrier separating blood from neural tissues. The necessity of BBB is to impede the passage of most pathogens and many toxic substances into the neural networks and pathways of the brain; however, low integrity is witnessed in aging people. One recent study has shown that with normal aging, BBB impairment occurs first in the hippocampus, invoking the interaction of harmful substances and inflammatory mediators into this critical region of learning and memory. It may be hypothesized that such impaired BBB function leads to hippocampal shrinkage, eventually resulting in cognitive decline.

2.5.8 Neurotransmitters

Aging is characterized by decreased synthesis of neurotransmitters, such as noradrenaline, glutamate, dopamine, and serotonin. Among these, decreases in dopamine might be most significant, as dopamine modulates motor recruitment and acquisition of new skills as one of the brain's reward chemicals. Normal aging is associated with the decline of dopamine-producing neurons and thus an impaired ability to learn from experience. However, recent findings show that when L-DOPA, a drug primarily used for the treatment of Parkinson's disease, increases dopamine levels, older adults learn as quickly as younger adults.

2.5.9 Spinal Cord

Although neuronal and neuroglial cell aging has very little effect on the function of the spinal cord, it is the changes that occur with age in vertebrae and intervertebral discs that result in increased pressure on the spinal cord itself and on the branching nerve roots, causing a decrease in the conduction of nerve impulses along the motor neuron and thus decreased muscle strength. The combined deleterious effects of impaired sensory and motor conduction are on the ability to move or perform the expected activities, increasing the risk of injury through poor coordination, poor balance, and last, poor motor control.

2.6 Age-Related Changes in the Peripheral Nervous System

Peripheral neuron regression (in terms of axon length), loss of mitochondria, and damage to the myelin sheath are all alterations typically accompanying aging. It has been proposed that increased concentrations of proinflammatory mediators inside the body may give rise to the aforementioned degenerative changes. An aging body is less efficient in removing toxic metabolites; this and the absence of a blood-brain barrier (BBB) around the peripheral nerves could cause damage to them.

Myelin loss would slow down the conduction of the impulses conveyed through those peripheral nerves by 5–10%. Normally, this slowed conduction would not really matter, but in the oldest diabetic patients, it becomes a contributing factor to diabetic neuropathy. This weakened repair capacity could result not only in impaired sensation and motor function but also in a subset of peripheral nerves that remain permanently unrepairable.

2.6.1 Short-Term and Episodic Memory

Signifying the first threat of age-associated neurological change is short-term and episodic memory loss. In someone who has dementia, nothing has changed concerning that person's other abilities; however, they forget how to cook because of the interference to their memory. Memory may also take the form of an annoying instance, such as forgetting to buy the milk listed on your shopping list. Episodic memory, defined as remembering personal events and when and how they happened, is diminished slowly in many older people.

2.6.2 Verbal Skills

Verbal communication skills stay behind, though people over 70 might have difficulties in using or remembering the word. The quick naming of common objects stays consistent until the age of 70 and then declines as the age increase.

2.6.3 Reaction Time

The gradual loss of neurons and the slight slowing down of certain impulsive signals interfere with fine changes in the spinal cord, which further translate into slower reaction times. This can be very dangerous in circumstances where faster reactions are imperative, such as swerving off the track to avoid oncoming traffic.

2.6.4 Depression

Neurotransmitters concerned with elevating mood (notably serotonin) diminish in concentration with increasing age, which may contribute to symptoms of depression. Depression can cause symptoms that may resemble dementia—pseudodementia. It often presents with extreme anxiety.

2.6.5 Emotional Reactions

Generally speaking, older adults are less likely to experience emotional eruptions compared with younger adults. This may be due to the relative structural integrity of some brain structures involved in emotions. Most studies of the amygdala—which is heavily implicated in impulsive behavior and emotional reactions—show little evidence of atrophy, or shrinkage, at a much slower rate than other brain regions. In addition, the amygdala also seems to maintain most of its functional activity into older age.

2.7 Neuroleptic Drugs

An increase in the effectiveness of neuroleptics, which include antipsychotics and antidepressants, in older individuals could be attributed to the overall decline in neuronal mass with age. Routine prescription doses for adults invariably lead to confusion or delirium and should be modified.

2.8 Brain Reserve and Cognitive Reserve

Neurons are unique in that the majority possess no ability to divide, in contrast to most other cells in the body; therefore, when some are lost through age or injury, they cannot be replaced. Brain reserve, often considered an internal redundancy of the brain, is thought to be present by most researchers. Brain reserve refers to the physical endowments of the brain with regard to brain mass and neuron count. Oftentimes, a bigger brain reserve favors a better outcome after brain insults and in various neurological diseases. Brain reserve does not always reflect variations in cognitive function—many people, despite advanced aging, lose brain mass. Hence, the term cognitive reserve was put forward. This means that a higher cognitive reserve can allow for a more effective use of brain reserve toward the manifestation of performance, which might occur through increased efficiency in functional neuron interconnectivity.

2.9 Brain Resilience

The brain has certain features that help compensate for these losses.

Redundancy: The brain has more cells than it needs for normal function. Redundancy may help compensate for the loss of nerve cells that occurs with age and disease.

Making new connections: The brain actively compensates for the age-related decline in nerve cells by making new connections between the remaining nerve cells.

Generation of new nerve cells: Certain regions of the brain, such as the hippocampus (related to memory formation and retrieval) and basal ganglia (coordinates and refines movements), may generate new nerve cells, especially following a brain injury or stroke. Individuals who have suffered from a brain injury or stroke, for instance, can learn new skills, as in the case of physical therapy. People can affect the pace at which brain function decreases. For instance, physical activity seems to decrease the speed of loss of nerve cells in parts of the brain accountable for memory. This form of exercise also helps in retaining the function of the remaining nerve cells. On the contrary, a consumption of two or more alcoholic drinks per day increases the rate of decline in the functioning of the brain.

2.10 Cardiovascular System

The circulatory system is the most vital delivery system of the body, with the primary task of providing blood supply and nutrients to organs and tissues of the body, bringing along digestion products out of alimentary tube matter, carbon dioxide to the lungs, and waste products of metabolism (like urea and uric acid) out of the kidneys for disposal. In addition, the circulatory system is heavily responsible for thermoregulation; in this case, we are concerned with the distribution of heat and blood supply to the inside of the body. The effectiveness of the circulatory system is a primary factor in our health and longevity, but it is limited by age, which in turn affects the functioning of other organ systems.

2.10.1 Changes

Arteries are innately elastic, flexible, and compliant to deliver optimum cardiac performance and uniform blood flow. During ventricular systole, the elastic arteries are stretched and distended as blood is pumped into the pulmonary and systemic circulations, which lowers resistance to blood flow. Age progresses, but vessels, particularly arteries, become less elastic through the rising stiffness and thickness of arterial walls.

The innermost wall of a blood vessel is the tunica intima, and it contains two main parts:

- Endothelium: A cellular monolayer.
- Lamina: A thin layer of connective tissue that supports the endothelium against the tunica media. It consists of elastin (elastic fibers) and collagen and exhibits considerable age-related variation.

The bigger arteries contain a high proportion of elastin, which makes them distensible in rhythm with the forceful ventricular contractions of the heart. Distensibility dampens the pulse wave and encourages a more laminar flow of blood into smaller arteries. Smaller arteries have lower elastic properties and a relatively lower elastin-to-collagen ratio in their walls.

The tunica media lies beneath the tunica intima and comprises layers of smooth muscle cells. This muscular layer is regulated by the vasomotor center in the medulla oblongata, the most caudal portion of the brainstem. The vasomotor center regulates systemic blood pressure by monitoring vasodilation and vasoconstriction.

Aging would create gradual thickening of the tunica intima and tunica media of large and medium arteries. Collagen fibers in the arterial wall would also increase in amount and concentration. Cross-linkage of collagen fibers decreases their normal capacity for flexibility as one ages. With aging and with continued stretching, elastin, which gives the arterial wall its elastic property, deteriorates and becomes more fragile. Calcification may occur to a varying extent of the age-worn blood vessels. These cumulative changes result in accumulating characteristics of poor quality and consequently enhanced arterial stiffness clinically manifested in terms of raised blood pressure.

2.10.1.1 Endothelium

The endothelium is the inner layer of the blood vessel walls, which comes into contact with the blood that flows through it. It is made up of a monolayer of squamous epithelial cells that appear smooth and regular in children and young people, thus minimizing resistance to blood flow.

With age, the endothelium takes on irregular shapes and becomes thicker due to the smooth muscle fibers becoming tunicate from the surrounding tissue. This results in a decrease in the elasticity and compliance of the artery, adding to the lumen size while increasing resistance to the flow of blood.

2.10.1.2 Atherosclerosis

Atherosclerosis, the most common form of blood vessel disease, results from damage to the endothelium, and the causes are varied. It may be due to:

- Toxins (e.g., cigarette smoke)
- High blood pressure
- Hyperglycemia

In the case of input being free from any kind of endothelial insult, the subsequent involvement of atherogenic factors triggers the binding of monocytic cells onto the compromised endothelium and leads to their migration into the tunica intima. Here, these monocytes differentiate into macrophages, which start to alter in function, increasing in diameter. These macrophages take up circulating damaged lipids and cholesterol, leading to their conversion into foam cells. The aggregation of these foam cells results in an atheromatous plaque that can occlude the vascular lumen. Atherosclerosis involving coronary arteries can thus lead to coronary artery disease. The rupturing of the plaque, a very common occurrence, activates the coagulum and may end up being a myocardial infarction. Likewise, acute atherosclerosis in the carotid or cerebral arteries renders the possibility of a cerebrovascular accident even higher.

2.10.2 Chemical Changes

2.10.2.1 Decreased Production of Nitric Oxide

The endothelial cells produce a range of biochemical mediators that modulate the luminal diameter of the blood vessels and thereby regulate blood flow. A key player in this process is nitric oxide, which the endothelial cells synthesize by converting the amino acid L-arginine. The nitric oxide then diffuses into the vascular smooth muscle layer, inducing a potent vasodilatory response that promotes adequate blood supply through the vasodilation of blood vessels.

Endothelial dysfunction with aging, as well as endothelial damage from other etiologies, can decrease the production of nitric oxide, which will subsequently decrease blood flow. Decreased nitric oxide bioavailability can cause, and may underlie, age-related vascular disease, including peripheral vascular disease and angina pectoris.

2.10.2.2 Increased Pro-inflammatory Chemicals

Age-associated circulating pro-inflammatory mediators are seen to rise with age. These mediators are proposed to be involved in vascular processes, such as arterial obstruction and blood-vessel calcification.

2.10.2.3 Impaired Angiogenesis

Angiogenesis, the rapid growth of new blood vessels, is a response to infection or injury and is regulated by numerous chemical signals and growth factors. As age advances, the rate of angiogenesis decreases, typically resulting in significant delays. This decline in angiogenic potential with age can be one factor for the decrease in wound-healing efficiency in older people.

2.10.3 Cardiac Changes

To compensate for the decreased elasticity and heightened vascular resistance of aging and atherosclerotic arteries, the heart's ventricles are required to generate greater contractile force. The myocardium adapts to this demand by hypertrophying. Studies prove that the thickness of the left ventricle rises by about 30% during the years spanning from 20 to 80. This goes hand in hand with a consistent reduction of myocytes, that is, of the critical heart muscle cells forming the myocardium, via apoptosis, or a process of cell death programming. The surviving myocytes experience vast morphological remodeling, commonly in the form of enlargement and habitually in aberrant shape. Furthermore, collagen deposition within the myocardium has a tendency to augment with advancing age. This, along with myocardial mass redistribution, generally results in a profound change in cardiac form, away from the normal ellipsoidal shape and in the direction of a spherical configuration. Deterioration in the heart's structural integrity, augmented by processes like hypertension, may result in calcification and fibrotic scarring of the cardiac valves. This often results in stenosis, or narrowing of the valves, that limits blood flow and thus cardiac efficacy. Stenotic valves often create turbulent blood flow, which is audible as a murmur on stethoscopic examination.

2.10.3.1 Heart Function

The overall decline in cardiac efficiency is due to changes in the blood vessels and the heart itself. Resting heart rate remains relatively stable with age when a person is lying down, but it generally decreases when sitting.

Maximal heart rate is the most apparent age-related alteration in cardiac performance and tends to decline linearly with age during exercise. Healthy young children can reach an approximate maximal value of 220 bpm after maximum exertion, but this value decreases with age, reaching "220 minus age in years." Therefore, at 60 years of age, the expected maximal heart rate will be about 160 bpm. This phenomenon is primarily due to age-dependent changes in the conduction system of the heart. The filling rate of the ventricles also decreases with age, due to some collagen build-up in the walls of the ventricles, which inhibits ventricular relaxation. Along with those, the regenerative potential of the heart becomes lessened with increasing injury or infection.

2.10.3.2 Cardiac Conduction System

A reduction in cellularity of the sinoatrial node begins with age after the fifth decade, with a 50–75% reduction in cell counts. The cellularity of the atrioventricular node is almost intact, while the His bundle or atrial bundle is affected by fibrosis and necrosis. These age-related changes can interfere with cardiac conduction and account for the decrease in maximal heart rate. Furthermore, the lesser population of pacemaker cells builds the risk for arrhythmias in older individuals, with both atrial and ventricular types being susceptible, the most common clinical manifestation being atrial fibrillation.

2.10.3.3 Blood Pressure

This gradual rise in blood pressure has been seen traditionally as a natural result of aging and has formed the basis for ignoring the presence of hypertension in older people.

Good circulation is increasingly difficult to achieve in older age because of a decrease in peripheral vascular elasticity and the accumulation of deposits in the vascular lumen. The increased peripheral resistance may be compensated for by an increase in systolic blood pressure. Similarly, the diastolic blood pressure increases due to age-related decline in cardiac output. Although this increase in blood pressure may compensate for changes that can interfere with adequate blood circulation, it creates new associated risks when blood pressure reaches levels considered high (>140 mmHg systolic and/or 90 mmHg diastolic). Whereas the overall prevalence of hypertension in the general adult population is approximately 16%, roughly 50% of individuals over 65 years have hypertension, which is a major risk factor for stroke, coronary artery disease, and congestive heart failure (CHF). Moreover, cardiovascular disease (CVD) was the leading cause of death among people with hypertension over 65 years compared to their younger counterparts.

2.11 Respiratory System

2.11.1 Chest Wall

In earlier years, the thoracic cage was more pliable. As one ages, rib calcification progressively increases, beginning with the anterior costal cartilages near the sternum, followed by calcification at the costovertebral joints. These changes lead to decreased chest wall compliance.

Age-related dehydration and reduced stiffness of the intervertebral discs have resulted in extra axial load compression, contributing to thoracic kyphosis in older people. Such curvature may extend beyond 50 degrees in some individuals, particularly among elderly women who may have osteoporosis or sarcopenia, constituting hyperkyphosis. Aging thoracic kyphosis reduces intervertebral and intercostal distances, resulting in reduced volume for the thoracic cavity. Along with these, a slow, age-linked decrement in the strength of respiratory muscles is noted, which can largely be linked to the loss of mass of the diaphragm and intercostal muscles. This phenomenon appears even more strongly for individuals whose lifestyle includes sitting down, whose muscles are not used, and whose activity is reduced to the point that soon they will experience loss of muscle mass, muscular atrophy, and weakening.

The outcome of this process involves labored breathing and inefficiency of the cough reflex; thus, one becomes prone to respiratory tract infections. Specifically, the age-related changes involving respiration are focused on elasticity and compliance of the chest wall, which lead to increased work of breathing or residual volume and functional residual capacity. A decline in the strength and function of respiratory muscles is also associated with these changes. All such factors lower the threshold for compensating an acute illness or respiratory failure in the aged patient. Another major effect of aging on the respiratory system is the stiffening of the trachea following calcification of its cartilages. This tightening reduces the cough and gag reflexes, increasing the risk of aspiration of different substances. Due to the weakening of the cough reflex, in some cases these aspirations are asymptomatic and are known as micro aspiration.

2.11.2 Nose

With age, there is a progressive loss of connective tissue in the nose, causing the nasal septum to deform over time, which will make it difficult to pass air.

The secretions of the mucous glands in the airways decrease, leading to the thickening of the secretions of this airway, which in turn makes the expectoration of these secretions more difficult and also favors their accumulation, resulting in chronic coughs. As a result of aging, the hairs of the nose thicken, which is why they also absorb more dust and fine particles, and airways narrow quickly, so nasal cavities need more frequent cleaning. Lung structure changes due to aging can be considered more limited to changes in the alveoli, and changes in the large airways are not significant. Alveoli lose their elastic capacity during aging and become dilated and remain in such a state during a phenomenon called "senile emphysema," which reduces the rate of ventilation.

2.11.3 Respiratory tract

Due to the extensive (85 square meters), warm, moist surface area directly exposed to the external environment, the respiratory system is especially vulnerable to infections and injuries caused by pollutants. This area would frequently encounter infectious agents emanating from different forms of pollution associated with human activity. Given that each inhalation potentially introduces novel infectious agents and irritants, the respiratory tract employs a sophisticated cleansing mechanism known as the mucociliary escalator to eliminate particulate matter. The inner lining of the bronchial tree is coated with mucus, which traps inhaled particulate matter, including dust and bacteria. Ciliated epithelial cells then propel this contaminated mucus away from the lungs. Upon reaching the pharynx, the mucus is swallowed, thereby transferring it to the acidic and sterilizing environment of the stomach. Dysfunction of the "mucociliary escalator" impairs effective removal of pathogens, mucus, and cellular debris from the lungs thus accentuating the risk of infection.

The cilia beat less frequently with increasing age, thus making the mucociliary escalator slower. Research studies that explored individuals across the age range of 19–81 years presented a truly prominent age-related decline in the clearance of inhaled particles. This phenomenon was partly attributed to the gradual reduction in the number of cilia and ciliated cells within the airways, as well as the toxic effects of cigarette smoke on these cells, which further impair particle clearance in smokers. In the younger portion of the population, the airways are extremely sensitive to mechanical stimulation-the inhalation of debris commonly generates a powerful cough reflex with which to expel the irritants. In the elderly, however, it appears that the sensory receptors governing the airways are less sensitive to stimulation, which may be blunting the cough reflex. This condition leads older individuals to be more susceptible to pathogens and irritants that access the deeper lung tissues, thus making them more prone to respiratory tract infections (RTIs). Even in the presence of cough reflex, lower inspiratory and expiratory muscle strength prevents its efficiency.

With advancing age, the upper airways tend to become calcified; therefore, the cross-sectional area of the upper airways becomes increased due to the increased diameter of larger airways, and thus, this will increase the volume of air space not participating in gas exchange with advancing age.

While the elastic and collagen fibers of lung tissue present in the alveolar septum do not appreciably decrease with age, the lungs do eventually lose elasticity, and their expanded state reduces lung pressure and volume. This change probably results chiefly from a gradual cross-linking or atrophy of the elastic and collagen fibers.

2.11.4 Changes to Alveoli

This basically refers to the structural and functional changes in the lungs with age. Lung tissue elasticity is reduced over time, as is airway compliance, leading to an increased diameter of the respiratory bronchioles and alveolar ducts. After age 50, the elastic fibers of the alveolar ducts begin to degenerate. This is when the ducts become dilated. This is followed by widening of the alveolar structure and decreased depth of the alveoli. In aging, this expansion of the air sacs results from destruction of the parenchyma walls and is significant due to the reduction of the general alveolar surface area.

In a healthy environment, macrophages reside in the alveolar environment and capture inhaled particulate matter. In older adults, however, the numbers of macrophages diminish in association with increasing proinflammatory neutrophils. As a result, macrophages and neutrophils in the aged lung become hyperactivated, releasing granules that contain enzymes and reactive oxygen species such as superoxide anions. This further pushes the environment of a chronic low-grade inflammatory condition into the lower respiratory tract, which, in turn, may exacerbate the deterioration of the alveolar structure. It is thought that the tenth decade of life is associated with an approximate 25% decline in alveolar surface area. These age-related changes have an accelerated and aggravated course in smokers and those exposed to other inhaled particulate irritants, leading to the severe state of emphysema, a characteristic of chronic obstructive pulmonary disease (COPD). Increased release of inflammatory mediators within the aged lung tissue may also enhance susceptibility to allergic reactions among older adults. Hence, older adults seem to be at a greater risk for multiple allergies (multiple allergy syndrome) and dying because of severe allergic reactions, including allergy-induced asthma.

2.11.5 Pulmonary Circulation

Increased pulmonary artery wedge pressure due to age has also been observed in healthy individuals without any cardiopulmonary disease. This increase may be primarily due to lesser compliance of the arteries and left ventricular hypertrophy.

2.11.6 Functional Changes

2.11.6.1 Lung Volume

Residual volume (RV) is the volume of air remaining in the lungs following a maximal forced expiration. It is typically around 1.2 liters at the age of 25. There is progression with age for either volume or decreased lung elasticity to augment RV. As with diminished elastic recoil of the lungs like air trapping during expiration, the average RV may usually exceed by about 50% for a normal 70-year-old, i.e., reaching a value of approximately 1.8 liters.

With advancing age, there is a decrease in vital capacity (VC) representation—the total volume of air forcibly exhaled following a maximally inspired volume. In an average 25-year-old male, VC is about 5 liters, decreasing to about 3.9 liters by age 65. Similarly, in females, VC drops from roughly 3.5 liters to about 2.8 liters during the same period. Progressively stiffening chest walls and weakening respiratory muscle strength are considered primarily responsible. With nonsmokers, VC is expected to decline by around 200 ml per decade.

Approximating 6 liters in the male population and 4.2 liters in the female population, the total lung capacity (TLC) is achieved at the last centile. Notably, total lung capacity (TLC) remains fairly constant throughout life. The loss of elastic recoil in the lungs is compensated by an age-related increase in chest wall compliance.

Tidal volume (TV) is the air volume exchanged during a single breathing cycle under normal, resting conditions. TV is about 500 ml and normally changes very little relative to age unless pathological processes occur. However, because chest wall stiffness increases and lung elasticity decreases with age, older individuals need to expend more energy during normal breathing. For example, a 60-year-old professional may require about 20% more effort than a 20-year-old.

2.11.6.2 Oxygen Saturation

Physiologic changes normally associated with aging in the respiratory system diminish the delivery of oxygen to the blood and hence decrease its saturation levels. Pulse oximetry indicates a saturation of 96–98% in healthy persons below 70 years of age at sea level, whereas a person above 70 years of age with saturation at 94% is still to be considered within this normal range.

2.11.6.3 Exercise Capacity

Aerobic capacity declines by 6–10% per decade. In the 6-minute walk test, a standard 6 minutes of walking, for distance covered, an 80-year-old person will cover about 200 meters less compared to a 40-year-old. This reduction in exercise capacity is mainly an age-related impairment attributed to the decreasing cardiovascular function. Other factors include changes in the respiratory system with, for example, increasing anatomical dead space or decreased vital capacity. On the other hand, a lack of exercise reduces respiratory efficiency since sedentary individuals lose strength and volume of more respiratory muscles considerably.

2.11.7 Infections

It is well known that older patients have a significantly increased incidence of pneumonia, both bacterial and viral, compared with younger individuals. Although much of this may be due to a general decrease in immune function, other specific factors may play a role. Pneumonia is commonly caused by aspiration of oropharyngeal secretions, and this aspiration is more common in older people. Perhaps even more importantly, normal mechanical tracheobronchial clearance by the mucociliary system is significantly slower in nonsmoking older people than in their younger counterparts. Finally, older individuals have higher rates of oropharyngeal colonization with gram-negative bacilli than younger individuals, possibly due to poor oral hygiene, decreased salivary flow, or difficulty swallowing.

2.12 Gastrointestinal Tract

2.12.1 Odor

Older age leads to the gradual reduction in the number of olfactory receptors, culminating in diminished smell. The research done in the United States estimates that significant impairment in olfaction is found in about 50% of the population between the ages of 65 and 80 years and in about 75% of the population over 80 years.

Olfactory decline, including the discrimination of odors, can result from age-related bone growth within the skull that compresses the olfactory nerve fibers. Although a localized taste deficiency is common among older adults, usually taste disorders or deficits are considered secondary to an initial olfactory deficit. Some studies argue that impaired sense of taste with aging may also be due to changes in taste cell membrane properties. The gradual erosion of smell and taste, in turn, reduces the appetite, which may lead to decreased food intake and, eventually, loss of weight and malnutrition. An inability to appreciate and enjoy food leads in turn to anxiety. Diminished taste for salt may lead to the increased consumption of sodium-laden foods, thereby worsening preexisting conditions such as hypertension. Encouraging older adults to replace salt in cooking with herbs or mild spices may help boost appetites.

2.12.2 Mouth and Teeth

The oral cavity, which includes the lips, tongue, salivary glands, and teeth, begins the digestive process in mastication, during bolus formation, and in deglutition. During aging, resorption of the mandibular and maxillary bones is coupled with a decrease in bone mineral density, perhaps compromising dental support structures and leading to gingival recession and greater susceptibility to root caries. Masticatory dysfunction may occur in edentulous individuals or those using ill-fitting dentures, with the possibility of low food intake and malnutrition ensuing as consequences. In contrast, the compensatory dietary modifications, which involve eating softer, heavily processed foods, provide minimal dietary fiber—an essential component for maintaining bowel regularity—thereby increasing the risk of constipation.

Xerostomia is a common problem among the elderly. Salivary output is considered to be reduced with advancing age after the age of 70. However, there still lacks a clear link in elucidating the correlation between the age-related acinar cell loss and salivary volume. Xerostomia is often caused by medications administered or sometimes caused by underlying medical disorders; diabetes mellitus being one common example. Xerostomia is even more common among those who take more than four prescription medications per day. A few of the most common classes of drugs that cause dry mouth are diuretics, antihypertensives, antibiotics, bronchodilators, and some antidepressants.

2.12.3 Swallowing

Bolus formation is followed by the initiation of a swallowing reflex in the oral cavity. A muscular contraction is initiated and triggered as the bolus makes contact with the posterior pharyngeal wall. This is the swallowing mechanism, whereby the bolus enters the esophagus through the upper esophageal sphincter. Age-induced physiological changes may interfere with this mechanism; the delay in the initiation of muscle contractions for starting swallowing leads to increased transit time through the pharynx and, thus, dysphagia may develop. This is clinically defined as an inability to swallow or feel obstruction from a bolus in the throat and to increase the risk of aspiration. The prevalence of dysphagia has been recorded to be as high as 26.7% among those aged 76 years and above.

2.12.4 Esophagus

Bolus formation is followed by the initiation of the swallowing reflex in the oral cavity. A muscular contraction is initiated and triggered as the bolus makes contact with the posterior pharyngeal wall. This is the swallowing mechanism, whereby the bolus enters the esophagus through the upper esophageal sphincter. Age-induced physiological changes may interfere with this mechanism; the delay in the initiation of muscle contractions for starting swallowing leads to increased transit time through the pharynx, thus dysphagia may develop. This is clinically defined as an inability to swallow or feel obstruction from a bolus in the throat and to increase the risk of aspiration. The prevalence of dysphagia has been recorded to be as high as 26.7% among those aged 76 years and above.

2.12.5 Stomach

With age, the stomach is less able to hold a large amount of food, mainly because its walls lose their elasticity.

Sometime, the stomach secrets its gastric juice, which has hydrochloric acid and pepsin as part of the digestive processes. The rates of secretion of gastric acid are usually similar to those between older and younger adults, but about 10–20% in the older counterparts see some decline in acid secretion, compared to less than 1% in their younger counterparts. This could, among other things, lead to the reduction in availability of certain drugs, for example, vitamin B12, and cause diseases such as chronic atrophic gastritis. Further, age reduces the number of mucous-secreting goblet cells in the stomach which leads to reduced production of protective mucus and a weakened mucosal barrier, thus exposing gastric lining to injury.

Normally, an alkaline layer of gastric bicarbonate ($HCO3^-$) and mucus protects the stomach lining from the gastric juice. However, studies have shown that aging is associated with a decline in $HCO3^-$ secretion. The diminished mucosal levels of prostaglandins associated with age compromise the gastric protection bestowed upon older individuals, thus predisposing them to mucosal injury including lesions and ulcers. The susceptibility to gastric damage in these people is further complicated by the almost universal use of NSAIDs in this population. To this end, proton-pump inhibitors (PPIs), which inhibit gastric acid secretion, are often prescribed along with NSAIDs to lessen this risk. The decrease in the speed of gastric emptying might be linked to age. A long time that food resides in the stomach may lead to the feeling of being full and increased somatic satiety signals and a decrease in hunger.

2.12.6 Small Intestine

The small intestine is responsible for digesting and absorbing nutrients, and it secretes large amounts of digestive enzymes with the help of accessory organs such as the pancreas and liver. The sites for digestive absorption within the small intestine are the jejunum and ileum. The lining of the intestine has folds that extend to microscopically small structures called villi, enlarging the absorptive surface area. While the heights of these villi have been found to reduce with increasing age, the actual impact on nutrient absorption does not seem to be clinically significant. It is observed that the production of lactase decreases as age advances, which is a predisposing factor for lactose intolerance in older age groups. This reduction is related to decreased activity of the LCT gene that encodes lactase. Aging is also associated with an increase in specific bacterial populations in the small intestines. This dysbiosis can lead to bloating and abdominal pain and causes malabsorption of some essential nutrients like calcium, folic acid, and iron, thus affecting the general health. Proton pump inhibitors (PPIs) have also been identified as the factors responsible for promoting bacterial overgrowth in the small intestine, as this will aggravate NSAID-induced small intestinal injury and contribute to the pathogenesis of systemic disorders like inflammatory bowel disease, diabetes, and autoimmune diseases.

Peyer's patches are aggregates of lymphoid tissue crucial for immune surveillance of the gut.

In doing so, they regulate the gut microbiota and inhibit the proliferation of pathogens. The number of Peyer's patches and lymphoid follicles present in the small intestine progressively declines as one ages, potentially resulting in dysregulation of the indigenous microflora.

2.12.7 Colon

Aging effects on colonic transit time stem mostly from diminished colonic motor function due to neuronal loss, whereas a compensatory decrease in neurotransmitter density and neuroreceptor density further compounds this abnormality. This physiological change induces a slowing of waste propulsion through the colon, which often present as constipation.

Deterioration of colonic mucosa and muscularis due to old age seems to play a role also in the peristaltic effectiveness. Weakened colonic walls may develop diverticula. On top of that, chronic straining may exert undue stress on already-weakened blood vessels, predisposing one to hemorrhoids.

Reduced capacity for the proliferation of digestive epithelium means its poorer ability to repair and regenerate. Quite pertinent is the increasing incidence of intestinal diseases associated with aging, of which age is paramount as a risk factor for colorectal cancer. Recent studies suggest that age-related changes in the intestinal epithelium, especially in the colon, include certain epigenetic modifications, especially in relation to DNA methylation. These epigenetic changes may also have a role in colon cancer development.

2.12.8 Sphincter Control

The loss of control of the internal and external anal sphincters in older people in the presence of essentially normal cognitive function is a most emotionally traumatic and humiliating experience. Fecal incontinence is consequently a major reason for admission of many otherwise healthy individuals to long-term care facilities. Recent studies have shown that the cause is loss of tone of the external rectal sphincter. Biofeedback techniques allowed the restoration of sphincter and bowel control in 70% of a group of patients studied.

2.12.9 Intestinal Microbes

Aging, as such, is accompanied with a change in the composition of the gut microbiota: an increased abundance of facultative anaerobic germs such as streptococci, staphylococci, enterococci, and Enterobacteriaceae. These bacteria are capable of flourishing extensively in environments rich in inflammatory responses. Age-related gut microbial profiles closely resemble those exhibited by individuals with inflammatory bowel disease and obesity. The integrity of the intestinal mucosal barrier built up by epithelial cells usually prevents colon-associated commensal microorganisms from accessing the tissue underneath. But the barrier function diminishes with age and becomes rather porous. In the same way, the decline of the inhibitory function of the mucosal immune system-related factors makes these individuals more liable to infection by GI pathogenic organisms, which carry the greatest mortality with respect to older adults. This population is at risk for *Clostridium difficile* gastrointestinal infection that can cause severe, potentially deadly dehydrating diarrhea. Advanced age (65 years or more) and exposure to antimicrobials are two major risk factors for this pathogen.

2.12.10 Peripheral Organs

With advancing age, atrophy and fibrotic changes in some tissues occur in the pancreas that produces four primary digestive enzymes. This leads to impaired exocrine function and diminished significance in the secretion of chymotrypsin and pancreatic lipase, thus impairing the digestive function of the small intestine.

The liver, a vital organ with over 114 functions, diminishes in size and blood flow with aging, causing a decline in functional capacity. This decline is demonstrated by a decrease in the synthesis and metabolism of proteins, capacity to detoxify substances, and less bile production and flow that consequently affect fat emulsification. Concentration is increased and the salt content of bile is low, contributing to increase in plasma cholesterol concentrations, especially in women. Then the ability of the liver to inactivate drugs quickly is impaired, raising the possibility of dose-related side effects. Therefore, while prescribing drugs to older patients, close monitoring of dosage assays should be performed.

2.12.11 Anorexia Nervosa

Food intake at reduced amount is an age-related phenomenon quite common to older adults, generally resulting from several factors dwelling complexly that bring down one's appetite. These are physiological changes, psychosocial factors, and effects of drugs. The major regulatory mechanism behind appetite is mainly based upon sensing by gastrointestinal receptors that are able to detect food presence, which will then stimulate the release of different kinds of hormones. This release that occurs throughout the day, namely pre-prandially, during eating, and post-prandially, is involved in the modulation of different behaviors in eating and volume as well as amount of food ingested. These hormones—including ghrelin, peptide tyrosine tyrosine (PYY), cholecystokinin (CCK), insulin, and leptin—are some of the key regulators responsible for this modulation.

2.13 Genitourinary System

2.13.1 Pre-renal Changes

Among the many prerenal changes that might affect renal function, a more significant and recognizable change involves the degeneration of the vasculature. Renal blood flow in young adults is around 600 ml/min; however, this value generally decreases by 50% in older individuals. This decrease is typically due to normative age-related changes in the vessels (see Sect. 2.1), which along with renal artery atherosclerosis tends to compound the vascular alterations and further lead to renal ischemia. The ischemia results in cellular necrosis, with fibrous tissue replacing the necrosed tissues, causing a mottled or granular appearance on the outer surface of aged kidneys. The afferent arterioles show evidence of hyaline and collagen deposition beneath the endothelium, contributing to luminal narrowing and decreased blood flow. The microvasculature of the kidney, including the glomerular capillaries, is gradually degenerating and undergoing fibrotic replacement. The age-related changes of a vasculature also include reduced nitric oxide production (potent vasodilators) (see Part 1 of this series), which contributes to further decline in renal blood flow.

2.13.2 Reduced Glomerular Filtration Rate

Reduced glomerular filtration rate (GFR) is the rate at which the liquids found at glomerular capillaries get filtered into the Bowman's capsule. GFR is a common parameter used to assess the progression of a particular kidney disease and is expressed in milliliters per minute. GFR values are usually at their peak in the early 30s, around 140 mL/min/1.73 m^2. Changes in the blood vessels due to aging bring about a gradual reduction in renal blood flow and therefore in GFR. In pure aging, the GFR falls by roughly 8 mL/min for each decade starting at 30 years of age. Thus, by the age of 90, the GFR usually falls to about 65 mL/min/1.73 m^2. A diminishing GFR means lower clearance for metabolic waste products. The main point that should be taken into account, however, is that some do not show a decrease in GFR with age, and indeed many people have been noted to have stable GFR for their whole life, suggesting that some other factors are there apart from aging, which favor GFR decline.

2.13.3 Renal Changes

After the age of 50, most of the reduction in renal mass and weight occurs. Normally, each kidney weighs between 250 and 270 grams in a person aged 20, while in a male or female of 90 years it would weigh between 180 and 200 grams. Estimated renal mass loss is 20% from 40 to 80 years of age. Only 3% of people in the tenth decade of life show normal renal histology. Collagen deposition increases progressively, together with chronic renal interstitial fibrosis. Nephrons continue to age and die, getting replaced by adipose or scar tissue. In a 70-year-old, nephron population numbers may decrease by 30% to 50%. Changes can thus be seen in the aged nephron and its fine structure.

Abnormalities of the glomeruli include a greater incidence of glomerulosclerosis, which would typically lead to progressive capillary collapse. Microscopic glomerular sclerosis is found in fewer than 5% of glomeruli of 20-year olds, increasing to about 30% by the age of 80.

2.13.4 Filtration Membrane Abnormalities

Some nephrons were found to exhibit chronic morphological changes, such as thickening and wrinkling of the glomerular filtration membrane and the Bowman's capsule. These changes work to reduce the effective filtrating surface area. At the same time, increased permeability of the filtration membrane allows for the passage of macromolecules, ranging from proteins to other substances, into the filtrate, thus causing proteinuria.

2.13.5 Tubular Defects

Renal tubules undergo progressive atrophy and are replaced by scar tissue—a process termed tubulointerstitial fibrosis. This seems to stem, among other factors, from an increased incidence of senescent cells; thus, the surface area for the absorption of important materials such as glucose, amino acids, and electrolytes is greatly diminished. The distal convoluted tubules show constriction and may also form diverticula. From these distal tubules, fluid-filled cysts may develop, which increase the susceptibility to renal infection and pyelonephritis.

2.13.6 Impaired Kidney Repair

In adult humans, the kidney has limited potential for proliferation, and it is estimated that only about 1% of all kidney cells retain the capacity to divide and replicate. This regenerative capacity further declines with age, thus reducing the capability of the kidneys to repair themselves. The other compounding factor in this advanced age is a decline in the effectiveness of chemical signals that duly regulate cell division and the processes of repair within the kidney.

2.13.7 Physiological Changes

The slower process of aging with respect to renal function may be considered as one major physiological change. In the absence of any other pathologies, beginning at the age of 65 years, the kidney function of such individuals may be reduced to almost 60% of a younger adult's functioning. Such slow deterioration poses great health importance, especially in the presence of chronic complications and blood circulatory disorders.

Conditions characterized by fluid overload and edema—including heart failure, hepatic disease, and progressive renal diseases such as diabetic nephropathy and hypertension—may be complicated by age-related declines in renal function. Among these conditions, there is a frequent practice of administering diuretics, thus leading to close monitoring and readjustment of therapy in view of gradual renal aging. Additional risk factors for kidney disease in older adults include obesity, diabetes mellitus, hypertension, ethnicity, and genetic predisposition.

Hence, renal age-related changes also compromise electrolyte homeostasis. The impairment of renal blood flow, along with an increased nephron number and decreased glomerular filtration rate (GFR), affects the kidneys' ability to maintain optimal electrolyte balance, particularly for sodium, potassium, calcium, and chloride. Electrolytes are again of utmost importance as blood pressure and nerve impulse transmission; hence elderly people are more prone to hypertension, hypotension, and its symptoms of dizziness.

On the other hand, sodium excretion efficiency declines with age. This could be caused by a reduction in GFR (that is, lowering the filtration of sodium-containing blood) accompanied by tubular degeneration and lessened hormone sensitivity-to aldosterone, as an example, causing sodium retention.

2.13.8 Decreased Acid-Base Balance

While pulmonary structures regulate blood pH, the kidneys perform most of the work with respect to acid-base balance because they can directly excrete acidic or basic molecules. Renal function declines with age, resulting in less clearance of acid-base metabolites and ions of some tubular damage origin. This particular decline with age poses broader risks for older individuals with diabetes because it puts them at risk for acid retention—the buildup of acidic molecules like ketones that can lead to potentially fatal ketoacidosis.

2.13.9 Decreased Creatinine Clearance

Continuous production of creatinine occurs in skeletal muscle, which is a low-molecular-weight compound. The concentrations of serum creatinine are generally steady because kidney creatinine clearance from circulation occurs at a rate equal to its production. By the time one reaches the age of 80, creatinine clearance by the kidney would have decreased by around 30%. Although, a person will find this incredibly high retention of creatinine in the serum due to a concurrent age-related decline in skeletal muscle mass, certain levels would be maintained in normal ranges.

2.13.10 Polyuria and Nocturia

Age-related nephron losses reduce the capacity of the kidneys to concentrate urine, requiring increased volumes of fluids to excrete metabolic waste effectively. Old age also goes along with decreased responsiveness of the renal tubules to the action of antidiuretic hormone, resulting in increased water retention in the collecting ducts and production of more dilute urine. With these impairments, there is resultant increased urine volume-symptomatic polyuria. In such geriatric patients, regular assessment of fluid balance becomes imperative without looking into signs of dehydration, followed by unrestricted access to fluids. Fluid intake at night increases the processing period and aggravates nocturia, which affects 80–90% of individuals over 80 years of age. Educating patients about using the toilet before sleep can help counteract this problem.

2.13.11 Impaired Elimination of Toxic Metabolites

Renal excretion or elimination of drugs concerns careful consideration. Thus, doses of certain water-soluble medications like antibiotics, amphetamine, and digitalis have to be changed according to renal function to prevent toxic accumulation. Elderly individuals may suffer unexpected toxicities from drugs as a result of the overestimation of glomerular filtration rate (GFR). Renal elimination may play an important role in this aspect, but there are also contributions from liver and other organ systems: changes associated with increasing age in such systems may also increase the risk of drug-related adverse events.

2.13.12 Decreased Insulin Clearance

Renal insulin clearance contributes to almost half of the total removal from systemic circulation, with glomerular filtration rate (GFR) that decreases with age due to nephron loss being the main impairment in the kidneys' ability to clear insulin. At the same time, insulin sensitivity also decreases with age in what could be a potential compensatory mechanism for the decrease in renal insulin clearance.

2.13.13 Changes in Erythropoietin and Vitamin D Biosynthesis

- Functionally related to vitamin D biosynthesis, erythropoietin or EPO is synthesized by both epithelial cells lining the nephron tubules and peritubular cells. Tubular degeneration often leads to downregulated EPO production, contributing to diminished erythropoiesis and subsequent anemia. Conversely, some reports indicate increased EPO secretion, perhaps related to age-induced resistance to the hormone. Furthermore, impaired vitamin D biosynthesis also reduces calcium and phosphate absorption in the intestine, which can lead to osteoporosis.

2.13.14 Post-renal Changes

With advancing age, the bladder's elasticity diminishes due to increased collagen deposition within its walls. This reduced elasticity and subsequent fibrosis can contribute to incomplete bladder emptying during micturition, particularly in males with benign prostatic hyperplasia. While the extent of age-related bladder changes remains a subject of debate, contemporary research indicates that significant alterations are infrequent.

2.14 Aging and Urinary Incontinence

With old age, urinary sphincter loses tone that may lead to urinary incontinence, which is one of the common age-related neurological incidents. Though common, incontinence is age related and not a concomitant effect of the aging process because some individuals will never experience it as they age.

According to studies, approximately 11.6% of those aged between 65 and 80 years suffer from urinary incontinence. This condition is reported to rise to approximately 35% among those older than 85 years and rises to an astounding 69% in its final age group, those older than 85 years living in a nursing home. Men have shown lower susceptibility to incontinence as opposed to women (26.6–35.0% vs. 12.6–24.0% in people aged 85 years or older) probably because of the effects of childbirth on the pelvic floor musculature. Psychological health and overall quality of life can be majorly affected by urinary incontinence.

2.14.1 Bladder

Urinary incontinence is seen in 17% of men and 23% of women over 65. In about half of women and a fifth of men this is due to stress incontinence alone. The ability of the bladder to hold more is reduced with age from around 500–600 ml in the group below 65 years to 250–600 ml above the age of 65 years. In younger people, desire-to-void sensation occurs with more than half filling but this often occurs later or sometimes never appears leading to overflow incontinence among many older people.

2.14.2 The Aging Urethral and Prostate

Conflicting data exist regarding the age-related changes in the female urethra. Some studies consider thin urethral walls with contraction, atrophy, etc. However, others say that no change in length occurs with age. Furthermore, alterations in pH with age can also disturb the vaginal microbial flora and increase susceptibility to urinary tract infections.

2.14.3 Prostate

Benign prostatic hyperplasia is a common condition, especially in older men, and is seen as nonmalignant enlargement of the prostate. The enlargement causes the urethra to be compressed steadily and eventually leads to difficulty in voiding. More than 90% of men have symptomatic prostatic hyperplasia with varying degrees of bladder neck obstruction and urinary retention by age 80. The cause of the hyperplasia is an increased concentration of dihydrotestosterone (DHT) in prostate cells. Two age-related changes account for the increased intraprostatic concentration of DHT: an increase in the number of androgen receptors on prostate cells mediated by estrogen, and a reduction in intracellular catabolism of DHT. One treatment option for benign prostatic hyperplasia is endocrine-based therapy aimed at decreasing intracellular concentrations of DHT with competitive steroid antagonists. Development of prostate cancer is also largely associated with enlargement of the prostate, which leads to compression of the urethra so that there is decreased flow rate of urine. Malignancy vs. benign prostatic hyperplasia associated with aging will warrant diagnostic evaluations such as PSA tests along with a physical examination of the prostate gland.

2.15 Reproductive System

2.15.1 Women

2.15.1.1 Ovaries

The number of ovarian follicles is gradually reduced throughout the lifespan of women. It reaches an accelerated phase during the fourth decade of life, after which it stabilizes at a very slow pace. The number and quality of ovaries declined with the reduction of estrogen production, which, in most women, results in menopause at about age 51. The aging process in relation to ovaries is primarily affected by genetic factors, though oxidative stress, aging, and environmental exposures do confer their share. Events identified as posing potential causative factors for the onset of premature ovarian failure (POF) include surgical interventions, radiotherapy, chemotherapy, autoimmune disorders, and infections due to mumps and cytomegalovirus.

2.15.1.2 Peri-menopause

Menopause is when menstruation and the capacity for reproduction stops in women. Hormonal fluctuations that lead to these changes begin early, even during the menstrual cycle phase. This can occur over a period from 2 to 10 years and is often characterized by increased menstrual cycle irregularity. Though there is still a possibility for childbearing in peri-menopause, conceiving does become harder. Symptoms related to peri-menopause closely resemble those of menopause. All of these symptoms are caused by hormonal fluctuations in the body, which trigger hot flashes, night sweats, mood swings, feelings of sadness, and other related effects.

2.15.1.3 Menopause

Quite a lot of women experience irregular periods in their cycles during perimenopause until they come to an end. Menopause signifies the cessation of menses for 12 successive months. About 95% of women experience it in their lives between ages 44 and 56 with a mean age of 50.7 years. Various factors that give rise to POF may result in the onset of early menopause. Since the production of eggs totally ceases, pregnancy without infertility treatment is out of question.

Hormonal changes in menstrual cycle are controlled by follicle-stimulating hormone (FSH), produced by the pituitary gland. FSH promotes the evolution of ovarian follicles. While developing, these follicles make and secrete estrogen. Women, both premenopausal and postmenopausal, will have elevated FSH levels; however, in postmenopausal women, FSH can no longer initiate follicular activity. When follicular activity comes to an end, estrogen production is reduced to low levels. Vasomotor symptoms, such as hot flashes, are related to increased FSH levels and decreased estrogen levels. Additionally, decreased estrogen levels lead to a fall in serotonin levels in the hypothalamus, inciting disturbances in the set point of the thermoregulatory center. Changes in these hormones—FSH, estrogen, and progesterone—are often associated with affective instability, poor cognition (memory and concentration), trouble with relationships, and low self-worth.

A vaginal time lapse refers to a period following menopause during which a person undergoes natural physiological changes, including a reduction in vaginal size and elasticity. Thinning of the vaginal epithelium and also the cessation of production of natural lubricating secretions create abrasions, bleedings, and infections. Lactobacilli, which produce lactic acid, become diminished, and this brings about a change in the pH of the vagina toward a lower value. An allusion can be made to the colonization of *Candida albicans* and other opportunistic microorganisms. All of these physiological changes accompanied by dyspareunia denote a condition suffixed under a term meaning painful sexual contact, hence rendering coitus very uncomfortable or painful and curtailing the drive for it. Studies show that between 27% and 60% of middle-aged women describe experiencing vaginal dryness and dyspareunia.

Another complaint that a menopausal woman succumbs to is urinary incontinence. Both the bladder and the urethra contain estrogen receptors; they are very sensitive to estrogen. Therefore, deficiency of estrogen leads to shrinkage of the urethra and as a result to urinary incontinence. Likewise, breast tissue responds to estrogen and most women will have lost some amount of the connective tissue that supports their breasts at this stage in their lives. On top of this, the process of skin ageing that results in thinning and loss of elasticity may strengthen these effects.

2.15.1.4 Fallopian Tubes

Impaired contractility of the fallopian tubes, coupled with a reduction in ciliated epithelium and mucus production, has been documented. These factors are implicated in the decline of age-related fertility, given that a significant proportion of conceptions rely on the proper function of this anatomical region for the transport of fertilized ova from the fallopian tube to the uterine cavity.

2.15.1.5 Uterus and Cervix

The endometrium, which is essentially the lining of the uterus, undergoes cyclic shedding, followed by a regenerative phase supported by estrogen during menstrual cycles. With the onset of menopause, estrogen production declines, and the integrity of this regenerative process becomes more and more compromised, until it completely ceases and menstruation is said to stop.

The myometrium, the innermost layer of the uterus, is composed of smooth muscle fibers and undergoes atrophy after menopause. Since estrogen is known to maintain the myometrium, it is assumed that decreased levels of estrogen may assist the noted loss in myometrial smooth muscle fibers. The thin serosa of the uterus, or perimetrium, appears to undergo comparatively fewer changes with aging.

The cervical or uterine neck consists of a smooth muscle layer with an overlying mucus-secreting cervical epithelium. Decreased cervical secretions during menopause affect receptivity to conception.

2.15.2 Men

2.15.2.1 Testicles and Vas Deferens

Men also undergo certain age-related modifications: primary among these would be declining testicular volume, often correlated with testosterone and sperm production; high volume is still possible in those men, keeping them fertile late into life.

Even though erectile dysfunction (ED) may prove troublesome, advanced age does not seem to affect the amount of sperm produced. Changes in flexibility can occur in the vas deferens responsible for sperm transport during ejaculation due to deposition of collagen and subsequent sclerosis of the vas deferens walls.

2.15.2.2 Prostate Gland and Seminal Vesicles

The decline in the secretory output of the seminal vesicles and prostate gland, which form the main constituents of semen, results in a reduced volume of ejaculate. Thus, with this concomitant decline in sperm count, sperm concentration is generally preserved to lessen the impact on fertility. And also, the drop in prostatic secretions will increase vulnerability to infections in the urinary tract because these secretions contain antibacterial factors.

Benign prostatic hyperplasia (BPH) is a very common condition of aging. It means a gradually progressive, non-cancerous enlargement of the prostate gland. Symptoms of BPH may overlap with those of prostate cancer. While the majority of men do not face such a drastic physiological and psychological metamorphosis, andropause is, nevertheless, accompanied by hormonal changes. In most men, serum testosterone levels begin to fall around the age of 30, with a mean yearly reduction of 1–1.4%. This decrease is considered to be related to the loss of the interstitial cells that produce testosterone, reducing the levels of free testosterone available in the blood.

2.15.2.3 Penis and Erectile Dysfunction

Reduced testosterone concentration could cause reduction of penis length during both flaccid and erect states. Libido loss and difficulty sustaining an erection adequate for orgasm are often the first indicators of oncoming andropause. Male subjects often remark that the frequency and rigidity of their erections have diminished. Smokers and those with underlying medical conditions such as diabetes, hypertension, or atherosclerotic disease carry a greater risk of ED.

2.16 Immune System

Changing with age, significantly almost every cell type of each component that together form the immune system is altered and, consequently, loses immunocompetence. The effective immune response is diminished with the number of mechanisms responsible for the clearance of foreign agents. Hence, it is described as a state of immunodeficiency. Aging does not spare innate defenses but shows very little collateral effect on adaptive ones.

The innate immune system itself is characterized by external and internal lines of defense: the skin and epithelial and mucosal linings of internal organs, and nonspecific white blood cells (leukocytes) and secreted molecules, including what are called antimicrobial agents (defensins per se) that drill holes in pathogen membranes. If an invading pathogen does breach the external barrier and the first line of defenses, then the second line of innate defenses is activated. The second line of innate defense is characterized by inflammation. Innate defense also depends heavily on cells that can phagocytize pathogens—neutrophils, monocytes, and macrophages.

2.16.1 Skin, Mucous Membranes, and Eyelashes

One of the most important roles of the integumentary system is to offer a protective barrier against the external environment. Thus, the skin is mainly composed of keratin, which is resistant to water and acts as an antimicrobial. The slightly acidic pH of 5.5 is attained with the help of lactic acid secretion, whereas the secretions from sebaceous glands and sweat glands co-operatively help in inhibiting bacterial growth.

Age-related changes in the skin occur with reduction in glandular secretion, thinning, and decreased elasticity; the skin will be less resistant to various forms of trauma, thus creating potential portals for pathogenic microorganisms. Though a natural defense, clinical interventions like intravenous cannulation may temporarily breach this barrier. Hence, such procedures should be indicated strictly when necessary, followed by prompt removal of the device and adherence to rigorous prevention and control of infection protocols.

Mucous membranes line the internal cavities, passages, and structures, providing mechanical defense through a thick epithelium. This protection is enhanced by mucus production, a highly effective means of trapping particulate matter, and pathogens present in the air. Aging will impair the structural constitution of the epithelial barrier as well as the functional ability of the mucosal immune response.

Eyelashes protect the eyes from particulate matter. They arise from special follicles, quite similar to hair follicles; however, with the progression of age, growth slows down and leads to decreased numbers of eyelashes.

2.16.2 The Innate Immune System Cells

2.16.2.1 Neutrophils

Phagocytic neutrophils defend from rapidly proliferating bacteria, yeasts, and fungi through the quick generation of reactive oxygen and nitrogen species and the expulsion of neutrophil extracellular traps. Neutrophils also play a vital role in the healing of wounds, being the first cell population to infiltrate the injury site; hence, they may remain in there for several days. With aging, the absolute number of neutrophils does not change, but their function is impaired. Impaired phagocytosis—the ability to engulf microbes—may result in accumulation of debris. Impaired chemotaxis—movement in response to chemical stimulation—means neutrophils take longer to arrive at the site of infection. Neutrophils secrete proteases to help them move through tissues: this too becomes less effective with age. Hence, the tissue damage and inflammation are more severe and more serious in older people.

2.16.2.2 Monocytes and Macrophages

Monocytes are leukocytes found in the spleen and blood that mediate inflammatory responses through differentiation into antigen-presenting cells (APCs) such as macrophages and dendritic cells. Macrophages mediate inflammation through the release of various inflammatory mediators like cytokines and chemokines that initiate the inflammatory cascade. Macrophages mediate phagocytosis and inflammation by activating other phagocytic cells when they encounter invading microorganisms. Macrophages also play an important role in wound healing, producing growth factors and secreting antigenic and fibrogenic factors. With advancing age, there is a sharp decline in macrophage function, and their phagocytic, killing, and wound healing capacity is reduced.

2.16.2.3 Dendritic Cells

Set within the skin, as well as other tissues and organs, are dendritic cells—leukocytes whose primary role is antigen presentation, a key step in activating T lymphocytes and initiating adaptive immunity.

2.16.2.4 Natural Killer Cells

Natural killer cells (NKCs) are non-specific cytotoxic leukocytes which play a crucial role in innate immunity. They recognize and kill the cells that are either virus-infected or malignant upon contact. NKC cytotoxic activity is suggested to be a potential biomarker for healthy aging, as diminished activity correlates with the onset of disease and susceptibility to infection. With increasing age, the absolute number of NKCs rises; however, the functional cytotoxicity is diminished. Zinc homeostasis changes may be partly responsible for the decline in natural killer cell (NKC) activity with age. There is evidence that zinc supplementation may improve NKC activity.

2.16.3 Adaptive Immune Response

- The principal components of adaptive immunity are B and T lymphocytes. Antigen-specific B and T lymphocytes mediate immunity against the particular antigen. Because of its specificity to the antigen, this immune response is said to be delayed on first exposure, usually within several days after activation of the innate immune response.

2.16.4 Thymus

- B and T cell precursors arise from the bone marrow; T cells, however, mature into immunocompetent lymphocytes within the thymus gland. This lymphoid organ, located above the heart, is most active during early childhood, supporting growth and immune function. It gradually shrinks over time, typically becoming fully atrophied by middle age. Thymic atrophy is a major and very early age-associated change that is linked to declines in immune function. It is further accompanied by a linear decline in the production of naive T cells continuing until it halts completely during the 50–60 years of age ranges. Further, there were thus reduced production levels of several immunoregulating hormones embedded in T and B cell differentiation, with some becoming undetectable in the plasma of those aged more than 60 years. One of the major tasks of the thymus is the conditioning of naive T cells, which are not yet exposed to antigens. These cells are changed from their quiescent state to the active state upon contact with foreign antigens. Another significant function of the thymus is to mediate central tolerance by "training" T cells with self-antigens and thus avoiding autoimmunity. In this selection phase, mature T cells are screened not to respond excessively against self-proteins. This selection process, however, becomes aberrant with age due to thymic atrophy, and this could add to autoantibody elevation in older individuals.

2.16.4.1 T Cells

Naive and mature T lymphocytes are to migrate to secondary lymphoid organs (including the lymph node and spleens), where the chance of meeting foreign antigens will be higher. T lymphocytes will be found in 65–85% of blood lymphocytes by recirculating daily in the lymph, blood, and lymph nodes to increase the chances of antigen exposure. After engaging with antigen, T lymphocytes may go through clonal expansion and can differentiate into cytotoxic T lymphocytes capable of killing target cells directly, helper T lymphocytes providing support to other immune cells, and memory T lymphocytes that stay inactive but respond quickly upon secondary antigen encounter. Activation of T cells requires their interaction with APCs presenting the antigen to them. APCs include dendritic cells: these cells, with their amorphous extensions, capture an antigen, phagocytize it, and then enter a lymph node and present bits of their captured antigen to T cells. Dendritic cells are quintessential for the activation of adaptive immunity. However, age-related changes affecting these cells not only weaken the defense against pathogens but also impair overall immunological function. An older adult displays a characteristic accumulation of memory T cells, Older adults typically exhibit an accumulation of memory T cells and a marked paucity of naïve T cells, resulting in a diminished response to novel antigens compared to younger individuals. Decreased T cell receptor diversity, due mostly to the frequencies of the latent CMV infection, is what underlies the age-associated decline in adaptive immunity. Because CMV is so prevalent in elderly populations, it has been implicated in the increased incidence of vascular diseases and overall mortality within this age group. By massively occupying the T-cell repertoire, CMV restricts the ability to respond to newer infections and thus increases vulnerability in older adults towards an array of pathogens.

2.16.4.2 B Cells

B lymphocytes develop and mature in the bone marrow and are activated by antigens, just like T lymphocytes. After activation, B lymphocytes differentiate into plasma cells which are responsible for the secretion of antibodies. These antibodies or immunoglobulins bind on to extracellular pathogens to neutralize them. A subgroup of B lymphocytes differentiate into "memory" B lymphocytes which respond to previously encountered antigens. Memory B and T lymphocytes circulate continuously throughout the body. The age-associated decline in the number of mature B lymphocytes produced in the bone marrow reduces the effective antibody response against infectious agents such as vaccines. This decline appears due to T helper cell dysfunction along with some intrinsic defects affecting B cell functions. The humoral component of immunity in the elderly is also compromised.

2.16.5 Autoimmunity

The generation and maturation of immune cells have to be stringently regulated so as to prevent autoimmunity when the immune system attacks the healthy host cells. Such regulatory contrivance may deteriorate with age. Autoantibodies ascend clearly with increasing age. Studies have shown that in individuals aged 101–106 years, there is a greater incidence of autoantibodies than in individuals aged 26–60 years. Rheumatoid factor, an autoantibody, was found to be present in 79% of samples obtained from individuals aged over 100 years. Dendritic cells, therefore, play a central role, not only in combating pathogens but also in ensuring that self-antigens remain tolerated, thus sustaining immunological homeostasis. Dendritic cells would normally not stimulate an immune response against circulating self-antigens, being worthy of maturation and T cell activation only against foreign antigens. Pathogens or tissue damage may promote aberrant maturation of dendritic cells that could subsequently initiate an autoimmune disease.

2.17 Endocrine System

2.17.1 Pituitary Gland and Growth Hormone Function

The pituitary gland, or hypophysis, is a key endocrine regulator often referred to as the "master gland" because of its control over many other endocrine glands. The pituitary is an organ consisting of two separate lobes: the posterior lobe, arising from the neural tissue of the hypothalamus, and the anterior lobe, derived from the epithelial cells that form the roof of the mouth.

The anterior pituitary synthesizes and secretes growth hormone (somatotropin), which is of paramount importance in the development of skeletal growth, muscle growth, and the internal organs. Somatotropin secretion is low in early childhood, but serum levels rise dramatically during adolescence, a time of great pubertal growth spurts. After the peak in secretion from around 25–30 years of life, somatotropin secretion begins a gradual decline in both sexes. For men, this is estimated to occur at about 50% every 7 years. However, there is great inter-individual variability in the actual rates at which somatotropin decline occurs.

The age-related decrease in somatotropin secretion reflects a decrease in the secretion of growth hormone-releasing hormone (GHRH) by the hypothalamus.

2.17.2 The Pineal Gland and Sleep Disorders

The pineal gland synthesizes melatonin, which is derived from the neurotransmitter serotonin, in the central region of the brain, also called the diencephalon. However, it acts as an internal biological clock as it secretes melatonin according to light exposure. Under well-illuminated conditions, melatonin production is reduced; just the opposite is true as the evening comes along—melatonin secretion increases as it prepares the body to be ready for sleep.

Calcification places the pineal gland under its growing burden, even before it comes into a person's life, for the younger children have some levels of calcification, which then increases with age. This therefore means that the levels of melatonin show a slow decline wherein an 80% reduction should be expected in level concentrations of melatonin in an individual aged seventy as compared to adolescents. These may include commonly prescribed medications for older adults, such as beta-adrenergic antagonists and non-steroidal anti-inflammatory drugs (NSAIDs).

Therefore, low levels of melatonin are associated with sleep disorders, the most important ones being insomnia in some older people. As sleep is a critical factor in how well one cognitively can process information and retain memories, sleep disturbances are likely to worsen age-related neurological changes.

- Studies have shown that even exposure to light—natural or artificial—during a bright morning can advance the circadian rhythm, shifting both the onset of sleep and the timing of melatonin secretion. In a similar way, extended-release formulas of melatonin have proved through therapy to enhance the outcome of sleep onset latency, sleep quality, daytime alertness, and overall quality of life in older adults aged 55 and above with insomnia.

2.17.3 Thyroid Gland and Metabolism

The thyroid gland functions significantly in metabolism control and homeostasis concerning blood calcium levels. They direct several physiological activities, which include:

- Metabolism of carbohydrates, lipids, and proteins
- Digestion
- Muscle and nerve function
- Maintenance of integrity and thickness of skins
- Maintenance of normal bone density
- Modulation of metabolic rate

The thyroid gland produces iodine-containing hormones such as thyroxine (T4, tetraiodothyronine) and triiodothyronine (T3), which are important in regulating the cellular metabolism. The amount of T4, which is secreted 15 times greater than T3, is converted into biologically active T3. T3 has a potency approximately three times that of T4.

In older individuals, there appears to be diminished hepatic clearance of T4; however, it can typically be compensated by a decrease in T4 secretion, which will lead to stable serum T4 levels. Serum levels of T3 and thyroid-stimulating hormone (TSH)—the latter produced by the pituitary gland—clearly decline with age. This reduction may contribute to the age-related decrease in basal metabolic rate observed in many middle-aged and older adults. The incidence of autoimmune reactions, targeting the thyroid gland, increases with age. Indeed, the presence of thyroid-specific antibodies is so common in older people that it is often classified as a normal age-related phenomenon. High-titer antibodies may signify an elevated risk for hypothyroidism due to autoimmune activity, which may affect as many as 5% of the population older than 60 years. Notable effects of this form of hypothyroidism include decreased metabolic rates, weight gain, and lowered core body temperature. Women are more at risk of autoimmune condition since autoimmune hypothyroidism is associated with the immune process, i.e., eight times higher risk, compared to men, which is consistent with the pattern seen in most autoimmune diseases.

- Caution has to be exhibited when interpreting results of thyroid function tests in the older adult population. Circulating thyroid hormone levels, especially the biologically active T3, may be decreased because of common chronic illnesses such as chronic obstructive pulmonary disease, hypertension, diabetes mellitus, and arthritis, in addition to dietary factors. This is referred to as nonthyroidal illness syndrome. Many of the drugs that are generally prescribed to chronic patients in older age groups, such as lithium or glucocorticoids, suppress thyroid function or decrease the biological activity of circulating thyroid hormones, leading to reduced metabolic rates. Calcitonin secretion changes. The thyroid, besides playing functions above, is also involved in calcium homeostasis. Calcitonin is released upon consumption of calcium and reduces the action of osteoclasts.

2.17.4 Parathyroid Glands and Hyperparathyroidism

The four parathyroid glands are located only on the posterior part of the thyroid gland. Their function is to secrete parathyroid hormone (PTH) as the concentration of blood calcium decreases. Since hypocalcemia impacts muscle contraction, nerve conduction, and coagulation, it shall be PTH's mandate to mobilize the reserves of calcium stored in the skeletal system. Specifically, PTH induces the indirect action of osteoclasts, causing the calcium from bone to enter the bloodstream.

A marked increase in serum PTH is usually found in older people. This state of hyperparathyroidism could be an important mechanism in the loss of bone mineral density in middle and older age. Many emerging studies also postulate an association of increased PTH with other age-related diseases, particularly cognitive decline and dementia.

2.17.5 Pancreas and Diabetes Risk

The islets of Langerhans, being endocrine components of the pancreas, regulate blood glucose homeostasis. Currently, beta cells in these islets synthesize and secrete insulin by increased blood glucose levels after carbohydrate ingestion. Beta cells secrete insulin upon stimulation by blood glucose, which was produced postprandially due to carbohydrate ingestion. Insulin binds primarily to cell surface receptors, helping them to absorb glucose from the bloodstream. Subsequently, within the cell, glucose is utilized or stored for production of energy or glycogen, respectively.

Other factors such as ethnicity, genetics, increased body mass index (BMI), and perhaps seniority are risk factors for type 2 diabetes mellitus. As age advances, an impairment with respect to insulin appears at the cellular level because it is related to the number of insulin receptors expressed on the cell's surface being lowered. This causes blood glucose concentration elevation, which corresponds to the progressive insulin resistance.

Fasting blood glucose levels are set to increase to the order of about 0.15 mmol/L per decade after the age of 20. They are the signs and symptoms of early diabetes, which sometimes go unnoticed until people grow older, and by themselves, they may not seem to constitute full-blown symptoms of diabetes.

It has been noted that with aging, less blood glucose stimulates insulin secretion from beta cells and, at the same time, an increase in insulin resistance typically occurring in cells of older individuals often encourages pancreatic compensation by secreting high amounts of insulin, leading to hyperinsulinemia. This compensation has a deleterious effect on beta cells that eventually succumbs to metabolic pressure.

The continual aging of the organism subjects further pancreatic beta cells to programmed cell death (apoptosis) and reduced pancreatic neogenesis, resulting in loss of beta cells from the pancreas. This loss then translates into reductions in the estimated secretion of insulin by as much as 0.5% per year of life. Also, with aging, the capacity of action of this latter facility, hepatic insulin clearance, increases, making less insulin available to receptor-cells thereby decreasing cell glucose uptake.

Such collective, age-related modifications in insulin production, clearance and responsiveness induce what could be called a pro-diabetic atmosphere in disposition, which may contribute to a higher risk of type 2 diabetes mellitus as age advances.

2.17.6 Belly Fat

Abdominal adiposity is a prevalent characteristic associated with aging, frequently observed in individuals with suboptimal dietary habits and/or sedentary lifestyles. Age-related endocrine alterations contribute to the increased deposition of adipose tissue in this region. These factors encompass changes in somatotropic function, autoimmune hypothyroidism, insulin resistance, and diminished levels of circulating sex hormones.

This deposition of fat in the abdominal region is linked to cardiovascular disease, hypertension, and type 2 diabetes. These disorders can occur singly or in combination as metabolic syndrome.

2.17.7 Adrenal Glands

A pair of endocrine glands called the adrenal gland is situated just above the kidney. Each gland has got two anatomically and functionally distinct regions, namely the inner adrenal medulla and the outer adrenal cortex.

2.17.7.1 Adrenal Medulla and Catecholamine Secretion

The catecholamines epinephrine (adrenaline) and norepinephrine (noradrenaline) are synthesized and secreted by the chromaffin cells of the adrenal medulla. They mediate the so-called "fight-or-flight" response when the body is made ready to either fight or flee from an actual or perceived threat or to confront a heightened arousal state. The physiological effects of the action of the epinephrine and norepinephrine would include:

- Striking up the heart rate
- Promoting vasoconstriction in cutaneous and visceral vasculature
- Raising the blood pressure
- Increasing blood flow to skeletal muscle groups
- Enhancing blood flow in the cerebrum
- Causing dilation of the pupils
- Speeding up respiration and dilating airways
- Stimulating hepatic glycogenolysis and hence increasing blood glucose.

Adrenal secretion of epinephrine diminishes in old age; however, plasma levels are maintained because renal clearance is also decreased. Studies suggest that in the elderly, the epinephrine response to acute stress is less vigorous compared with young adults.

2.17.7.2 Adrenal Cortex, Aldosterone, and Cortisol

- Derived from cholesterol by the adrenal cortex, there are several steroid hormones, of which the most significant products are aldosterone and cortisol.

Aldosterone

Aldosterone, a mineralocorticoid hormone, plays a vital role in the regulation of plasma sodium and potassium levels and therefore affects the maintenance of fluid balance and blood pressure. Studies have shown an age-related reduction in serum aldosterone concentration, limiting the ability of the body to conserve sodium.

The decline in aldosterone secretion may thus account for some of the light-headedness related to orthostatic hypotension reported by many elderly persons on standing. Studies have shown serum levels of aldosterone to decrease significantly in elderly subjects during postural changes from the supine to the standing position.

With sodium being responsible for water retention in the cardiovascular system via osmosis, lower plasma sodium concentration (hyponatremia) may cause a decrease in blood volume and resultant hypotension. Numerous drugs commonly used by the elderly population, such as opioids, NSAIDs, diuretics, and antidepressants, may exacerbate hyponatremia. There is also the possibility that an age-dependent increase in the secretion of atrial natriuretic hormone (ANH), a potent diuretic from the heart, could compromise blood volume and blood pressure further.

Cortisol

Cortisol is a glucocorticoid that is released primarily in biological stress, including injury or starvation. This hormone has its inherent anti-inflammatory effects and plays a major role in the catabolism of protein and lipids.

Studies of age-related differences in cortisol concentrations have given contradictory results. Initial reports suggested an increase of 20–50% in mean cortisol production at 20–80 years of age; more recent findings have indicated that such an increase does not hold for everyone; in some people, secretion may decline with aging, whereas for others, it remains fairly stable.

There would seem to be a relationship between high levels of cortisol, low bone mineral density, and a greater risk of bone fractures. In addition, high amounts of cortisol can cause the death of hippocampal cells, culminating in atrophy of that region, which is linked to age-related cognitive dysfunction. Age-related rises in cortisol levels were also said to be implicated in the deterioration of memory and sleep patterns.

2.18 Musculoskeletal System

As individuals grow older, degenerative changes usually occur in muscle strength, possibly due to anatomical and physiological adaptations in skeletal muscle tissue. This age-associated wasting of muscles, or sarcopenia, is characterized by a decrease in muscle mass, velocity of contraction, and force production. Sarcopenia can severely interfere with activities of daily living, such as getting up from a chair, doing household tasks, or taking care of oneself.

Muscle mass and strength are usually maximized in the third to fourth decade of life and generally begin to decline thereafter, a process that accelerates after the age of 60. At this advanced age, the loss of muscle tissue may have been so great that the limbs of those few with limited mobility appear grossly slender. The atrophy of intercostal muscles may create deep intercostal grooves, while atrophy of facial muscles may lead to facial ptosis.

The extreme loss of muscle tissue into the later years is termed senile sarcopenia and it becomes associated with increased frailty. Although frailty is multifactorial, musculoskeletal deterioration due to sarcopenia is its main component, and both have now been associated with increased weakness and fatigue and a higher risk for adverse events such as falls that lead to morbidity.

There are two main types of muscle fibers:

- Type I (slow-twitch) fibers, used primarily for endurance activities such as walking for long durations
- Type II (fast-twitch) fibers, which are primarily used for short-duration and high-intensity activities such as sprinting

Sarcopenia has a greater effect on changes in the quantity and function of fast-twitch fibers than slow-twitch fibers. Slow-twitch fibers appear to be relatively spared by aging; indeed, some studies suggest that those fiber types maintain or even increase the concentration of some metabolic enzymes, which may help minimize the decline in fast-twitch fiber function.

Neurodegeneration or loss of motor neurons and the degeneration of neuromuscular junctions, which are the synapses connecting motor neurons to skeletal muscle, are also proposed causes of sarcopenia. These processes reduce excitability and mass.

In turn, the development of sarcopenia is influenced by the age-related decline in the blood levels of the anabolic hormones, beginning in the middle phases of life, with the principal hormones identified to be somatotropin (growth hormone), testosterone, and testosterone-like hormones. Considering the fact that skeletal muscle uses high amounts of energy, sarcopenia is perhaps one of the prime factors causing the slowing of metabolism with aging. Lean muscle mass is lost on average at a rate of 3–8% per decade after the age of 30, leading to the initial decline in the basal metabolic rate after approximately age 20. Assuming constant caloric intake, an increased risk for storage of those excess calories as body fat becomes evident. In addition, this may further aggravate insulin resistance in the elderly, where skeletal muscle wasting contributes to progressive loss of support in bones and joints, ultimately leading to postural changes commonly observed in older adults.

Muscle wasting in the skeletal part brings about progressive loss in supporting bone and joint, thereby leading to postural changes in older people. It contributes further to increased risk for pathological conditions in the joint system, mainly osteoarthritis, as well as chances of falls and fracture.

2.18.1 Bones

Bone is principally made up of:

- The inorganic component, calcium phosphate (hydroxyapatite)
- The organic component, type 1 collagen

Calcium phosphate crystals constitute the bone matrix and confer mechanical strength to osseous tissue. The skeletal system functions as a substantial calcium reservoir, storing approximately 99% of the body's total calcium. Insufficient calcium or vitamin D, essential for intestinal calcium absorption, can result in decreased bone mineral density and a heightened risk of osteoporosis and fragility fractures. With advancing age, intestinal calcium absorption diminishes, and circulating vitamin D concentrations decline, thereby limiting calcium bioavailability for bone maintenance. Collagen serves as a structural scaffold for calcium phosphate crystals and contributes to bone integrity by preventing fractures. Certain genetic mutations can disrupt collagen synthesis, predisposing individuals to osteogenesis imperfecta, a condition characterized by skeletal fragility.

The bone, analogous to the muscle tissue, is a dynamic entity undergoing continuous remodeling via deposition and resorption. This process is mediated by two principal bone cell types:

- Osteoblasts: Specialized cells responsible for bone matrix deposition and mineralization.
- Osteoclasts: Multinucleated cells that resorb bone tissue, releasing ionic calcium into systemic circulation.

Osteoblast activity is augmented by mechanical loading, particularly weight-bearing exercise. During young adulthood, osteoblast and osteoclast activities are typically balanced, maintaining bone mineral density. Conversely, physical inactivity results in diminished osteoblast activity and subsequent bone loss. Age-related sarcopenia (loss of skeletal muscle mass) further reduces the mechanical load on bones, contributing to decalcification. Consequently, maintaining mobility and physical activity is crucial for preserving bone health in older adults.

2.18.2 Changes in Bone Density

Skeletal development is largely finished by early adulthood, and around 90% of peak bone mass is achieved by age 20 in males and age 18 in females. Accretion is noted in both sexes until about age 30, at which time peak bone strength and density are attained. Thereafter, loss of bone density commences with advancing age.

Women are more susceptible to bone demineralization and osteoporosis due to natural decline in estrogen with perimenopause and postmenopause. Studies show that women lose bone in the forearm at a rate of 1.5–2 times compared to men during a 10-year period. Bone loss continues with aging for both sexes and may allow males and females to maintain approximately 50% of their peak bone mass by the time they reach 80.

2.18.2.1 Osteoporosis

Most of the skeletal loss that occurs with increasing age also leads to osteoporosis, which is typified as having porous, spongy bones. This condition has been divided into two main types:

Type 1 osteoporosis results from rather declining estrogen levels. It is mainly prevalent among premenopausal and postmenopausal women.

Type 2 osteoporosis is also known as senile osteoporosis, and it is said to affect both sexes, namely men and women. This is thought to occur due to the falling number and activity of osteoblasts in them. To add insult to injury, they produce elevated amounts of pro-inflammatory cytokines like interleukin-6 (which is found to increase with aging) that favor osteoclastic activity, ultimately resulting in demineralized bones.

The vertebrae are predominantly developed osteoporotic culprits, with great proneness to microfractures. These microfractures usually result in the disintegration of the vertebrae under body weight into compression and fragile changes. These essentially contribute to the exaggeration of spinal curvature in most cases found among the elderly.

There are also many causes of age-related bone loss and the development of senile osteoporosis.

2.18.2.2 Fracture Risk

Age-related reductions in bone mass have been linked to a greater tendency to sustain fractures, particularly of the hip, rib, vertebra, arm, and forearm bones. Bone fragility is influenced not only by the loss of mineral density but also by the depletion and structural changes in collagen—most notably affecting its role as the key component in bone cohesion. As collagen degradation increases, fracture risk becomes significantly elevated.

Immobility, as in prolonged hospitalization, is a well-known risk factor for fractures. Age increases the likelihood of occurrence of fractures, and, in particular, this aspect makes such occurrences bring along a long period for healing, especially among the elderly.

Osteoporosis affects nearly 5% of the population over 50 years and is often localized in the femoral neck, making fractures of this region a common occurrence. The femoral neck is crucial since it bears all vertical weight on it. Fractures of the femoral neck are serious and can be life-threatening, increasing in number after the age of 60 years, predominantly affecting females than males during this period.

2.18.3 Joint Changes

Synovial cartilage provides compressive resistance and frictionless articulation between the osseous components of synovial joints. As a result of aging, there is a reduction in both the number and the metabolic activity of chondrocytes, the cells responsible for synthesizing and maintaining the cartilage matrix, which would compromise the impact-absorbing properties of the tissue. Thus, aging may bring about thinning of the articular cartilage. The resulting cartilage loss renders the joints of older individuals more susceptible to mechanical trauma, which finally leads to a direct bone apposition—the significant cause of pain in osteoarthritis.

2.18.3.1 Osteoarthritis

Osteoarthritis is the most common arthropathy in the world. Epidemiological studies in the United States show that about 10% of men and 13% of women over the age of 60 years suffer from symptomatic osteoarthritis of the knee. Approximately 8.5 million people in the United Kingdom suffer from osteoarthritis-related joint pain. This creates a huge burden on the healthcare system as many of these patients require expensive joint replacement surgery, especially of the knee, hip, and lumbar spine.

The articular capsule has an external layer of elastic ligaments anchoring the joint. Stiff ligaments prevent dislocation but allow free movement. Age-related degradation of collagen and elastin in these ligaments reduces its elasticity, causes stiffness, and decreases mobility of the joint. Certain joints are more prone to such changes; for instance, women in the 55–85 age cohort may experience up to 50% decrease in ankle flexibility and range of motion. Besides aging, various factors such as genetic predisposition, gender, obesity, and previous injury to the joint may contribute to the pathogenesis of osteoarthritis. Still, the most significant factor is age.

2.19 Skin

The skin, often defined or thought of as the integumentary system, is the organ that is considered more visible and apparent with aging. Having an average surface area of 1.67 square meters and a weight of 4 to 5 kilograms, the skin constitutes the largest organ in the body. It functions as a strong and durable barrier. It is vital for wrapping and protecting the internal environment of the body against different threats: dehydration, thermal dysregulation, and infection due to pathogens.

2.19.1 Skin Structure

The skin consists of two main layers, the epidermis and the dermis. The epidermis, the outermost layer of the skin, acts as a barrier against external aggressors. It comprises keratinocytes, which produce keratin—a protein that makes the skin waterproof and resilient—and melanocytes, which synthesize melanin, the pigment responsible for skin color and photoprotection. There is no blood supply going to the epidermis, but immune cells are present to aid in fighting infectious agents and pathogens.

The dermis, the deeper and always thicker layer, is responsible for structural support and sensation. Dermal fibroblasts synthesize collagen and elastin fibers to provide strength and elasticity to the skin. Sensory receptors in the dermis respond to pressure, pain, and temperature, while a vascular system delivers nutrients and expels metabolic waste. The sebaceous glands help in moisturizing the skin, softening the hair, and clearing the pores by secreting an oily substance known as sebum and are distributed over the entire body except for the palms of the hands and soles of the feet. Other contents found in the dermis are sweat glands and hair follicles.

Beneath the dermis is the hypodermis, known as the subcutaneous tissue. It is the deepest layer, anchoring the skin to the immediately underlying fascia (connective tissue surrounding skeletal muscles) and is also referred to as superficial fascia. The hypodermis starts out mainly filled with adipocytes that exhibit insulating properties and aid in thermoregulation.

2.19.2 Functions of the Skin

The skin, as well as sweat glands, hair, and nails, form a functional unit involved in carrying out crucial functions, including:

- Thermoregulation
- Storage and Synthesis
- Sensation
- Protection

Thermoregulation: It regulates changes in the internal temperature of the human being when there is a change in the outside temperature. The dermal blood flow within the skin is an important factor related to the body, acclimatizing it to other temperatures or other temperature variations. An average daily sweat gland would put out an average of 500 ml a day to accomplish this thermoregulation. It should be noted that colognes would initiate vasodilation of the cutaneous blood vessels by the nervous system when temperatures get hot enough to trigger sweating. The evaporation of sweat acts to cool and prevent the body from being overheated. In cold environments, the opposite occurs, as there will be vasoconstriction in the skin, causing warm blood flow to be redirected away from the body's surface, reducing heat loss.

Storage and Synthesis: The skin serves as a reservoir for lipids and water. The cholesterol molecules that come in contact with sunlight are converted into a vitamin D precursor, which is then converted to vitamin D, needed for calcium absorption in the intestine. Collagenases are also synthetic, produced by cells in the skin, which are enzymes used for normal turnover of collagen.

Sensation: A good range of nerve endings is found in the skin, assembling them as a general type called mechanoreceptors which are also sensitive to touch, pressure, and vibration. Heat, cold, and pain are stimuli to which these receptors give responses.

Protection: It provides well-structured protection by the stratum corneum, consisting of many layers of dead, flattened cells, glycolipids, and greatly keratinized cells.

2.19.3 Intrinsic and Extrinsic Skin Aging

Aging in skin development occurs because of intrinsic and extrinsic pathways. Intrinsic aging is an innate process that is time-dependent and is manifested by the skin itself. The process involves the actions of reactive oxygen species (ROS) combined with decreasing dermal mast cells, fibroblasts, collagen production, and an epidermal-dermal junction flattening. The typical findings of intrinsically aged skin would be a smoother, relatively fairly unblemished, pallid, dry appearance, and a reduction in fine lines.

Extrinsic skin aging is caused outside the body by:

- Tobacco
- Dietary excesses
- Chemical exposures
- Physical trauma
- Ultraviolet (UV) radiation

Most importantly, long-term, unprotected UV radiation exposure is said to be responsible for extrinsic aging of the skin. It is believed that 80% of the facial skin aging can be accounted for by chronic and low amounts of UV exposure. Actinic accretion changes the epidermis, finding irreparable fang in the cellular DNA, proving useful for increasing the production of ROS. Within 30 minutes of UV irradiation, the concentration of hydrogen peroxide, one of the most potent ROS, in human skin may increase by more than 100%. There is also acute collagen loss concomitant to the effect of UV exposure on collagen synthesis.

It also triggers melanocyte proliferation, causing increased pigmentation of the skin. Melanin is a natural protectant against the cumulative damaging effects of UV radiation, which accounts for the higher incidence of skin cancers in individuals with fairer skin than in people with darker skin. The same holds true for basal cell carcinoma; it occurs almost exclusively in individuals who have fair skin and have been exposed to sunlight.

Extrinsic aging skin-wise presents with coarse deep wrinkles, rough texture, telangiectasia, irregular or mottled pigmentation, sallow or yellow complexion, and elastic loss. Extrinsic aging varies with the skin type, that is, lighter skin tones are more susceptible to extrinsic aging than darker skin tones.

2.19.3.1 Epidermis

The epidermis, which is the protective outer layer of the skin made up of keratinized squamous epithelium, contains in its outermost part the stratum corneum, a superficial barrier of terminally differentiated cells. Below are several strata of epidermal cells that give way to the basal layer, characterized by rapid cell division, distally located to the basement membrane and dermis. The epidermis hosts keratinocytes, which synthesize keratin, and melanocytes, which produce melanin. Langerhans cells—dendritic cells that act as immune sentinels—are also available to safeguard the body from the entry of foreign microorganisms through the skin. Melanocytes and Langerhans cells undergo age-related decline in numbers.

The epidermal tissue does not possess its own vascular supply; therefore, it obtains its nutrients through diffusion from the underlying dermis. An important feature of intrinsic skin aging is that epidermal and dermal surface areas of contact have been reduced due, mainly, to the progressive flattening of rete ridges, epithelial projections that interdigitate below with the connective tissue. This changed situation reduces the dermal papillae, which are richly endowed with capillaries, thus restricting the delivery of nutrients, metabolites, and oxygen to the epidermis. It is also the decrease in surface area at the dermal-epidermal junction that will reduce the resistance to shear stress. Further, age will induce impairment of the epidermis due to progressively declining cell proliferation, and a report states that cell production drops by at least 50% from the age of 20 to 70.

Excessive transepidermal water loss is prevented by the stratum corneum, which functions as a barrier. Unlike the stratum corneum, its thickness does not change significantly with age; however, its turnover rate slows down over time, leading to increased roughness and dryness. Dry skin (xerosis) is a characteristic feature of aging skin and is a precursor to irritant dermatitis. Its effects slow healing, as mitosis of the basal layer of the epidermis slows down as well.

- Lastly, we have a decline in hormones and signaling molecules critical to skin maintenance and repair with age, along with a decreased density of their receptors. For example, there is a decrease in density of vitamin D receptors on epidermal keratinocytes during aging.

2.19.3.2 Dermis

Blood capillaries within the dermis provide oxygen and nourishment to all skin cells. It consists of an extracellular matrix with a dense meshwork of collagen fibers and elastin, which confer strength, elasticity, and flexibility to the skin. The important cells found in the dermis are:

- Fibroblasts: These synthesize collagen, elastin, and other structural components of the matrix.
- Mast cells: These are immune cells that release histamine.

The skin begins to lose volume due to aging; by the age of 30 itself, the skin loses about 20% of thickness. The number of mast cells decreases by about 50% and the blood flow is reduced by 60%. Hence, the skin cannot respond readily to injuries or infections.

Collagen is the most abundant protein in the body and gives strength and support to the skin.

The collagen content of the dermis decreases by 1% per year throughout life. In addition, the structure of the collagen itself becomes altered in older skin, where there are random fragments of irregular fiber, unlike the uniform, organized bundles of fibers laid down in youths with an extensible interwoven architecture with elastin fibers, helping the skin return to shape after deformation.

Evidence for decreased fibroblast activity includes: These cells show visible signs of aging, exhibit a decreased number of epidermal growth factor receptors, and show a concomitant reduction in collagen synthesis. Atrophy of collagen bundles also occurs, while there is an increase in the expression of matrix metalloproteinases, which are matrix-degrading enzymes. Consequently, the quality of collagen is altered to poorer grade, giving rise to impaired wound healing.

As the collagen fibers begin to tear down, cross-link, and stiffen, they lose their capacity to bind water, and the skin ceases to be elastic, hence becoming wrinkled. It seems that wrinkles are the result not so much of breakdown of elastin fibers, as was once believed, but of decreased collagen and mucopolysaccharide ability to hold water.

Aging skin is marked by diminished perfusion and vascularity. These changes particularly affect the upper dermis, especially the papillary regions. There has been a marked decrease in the cutaneous vascularity with a concomitant shrinkage of the dermal papilla capillary loops, leading to skin pallor, diminished nutrient exchanges, and impaired thermoregulation.

2.19.3.3 Hypodermis

The hypodermis is made up mostly of fat and serves as an insulator and shock absorber. As a person ages, subcutaneous fat is lost and the skin becomes thinner and more susceptible to shock. The loss of subcutaneous fat will reduce the volume of this layer, and hence the insulating effect of the hypodermis on conductive heat loss is impaired. The distribution of subcutaneous fat also changes: it decreases in parts of the face and hands but increases in the thighs and abdomen. The reduction of fat in bony areas increases the risk of pressure ulcers (Box 2.2) and fractures.

2.19.4 Loss of Protective Function

The skin has a very important role in protecting against mechanical damage by deforming and then returning to its original shape when tension or weight is applied. Human skin has a great degree of elasticity that can extend much more than its initial state. An ideal elastic substance has the quality of completely recovering its original shape after the unloading of an applied force. Failure to recover leaves what is called residual deformation. Compared with that of older adults, children's skin is generally more elastic and stronger, withstanding strains better in strength and elongation. With age, the levels of stiffness, thinness, decreased elasticity, and cell laxation resistance become higher. Many sensory receptors—such as Pacinian corpuscles, Meissner corpuscles (primarily pressure receptors), as well as those responsible for sensing pain and temperature—decline in sensitivity and decrease in number with age. A similar decline is seen in the sensory nerve endings existing in the different layers of skin, epidermis, and dermis. This is why older adults often experience a reduced ability to perceive environmental changes, which increases their vulnerability to injury.

With age, the sebaceous gland activity reduces and produces less sebum. This production of sebum also leads to a corresponding decrease in the protective acidic barrier against infections. The protective resistance becomes less, increasing the infection rate in older adults against the skin. Various organisms can cause primary bacterial infections of the skin and soft tissues such as virus (shingles), bacteria (cellulitis), and fungus (icterus).

2.20 Characteristics of Aging Skin

2.20.1 Wrinkles and Sagging

Many factors cause rhytides, which include gravity, decreased subcutaneous fat, and dynamic motion by the facial musculature working against expression lines, leading to deeper furrows formed in the forehead and glabellar areas, periorbital area, and nasolabial fold. Other clinical features of aging skin are xerosis, diminished tanning, and descent. All of these conditions are most pronounced on the face, the area of the integument most exposed to environmental factors. Accumulation of lipofuscin—the age pigment—in the facial muscles attests to age-related cellular damage. Subsequent cellular damage, along with impaired neuromuscular coordination, aggravates the formation of rhytides.

Reduction and altered distribution of facial adipose tissue, which have an inclination to deposit in particular regions of the nasolabial folds and submandibular region, together with gravity, lead to ptosis and sagging of the skin.

2.20.2 Changes in Hair and Nails

Most probably, as one ages, the density of chest, armpit, and pubic hair will decrease, although males often grow more hair in other parts of their bodies, such as eyebrows, ears, and nostrils. Hair also becomes drier due to reduced secretion of sebum by the sebaceous glands. Hair graying, considered genetically controlled, seems to result from a decrease in hair melanocytes that can no longer color the growing hair in the follicle. It decreases due to some dysfunction in signaling by melanocyte stem cells, which can no longer maintain their production of melanocytes or, at least, might have become unable to do so. What has been demonstrated is the fact that hydrogen peroxide, synthesized by the hair follicle, gets progressively higher over time, which causes the loss of hair color. Different follicles gray at varying speeds, hence fast and slow progress spans a couple of decades. In comparison, white hair grows thicker and rapidly than pigmented hair. A reduction in the growth rate of nails is observed with old age. Ridges develop in the nails along with their becoming brittle with falling levels of lipophilic sterols and fatty acids.

2.20.3 Skin Lesions

As we age, the number of melanocytes decreases; however, localized increases can occur, resulting in the appearance of mottled hyperpigmentation known as "liver spots" found on the dorsal surfaces of the hands. Benign skin lesions including seborrheic keratoses or solar lentigines, generally known as "age spots," appear from the third to the fifth decade of life; thereafter, the incidence increases. Additionally, skin cancers become more likely as sun damage accumulates with aging.

Cherry angiomas are benign vascular proliferations of the skin that most often appear in older adults. They appear as round to oval, bright red papules or punctate macules that are dome-shaped, usually found on the trunk or proximal aspects of the limbs. Newly formed capillaries are present in these lesions, along with prominent endothelial cells arranged in a lobular configuration within the papillary dermis. Initial lesions grow as flat, red spots resembling petechiae, gradually enlarging into red papules from 1 to 5 mm. The lesions are usually not bothersome and may bleed after injury.

2.20.4 Senile Purpura

Less than 10% of people over the age of fifty exhibit signs of senile purpura, a condition that, while common and innocuous, still remains idiopathic. It is characterized by recurrent development of contusions in irregular shapes and dark purple colors. These usually have dimensions of about 1 to 4 cm and are frequently found along the forearms due to trivial trauma, very much unlike bruises. Also different from normal bruising is the fact that there are no characteristic color variations in these lesions. It may take as long as three weeks to resolve. Factors that predispose include sunlight, corticosteroids administered orally and applied topically, and anticoagulants.

For that matter, although some aging-related dermatoses can be quite uncomfortable, they are generally not disastrous or life-threatening for older adults. Typical dermatoses among elderly individuals would include eczema, psoriasis, infections, and pruritus, the bulk of which can be credited to their xerosis and related pruritic conditions. The lower limbs which appear dry and desquamated would be a result of dehydration coupled with diminished sebaceous activity and atrophy of sebaceous glands and microcirculation changes that favor injury, infection, and rashes underneath.

Senile purpura is a disorder that has been known to be caused by the thinning of dermal tissues and increased vascular fragility due to aging. The erosion of superficial vessels can be caused by even minor trauma. The resulting blood then leaks into the surrounding dermis and gives rise to senile purpura.

2.20.5 Visual System

2.20.5.1 Eye

Visual function is subject to age-related alterations that affect both internal and external ocular structures. In general, the decline is gradual and linear, and most noticeable alterations begin to occur in the third decade.

In advanced age, atrophy of the retro-orbital fat, which usually cushions and protects the eye, can cause enophthalmos (depressed position of the globe within the orbit). It may also be attended with a thinning of the tissues of the eyelids along with the levator palpebrae superioris muscle so that it could also result in ptosis (drooping of the eyelids). In severe situations, ptosis may affect the visual field.

The combination of enophthalmos with ptosis may disrupt the moisture retention of the cornea by tarsal conjunctivas, thereby predisposing to the formation of a pre-corneal air space, especially at night. This will, in turn, make the cornea more prone to break down at the epithelial level.

Entropion (inward misdirection of the eyelashes) may occur in susceptible subjects, with laxity of the eyelid support muscle deprived of functional support by ptosis, resulting in corneal abrasion and subsequent scarring. On the contrary, great weakening of lower eyelid support muscles can lead to ectropion (eversion of the lid margin), producing corneal drying and irritation. Both entropion and ectropion could be treated symptomatically using anti-inflammatory ophthalmic solutions or artificial tears into their confinement; nevertheless, surgical correction at either end of lid pathology addresses laxity more directly as a therapeutic approach.

Lacrimal secretion diminishes with aging and changes in the composition of the tear film, making it less effective at wetting the eye and more unstable. These changes contribute to dry eye syndrome—a condition affecting nearly 14% of adults over 65. Symptoms such as irritation, a sensation of a foreign body in the eye, and pain can interfere with daily activities like reading and watching TV. Chronic irritation may blunt corneal sensitivity, impairing the eye's ability to detect injury or infection.

2.21 Vision Changes

2.21.1 Presbyopia

Lifelong cell division in the human eye lens continuously generates new cellular layers that accumulate at the lens periphery. With a confined ocular volume, this type of lens does not grow as it should with age. Thus, newer cells generated get compressed inside the existing mass thereby leading to lens density and less intrinsic flexibility over time. It gradually reduces the lens' ability to alter its shape and focus light effectively onto the retina.

Presbyopia is the term used in the medical literature which explains this general age-related vision impairment associated with challenges in focusing on near objects. It is most often an impediment to reading from very close distances. Usually, it comes in at about the fourth or fifth decades of living. Inherent in the development of presbyopia is a reduction of accommodative amplitude of the crystalline lens. The nearest point where an object becomes visible is about 10 cm away at 20 years, advancing to beyond 100 cm away at age 70.

Aging continues to add on to the continued density due to the continuing production of lens cells. Such an accumulation of lens materials could give rise to specific wavelengths of light that manifest yellow color in the lens, affecting its contrast sensitivity, as well as color discrimination and differentiation.

Patients in whom the concentration of lens proteins is beyond a certain threshold level, precipitation takes place, giving rise to cataracts. They usually manifest clinically as glare and halo effects when a person looks at bright light sources. The central part of the lens, which is denser than the rest, is where age-related cataracts are most common.

2.21.2 Cataracts

Cataracts can make it difficult to see in certain situations, for example, when driving at night. They can also interfere with the ability of certain wavelengths of light to enter the eye, thereby reducing color perception: People with cataracts may wear rough clothing because of their color vision.

2.21.3 Pupil Changes and Poor Night Vision

Pupillary function includes regulation of the quantity of light entering the eye. With advancing age, pupillary diameter diminishes, consequently reducing light transmission. Furthermore, the capacity of the pupils to adapt to variations in light intensity is negatively impacted by age, such as during the transition from a brightly illuminated environment to one of darkness. Dark adaptation is dependent on the regeneration of the photopigment rhodopsin by the photoreceptor cells of the retina. This regenerative process is significantly slowed with age, contributing to impaired night vision. These changes increase the risk of falls and other accidental injuries in older adults; they may stumble or fall while transitioning between a well-lit bathroom and poorly lit stairs while ascending or descending.

2.21.4 Posterior Vitreous Detachment

The eye consists of two chambers: an anterior and a posterior chamber. The anterior chamber is separated from the posterior chamber by the lens, and the aqueous humor is the clear watery fluid in the anterior chamber. The posterior chamber contains the vitreous body, which is jam-like. With age, the vitreous body loses part of its gel-formed structure and becomes liquid. In some cases, the fluid-filled cavity may collapse, contract, or detach from the retina, which is termed as posterior vitreous detachment. This is usually felt through discrete opacities or translucent patterns visualized within the field.

2.21.5 Age-Related Macular Degeneratio (ARMD)

Age-related macular degeneration (ARMD) occurs when cone photoreceptor cells in the fovea begin to degenerate, allowing high-acuity color vision to diminish. This degeneration is likely related to alterations in the retinal pigment epithelium (RPE) cells that provide much support to photoreceptors.

ARMD presents in two types: dry (atrophic), accounting for 90% of cases, and wet (exudative), constituting only 10% of cases. In dry ARMD, a gradual impairment of vision in a bilateral pattern results due to degeneration of the RPE. In contrast, in wet ARMD, neovascularization under the retina, where new blood vessels develop between the photoreceptor layer and the retinal pigment epithelium, along with the leakage of serous fluid, is evident. Wet ARMD progresses at a faster pace along with poorer vision.

Drusen is the typical characteristic of ARMD that appears as pale yellowish-white deposits accumulating at the surface of the retina. Disruption of normal retinal function caused by this promotes visual disturbances and lowers visual acuity. Increased age also brings about a significant increase in the quotient of drusen, primarily in those beyond 60 years. It is one of the leading causes of visual impairment, accounting for nearly half of all cases among individuals aged 75 and older.

2.22 Auditory System

Taking into account auditory perception, which is the paramount function of the ear, the ear also serves a secondary purpose in maintaining equilibrium. Presbycusis stands out as the most common hearing deficits in humans. Statistics show that approximately one-third of persons aged between 61 and 70 years have difficulty in speech comprehension against background noise, the number rising to about 80% for persons beyond 85 years of age.

2.22.1 Outer Ear

The auricle (pinna) serves to capture and funnel sound waves into the external auditory canal and onward to the tympanic membrane. With aging, the auricle tends to show signs of increased size, along with the proliferation of external hairs over the tragus and antitragus. Such facial changes are frequently noted in men. In both sexes, the auricle becomes dry and scaly with age.

The external auditory canal produces a yellowish substance called cerumen, which helps keep the canal moist and mildly antiseptic, thereby helping in preventing infections. With aging, the self-cleansing ability of cerumen may become less effective.

Reduced activity of the ceruminous glands with increasing age results in decreased production of cerumen. This may throw the ear into the dry and infected category. Improvement in circulation through bilateral age-related changes in cartilage that forms the walls of the external auditory canal may also lead to loss of elasticity, degeneration, and probably collapse of the canal. The conjunction of a dryer environment and possible collapse renders the ear further obstructive to cerumen, often leading to conductive hearing loss. Older patients may require cerumenolytics prior to managed removal of impacted cerumen by means of microsuction in an audiology clinic or irrigation in a general practice. The space between the outer ear and the inner ear contains the tympanic membrane and an air-filled cavity with three auditory ossicles: the malleus, incus, and stapes. The outer ear captures sound waves which cause the tympanic membrane to vibrate. The vibrations are then transmitted and amplified through the ossicles into the inner ear. The tympanic membrane shows age-related changes such as decreased vascularity, thinning, and increased rigidity. Further complicating sound wave amplification are stiffening, calcification, and reduced flexibility of the synovial joints between the auditory ossicles.

It equalizes pressure on the tympanic membrane to prevent damage from pressure imbalances—a function that may be linked to age-related curvature of the Eustachian tube. This will cause difficulties for the Eustachian tube to open on swallowing, making it more possible to have pressure imbalance.

2.22.2 Inner Ear

The parts of the inner ear are made up of a coiled structure called cochlea that performs auditory transduction, whereas vestibule and semicircular canals are responsible for balance. Sound waves generated by the movement of the stapes travel through the fluid and, at the base of the cochlea, come into contact with specialized hair cells which serve as sensory receptors transducing the generated mechanical stimuli into electrical impulses that are transmitted through the cochlear nerve and interpreted in the brain as sound. A typical phenomenon is that sound perception is highly acute in childhood but gradually declines with age.

2.22.3 Presbycusis

Presbycusis, or age-related hearing loss, is the predominant form in most cases, and currently, there are few effective preventive or restorative interventions available. Presbycusis is the term used to describe this condition and has various meanings: refers to older adults who experience reduced hearing sensitivity due to aging. These include general aging effects, but the progression is always influenced by factors such as high-intensity noise exposure, cardiovascular disorders, or nerve injury. Pathophysiological processes generally include hair cell and neuron degeneration in the cochlea.

In addition, individuals with auditory trauma may suffer chronically from prolonged noise exposure. Notably, agerelated hearing loss has also been reported in isolated, non-industrialized regions of Africa and India, highlighting the multifactorial etiology of presbycusis. Factors associated with hastening presbycusis are genetically inherited, with increased free radicals and toxins. There are also decreased vascular perfusion reaching the inner ear. This age-related decline in the body's abilities is further exacerbated by a progressive slowing of central auditory processing.

A lack of hearing acuity at higher frequencies is typical of presbycusis because it is in high-frequency sounds that most of the phonemes for speech are present. As a result, older people often find it much more difficult to follow and participate in conversations with competing background sounds, especially if that sound comes from a television or music. These types of auditory processing address barriers to socializing and contribute to loneliness and social isolation.

2.22.4 Tinnitus

Tinnitus is defined as an auditory perception often described by people as a ringing, buzzing, humming, or hissing sound without any external stimulus. Certain patients may even describe the sound as having a musical quality. The causes of tinnitus are myriad, including:

- Certain drugs that are ototoxic (like gentamicin, for example)
- Spasms of the middle ear muscles
- Damage or loss of cochlear hair cells
- Changes in blood circulation in the inner ear

Interruption in sensory signal transmission to the auditory cortex may form the underlying pathophysiology for the genesis of tinnitus. Just as after an amputation, certain sensations may be felt in a phantom limb; consequently, individuals may also report the feeling of tinnitus after the sectioning of the cochlear nerve. An association between presbycusis and the death of the sensory hair cells means reduced auditory input to the brain, which may predispose the occurrence of tinnitus in the old age. Of course, as mentioned before, presbycusis may accelerate due to the chronic exposure to high sound levels, increasing the chance of developing tinnitus. Audiologists are becoming increasingly alarmed by trends of considerable numbers of young people attending loud concerts and using headphones at high volumes for long periods of time, which may lead to a more rapid onset of hearing loss and, consequently, a greater likelihood of earlier onset auditory dysfunction and deafness.

2.23 Strategies for Maintaining Physiological

2.23.1 Performance with Aging

2.23.1.1 Primary Prevention

The aim of effective strategies in primary prevention is to delay or prevent the age-related decline in functional status, and through this, the functional status is maintained and the life span extended. This works by targeting biological factors contributing to functional loss in the aging process. Examples include maintaining vascular function through the preservation of nitric oxide bioavailability, prevention of cardiac fibrosis to preserve diastolic function, and maintenance of glomerular integrity to preserve renal health. Early implementation in life is important for maximum longevity benefits.

2.23.1.2 Secondary Prevention

Secondary prevention targets middle-aged and older adults who have already suffered some physiological dysfunction, as a means to delay functional limitations and age-related syndromes like frailty. Such interventions seek to identify the root causes of functional decline and must prove effective for individuals with impairments in later life.

2.23.1.3 Tertiary Prevention

Tertiary prevention involves interventions in the management of complications among people with established diseases to enhance the quality of life. This involves rehabilitation, follow-up care, and medical advice that help patients regain normal function and manage complications. Examples include monitoring of blood sugar for diabetics and the provision of psychological support that helps the patients adapt to chronic conditions. Tertiary prevention is important in maintaining quality of life and encouraging independence among older people as well as reducing medical costs.

2.24 Lifestyle-Behavioral Strategies

To maintain physiological function with aging, lifestyle-behavioral strategies include regular physical activity, healthy eating, cognitive stimulation, and preventive practices such as not smoking and scheduling regular check-ups. Much evidence puts forth the positive impacts of physical activity and diet on various physiological functions.

2.24.1 Phyical Activity

Physical activity is any activity of muscles that is associated with a high energy expenditure compared to a resting state, performed in the form of regular and planned movements which can include activities of daily living. Regular physical activity is one of the most evidence-based lifestyle strategies for maintaining function as we age. More occupational or recreational physical activity, and higher levels of structured exercise, generally maintain better body function despite advancing age. While there are several barriers to physical activity in older adults, exercise has positive effects on life expectancy by reducing the incidence of diseases and the natural and unnatural complications of aging. Prior consistent physical activity lessens or delays the age-linked degeneration of cardiorespiratory fitness, glucose insulin management, neuromuscular competence, cardiovascular health, and cognitive performance; it has been successfully used for the treatment of functional capacity improvement in older persons. These are maintained at higher levels in physically active individuals who continue activities regularly and over the long-term compared to age-matched sedentary peers. Given that changes in motor function with age predict future morbidity and mortality, higher levels of physical activity are associated with reduced rates of age-related decline in several neuromuscular functions: distance walked, stair climbing, walking speed, and body movements. The greater the volume of the physical activity, the better one's health is likely to be, and the lower one's disease risk. Thus, even when one had not been consistently active in youth, the increase of activity later in life leads to a gain in health status similar to that achieved by a person who was consistently active since youth. This will delay the beginning of decline in physical functions, such as cardiorespiratory fitness and muscle strength, by approximately 30 years compared to healthy, inactive adults. Epidemiological analyses indicate that even moderate levels of physical activity, such as just half of the recommended 150 minutes per week, have a significant impact on life expectancy.

Cellular and molecular mechanisms underpinning the benefits of regular physical activity to physiological function involve slowing or reversing one or more fundamental mechanisms of aging. Regular exercise suppresses oxidative stress by preventing or reversing the age-related rise in superoxide production from several sources including the major oxidant enzyme NADPH oxidase, dysfunctional mitochondria, and uncoupled endothelial NO synthase. Lower superoxide concentrations due to chronic exercise in turn reduce superoxide reacting with NO and hence increase NO bioavailability. Exercise also reduces aging-induced oxidative stress by stimulating antioxidant enzyme defenses and, in part, inhibits inflammation by suppressing the activation of a key pro-inflammatory transcription factor, nuclear factor kappa B.

Regular exercise also promotes mitochondrial "health" and function by intermittently engaging energy-sensing pathways that increase oxidative metabolic capacity. Other mechanisms thought to contribute include the prevention of genome instability effects, maintenance of telomere length and telomerase, improvement of protein homeostasis, increase in viability/function of stem cells, epigenetic changes, and release of signaling molecules from active skeletal muscle.

Improved cognitive function following regular physical activity is partially related to neural growth related to increased levels of growth factors that include brain-derived neurotrophic factor (BDNF), vascular endothelial growth factor (VEGF), and insulin-like growth factor (IGF).

Conceptually, functional fitness embodies the level of physical ability or capacity needed to execute daily tasks without unnecessary fatigue. With this approach, however, aging can be said to weaken an individual's physical fitness—strain, endurance, agility, and flexibility—which can make the activities of daily living and normal functioning compromised among the older people. It is a process that characterizes normal and widespread changes that occur in the human body. As we grow older, composition of the body changes, where muscle mass and bone mass can be lost along with diminished physical capacity over the years.

Muscles account for around 40% of the entire body; muscle cells represent about 75% of the mass from cell sources. The muscular system contributes almost 25% to total protein biosynthesis in the body. Skeletal muscle is considered the kind of tissue responsible for voluntary movement. Aging is a gradual decreasing space of the mass and strength of muscle, where evidence of the strength of muscle is actually a direct effect of muscle mass.

Physical activity is well known and important for independent living, prevention of chronic health problems, and quality of life. If older adults do not participate in a physically active lifestyle, they are at risk of 40% and 10–40% decrease in muscle mass and joint mobility, respectively, depending on their body part, while the loss of muscle strength is 30% related to the decrease in muscle mass. Moreover, during the aging process, there is a loss in muscle strength at a rate of around 12–14% per decade after the age of 50 years. If the level of physical activity is not adequate, not only is muscle function affected, but other systems of the body, such as the cardiorespiratory system, are also prone to change, and from the age of 40 onwards, a marked decline in aerobic capacity has been observed, such that at 65 years of age it has a capacity that is approximately 30% lower.

2.25 Causes of Diminished Strength and Muscle Mass with Aging

2.25.1 Reduced Number of Muscle Fibers

Pathophysiology of strength and decreased muscle mass with aging is complex.

Reduced muscle mass is due to a reduction in the number and size of muscle fibers. If the size of the muscle fiber reaches a minimum 'critical' size, then apoptosis is initiated. Other causes of apoptosis with aging are denervation and loss of neurons. Loss of muscle fibers causes a decrease in strength capacities, a decrease in muscle metabolism, and an increase in the risk of muscle injury. The rate of muscle protein synthesis decreases with aging, and the capacity for muscle repair also decreases with age.

2.25.2 Hormonal Changes

This catabolic situation affects muscle and bone tissues due to deficits in anabolic hormones such as growth hormone and insulin-like growth factor that are implicated in this condition. Also, hormonal changes in menopause, which begins between the ages of 45 and 55, lead to specific changes in the human body with a decrease in muscle mass and strength. The loss of muscle mass and strength is also related to increased catabolic factors, for example, inflammatory cytokines. TNF-α and interleukin-6 have supported the loss of muscle mass. The complications, malignancy, chronic obstructive pulmonary disease, congestive heart failure, inflammatory bowel disease, and rheumatoid arthritis, further contribute to the loss of muscle mass and strength with aging. Other diseases associated with periods of incapacity—such as deep vein thrombosis, pulmonary embolism, myocardial infarction, pneumonia, or surgery—also increase the risk of strength and muscle mass loss in older adults.

2.25.3 Changes in Appetite

One of the main causes of age-related decline in strength and muscle mass is decreased physical activity. As people grow older, this is a usual phenomenon. Also, with insufficient intake of nutritional factors, loss of appetite is a growing concern with aging. In such circumstances, the overall effect falls on the muscular system with muscle loss.

2.25.4 Syndrome Sarcopenia

Among these changes, one of the most prominent is sarcopenia, which has been defined as the age-related loss of skeletal muscle mass, which is associated with a decline in strength and aerobic capacity and, consequently, functional capacity. Sarcopenia is also associated with a decline in bone mineral density and basal metabolic rate, and an increase in body fat content associated with aging. The definition includes low muscle mass, low muscle strength, and poor physical performance. A diagnosis of sarcopenia may thus be made in cases where there is low muscle mass and at least one of the other two criteria exists. This means that aging reduces the capacity of older adults to perform aerobic activities like walking and running due to a decline in maximal oxygen uptake of about 0.5–1.0% per year. Falls, which are partly contributed by reduced muscle strength, balance, and mobility, have also been shown to increase by 35–40% after age 60. It may be possible to prevent sarcopenia and a significant set of associated disorders, including type 2 diabetes, coronary artery disease, hypertension, osteoporosis, and obesity, through exercise and physical training, especially resistance training.

2.26 The Effects of Aging Changes on Performance

Changes of aging affect functional capacity to some extent, yet the extent to which older adults are physically active through their lifetime is debated. The common age-related changes affecting physical activity include decline in visual acuity (with corrective lenses), hearing loss, joint pain, reduced range of motion of joints, muscle atrophy, and sometimes edema.

With aging, the role of physical activity becomes more vital for reducing potential loss in strength, flexibility, endurance, and balance. Functional capacity prevents injuries and falls, isolation, dependency, and depression and determines the ability to carry out activities that provide a better quality of life. The onset or progression of a medical condition can result in increased risk of physical function decline.

National Evidence-Based Recommendations and Resources Current physical activity recommendations for older adults are 150 minutes per week (30 minutes continuously) of moderate-intensity aerobic activity or 75 minutes of vigorous-intensity aerobic activity. Shorter bouts of at least 10 minutes several times a day for those with less endurance can help meet the overall 30-minute goal. Recommendations also include at least 2 days per week of muscle-strengthening exercises for all major muscle groups: legs, hips, back, abdomen, chest, shoulders, and arms. Balance and coordination activities should be done three or more days a week to prevent falls. It is best to do exercises with a frequency, intensity, and duration that are appropriate for the individual's abilities and goals. Strength and balance can enhance a person's ability to get around safely at faster speeds and for longer distances. However, less than 12% of older adults are recommended aerobic and muscle-strengthening physical activity.

Older adult should be advised to gradually increase their physical activity volume, as well as the frequency of said activities, from their current baseline. It has also been observed that a health screening by the clinician before joining an exercise should be mandatory, yet some research studies opine that the same must not create any obstacle.

2.27 Common Barriers to Exercise Among Older Adults Agism

A pervasive bias among health professionals, as well as older adults and their families, is that age is often a barrier to physical activity. These negative aging stereotypes can shape the level of activity an older person undertakes; the type of activities selected; and the supportive products, environments, and services available, such that older adults, their families, and health care providers may question their capability to be active and whether it is safe or acceptable to do so or may believe that physical activity should be reduced.

2.28 Motivation to Be More Active

Physical activity recommendations can be overwhelming for older adults. The philosophy of "any activity is good" and starting slowly and gradually over time provides reassurance. Help motivate older adults to change their current behaviors that put them at risk of deterioration or potential harm. Motivational interviewing (MI) focuses less on correcting or convincing people to change behavior, but rather understanding behaviors and problem-solving in a collaborative manner.

There are four generally accepted techniques for MI:

1. Engaging
2. Focusing
3. Motivating
4. Planning

Engaging a person creates a foundation of rapport and mutual respect and builds trust. Focusing techniques offer strategic direction by identifying a goal. Motivating strategies focus on the individual's reason and/or readiness for change. Planning focuses on the process that facilitates and sustains change. Key points of MI are not attempting to convince an individual to change their behavior, but rather to try to understand an individual's current motivation, actually listening, and empowering the individual to make the changes that are desired.

2.29 Risk and Fear of Fall

A realistic and common concern among older adults is the risk and fear of injury from falls. Rather than restricting activity, which inevitably leads to further disability and decline, it is better to focus on the root causes of the falls. An evaluation following a fall or near fall is valuable as it identifies future risk and an opportunity to outline an individualized fall prevention plan. Previous falls are the most powerful predictor of future falls. Fall risks are often best addressed using a team. Physical therapist (PT) specialize in the in-depth assessment and treatment of falls.

2.30 The Effects of Physical Inactivity and Physical Activity on Selected Medical Conditions

Physical activity is a contributing factor in the reduction of chronic medical conditions, including cognitive impairment, cardiorespiratory disorders, and a wide range of musculoskeletal disorders. Physical activity and exercise can be effective in the primary and secondary prevention of chronic diseases that lead to physical impairment, disability, and premature death, and can lead to improved quality of life, successful aging, and reduced health care burden.

2.30.1 Cognitive Dysfunction

Regular physical activity is associated with a decreased incidence of cognitive impairment and functional impairment. The theory for this is explained by cross-stimulation of neuroplasticity with an environmentally enriched physical activity. Some other proposed mechanisms include enhanced cerebral blood flow, reduced cardiovascular and metabolic risk factors, prevention and treatment of depression, and improved sleep quality. Besides, exercise and physical activity enhance hippocampal volume and white matter integrity. Home-based exercises like walking, which are characterized by high adherence rates, are safe, effective, and can delay cognitive decline and improve ADL and physical fitness in dementia patients.

2.30.2 Falls

With the advancement of age, there is the likelihood of an increased incidence of unintentional falls, which is linked to the reduction of muscle strength, dynamic balance, and the speed of movement. Low levels of physical activity among older adults are associated with an increased risk of falls, but the relationship between physical activity and increased risk of falls is complex. The increased risk of falls is often attributed to physical limitations rather than directly to low levels of physical activity. However, increased physical activity reduces fall-related injuries by 32–40%. With advancing age, the likelihood of unintentional falls increases, often linked to reduced muscle strength, impaired dynamic balance, and slower movement speed. Low levels of physical activity among older adults are associated with a higher risk of falls, though the relationship is complex. The increased risk is typically attributed to physical limitations rather than inactivity alone. However, regular physical activity has been shown to reduce fallrelated injuries by 32 to 40 percent.

While physical exercise may, in rare cases, contribute to fractures—particularly from high-impact or risky activities such as cycling—there is limited evidence suggesting that older adults face a significantly increased risk of injury from physical activity itself. Despite this, fear of injury remains a common barrier to participation. Importantly, physical activity helps prevent osteoporotic fractures by improving bone density and muscle strength.

2.30.3 Musculoskeletal System

Age-related chronic musculoskeletal pain can be a barrier to physical activity among older people. This is because musculoskeletal pain is highly associated with reduced physical function in older persons. For instance, 37% of arthritic individuals are physically inactive. However, strong muscle strength around the joint can be a very decisive factor in preventing the onset of osteoarthritis. Among the older people, musculoskeletal pain is often mentioned as a hindrance to physical activity. This may be overcome when an appropriate physical activity program is prescribed for the improvement of muscle mass and strength that protects the joint complex and prevents the pain and dysfunction associated with musculoskeletal disorders. Common activity-related musculoskeletal injuries include acute strain, overuse/repetitive strain, sprain—mostly occurring in the lower body—and falls or overexertion. Prevention of these injuries or reducing them is possible through proper selection of safer types of physical activity. Planning individualized exercise approaches should include educating the patient on strategies to prevent specific injuries, such as proper warm-up techniques before beginning exercise.

2.30.4 Frailty

Frailty is a condition of vulnerability, operationally defined as a syndrome meeting three of the following five phenotypic criteria: low strength, low energy, slow gait speed, low physical activity and unintentional weight loss. It is one of the major syndromes of aging, with a prevalence of 7–16% in older adults aged 65 years and older.

2.31 Physical Activity Assessment

The first step is measuring the current level of motor activity. According to the different methods employed, assessment methods can be divided into self-report questionnaires, diaries, direct observation, and wearables. Whichever physical activity assessment method is used, it should be determined and measured based on several aspects: type, intensity, frequency, time, frequency of physical activity participation, and the costs and limitations of the subject, which should be objectively noticed and assessed.

There are several survey instruments to assess the level of physical activity in community-dwelling older adults. The Physical Activity Scale for Older Adults, the Community Healthy Activity Pattern for Older Adults questionnaire, and the Yale Physical Activity Survey have been studied in various populations of older persons and have been reported to be associated with relationship-based performance.

Wearable monitoring devices can be useful for obtaining objective measures of physical activity. In addition, these activity tracking devices can be useful to promote behavioral changes to maintain a physically active lifestyle by self-monitoring and goal-setting. Common devices include pedometers, accelerometers, heart rate monitors, and wristbands with mobile apps. Pedometers are traditionally used to measure step counts and allow for different levels of physical activity to be categorized as very active (>10,000 steps per day), moderately active (5000–10,000 steps per day), and sub active (<5000 steps per day). With advances in mobile health technology, accelerometers in smartphones, smartwatches, and other wearable devices can provide enhanced activity-related data, including heart rate (HR) monitoring, profiles of physical activity throughout the day, and activity intensity (e.g., moderate to vigorous). Technologies such as pedometers or other wearable devices or fitness apps can provide physical activity feedback directly to the user. Technology can be used alone or in combination with other strategies, such as goal setting and coaching, to encourage and maintain increased physical activity. Technologies can also be used to provide guidance to individuals remotely via text messaging, telephone, or over the Internet. Telephone and Internet delivery strategies can provide guidance to individuals through trained peers or through interactive voice response systems.

2.31.1 Types of Physical Activities

2.31.1.1 Aerobic Activity

In aerobic activity (also called endurance or cardio activity), large muscles move rhythmically for a sustained period of time. Aerobic activity increases the heart rate and makes breathing harder. Aerobic physical activity has three components: intensity, frequency, and duration. Intensity describes how hard a person is trying to perform the activity. The intensities most often studied are moderate (equivalent to the effort of a brisk walk) and vigorous (equivalent to the effort of a jog or run). Frequency describes how often a person does an aerobic activity. Duration describes how long a person does an activity for each session.

2.31.1.2 Muscle-Strengthening Activity

Muscle-strengthening activities, which include resistance training and weightlifting, cause the body's muscles to work or hold against applied force or weight. These exercises often require lifting rather heavy weights to strengthen key muscle groups. Although body-weight exercises may not qualify as traditional resistance training, they still involve external forces—such as the ground or floor—and rely on the individual's own body weight to create resistance, yet in all cases, it would tend to train with all muscle groups over a 7-day period. Resistance training has three key elements: intensity, frequency, and sets and repetitions. Muscle-strengthening activity intensity is based upon how much the muscle has to work in relation to its maximum potential to move the weight. Frequency is the number of days per week that muscle-strengthening activity is performed. Sets and repetitions refer to how many times a person performs a muscle-strengthening activity, such as lifting weights or doing a push-up (in comparison to how long aerobic activity is done).

The effects of muscle-strengthening activities are limited to the muscles that are doing the work. It is important to work all the major muscle groups in the body—legs, hips, back, abdomen, chest, shoulders, and arms.

2.31.1.3 Bone-Strengthening Activities

Bone-strengthening activities (sometimes referred to as weight-bearing or resistance exercises) exert a force on the bones of the body that stimulates bone growth and increased density. This force is usually created by impact with the ground. Bone-strengthening activities can also be aerobic and muscle-strengthening in nature.

2.31.1.4 Balance Activities

These types of activities can enhance the ability to resist forces from within or outside of the body that may cause a loss of balance and a fall, while the person is stationary or moving. Also, the strengthening of back, abdomen, and legs muscles will enhance balance.

2.31.1.5 Multicomponent Physical Activity

Multicomponent physical activity programs include a combination of balance, muscle strengthening, and aerobic physical activity. Additionally, these programs may also include walking, coordination, and physical function training. Recreational activities such as dance, yoga, tai chi, gardening, or sports can also be considered multicomponent because they often incorporate different types of physical activities.

2.31.2 Intensity of Physical Activity

Absolute intensity and relative intensity are two ways to assess the intensity of physical activity.

2.31.2.1 Absolute Intensity

The amount of energy expended during the activity, regardless of the individual's cardiorespiratory fitness or aerobic capacity. Absolute intensity is expressed in metabolic equivalents of task units (METs).

- 1 MET is equivalent to resting metabolic rate (energy expenditure while awake and sitting still).
- 3 to 5.9 METs are equivalent to moderate-intensity activities (including brisk walking at 2.5 to 4.0 mph, playing volleyball).
- 6 or more METs are equivalent to vigorous-intensity activities (including running, carrying heavy groceries, or participating in an intense fitness class, swimming, or cycling).

Low-intensity physical activity is especially beneficial for sedentary people, but the greatest benefits of physical activity come from moderate-intensity or vigorous-intensity activities. For adults, a general rule of thumb is that 2 minutes of moderate-intensity activity is equal to 1 minute of vigorous-intensity activity.

2.31.2.2 Relative Intensity

The level of effort required to perform an activity compared to a person's capacity. For a given absolute intensity, the relative intensity will be greater for someone with a lower aerobic capacity than for someone who is more fit. Relative intensity can be measured using a scale of 0 to 100. It is rated on a scale of 10, with sitting at 0 and the highest possible level of effort at 10. On this scale, moderate-intensity activity is a 5 or 6. Vigorous activity starts at a 7 or 8.

The talk test is a simple tool that can be useful to distinguish between moderate and vigorous levels of physical activity. While one is engaged in moderate-intensity aerobic activity, a person would be expected to be able to converse in a comfortable manner. In contrast, vigorous activity makes it difficult to speak more than just

Table 2.1 Types of activities based on intensity

Low-intensity physical activity	Moderate intensity physical activity	High-intensity physical activity
Making a cup of tea	Walking for health	Aerobics
Moving around the house	Water aerobics	Swimming
Walking at a slow pace	Cycling	Cycling fast or on hills
Cleaning and dusting	Dancing for fitness	Soccer
Vacuum cleaning	Pushing a lawn mower	Walking uphill
Making the bed	Hiking	Dancing for fitness
Standing up		Martial arts

a word or two at a time before the need to catch a breath arises.Relative intensity in older adults is not a better guide to absolute intensity because aerobic capacity changes with age, peaking in adulthood and then declining in old age. For example, some activities, such as some types of yoga or tai chi that are considered low on the absolute intensity scale may be considered moderate or vigorous for older adults (Table 2.1).

2.32 Physical Activity for Older Adults

The benefits of regular physical activity accumulate throughout life and are especially important for healthy aging. Adults aged 65 years and older gain substantial health benefits from regular physical activity, even if they are unable to meet the recommended guidelines. Older adults who are physically active tend to be more likely to participate in activities of daily living and have better physical function (even if frail). They have less chance of falling, and when they fall, they are less likely to hurt themselves. Since most adults sit around for a big portion of the day, it all goes back to what the adults' guidelines began with—move more, sit less throughout the entire day. Light or better yet, moderate-intensity physical activity may bring important benefits when sitting is replaced with this type of physical activity. Multimodal physical activity is important for older adults. Multimodal physical activity is a mix of aerobic, muscle strengthening, and balance exercises. All three features are necessary for this age group due to the threat of falling; strength and balance are required for the population to avoid this.

2.33 Guidelines for Adults with Chronic Health Conditions and Adults with Disabilities

For adults with chronic diseases or disabilities, at least 150 (2 hours 30 minutes) to 300 minutes (5 hours) per week of moderate-intensity or 75 minutes (1 hour 15 minutes) to 150 minutes (2 hours 30 minutes) per week of vigorous-intensity aerobic physical activity, or an equivalent combination of moderate- and vigorous-intensity aerobic activities is recommended. Aerobic activity should preferably be spread throughout the week.

For adults with chronic diseases or disabilities, moderate- or vigorous-intensity muscle-strengthening activities involving all major muscle groups should be done for two or more days per week, as these activities provide greater health benefits.

When adults with chronic conditions or disabilities are unable to meet the key guidelines above, they should engage in regular physical activity according to their abilities and avoid inactivity. Adults with chronic conditions or symptoms should be under the care of a physician. People with chronic conditions can consult with a health care professional or physical activity specialist about the types and amounts of activity appropriate for their abilities and chronic conditions.

2.34 Physical Activity and Injury Risk Management

Physical activity is generally safe for most people, and for most individuals, the health benefits of regular physical activity substantially outweigh the risks. While injuries can happen, it is possible for people to reduce the chances of injury by using proper protective equipment, choosing safe environments to perform activities, following policies and rules that ensure safety, and making responsible decisions regarding physical activity participation. It has also been proved through studies that those who are in good physical shape tend not to get injured as much as those who are not fit. Therefore, regular engagement in physical activity over a period may result in lower risks of injury. It is also recommended that the frequency, duration, or intensity of physical activity be progressively increased to further reduce the risk of injury.

Box 2.1 Key Recommendations for Safe Physical Activity

- To exercise safely and decrease the risk of injuries and other negative outcomes, it is necessary that:
- People ought to consider the risks involved but know that most people can safely engage in physical activities.
- People ought to select physical activity in accordance with their fitness level and health goals; certain activities present a lower risk.
- Gradually, individuals should increase their level of activity and strive to meet the recommendations set forth or some health outcome. Those who are more sedentary should start with low-intensity activities and gradually work toward more frequency and duration.
- Be safe while exercising by using proper equipment, selecting safe places, following rules and policies, and making sensible choices about when, where, and how you are active.
- Anyone facing a chronic disorder or symptom is advised to seek medical help. Those with preexisting medical conditions and those with persistent symptoms need to discuss suitable exercise regimens with a qualified healthcare practitioner or therapist to arrive at decisions regarding safe and beneficial activities and intensities.

2.35 Designing an Exercise Program

WHO has come up with specific guidelines in 2020 for people over 65 years of age that recommend a mix of both aerobic exercise and strength training.

The dose response of health benefits indicates that, for adults and older adults, at least 150–300 min/week of moderate-intensity aerobic physical activity or 75–150 min/week of vigorous-intensity aerobic physical activity can confer the best health benefit.

- Muscle-strengthening activity should be performed in at least 2 days but preferably on all days of the week, at moderate or greater intensity and incorporating all major muscle groups.
- For older adults, multicomponent physical activity with a focus on functional balance and strength training should be done for three or more days a week to improve functional capacity and to reduce the risk for falls.
- To maintain bone and muscle strength, strength training should be performed 2–3 days per week on nonconsecutive days, with at least one day of rest between sessions. The intensity of the exercise should be gradually increased over time.

2.35.1 Nutrition

As we age and physiological changes occur in various organs of the body, including the digestive system, the possibility of nutritional deficiencies and related problems increases. However, lifestyle, proper nutrition, and healthy eating habits can have an even greater impact on longevity and improve chronic diseases than genetic factors. Healthy eating habits not only help improve nutritional status but they can also reduce the risk of disease.

Proper nutrition plays a crucial role in determining energy levels and quality of life. Consequently, the nutritional status of older individuals significantly impacts the frequency of visits to healthcare providers. Nutrition has a profound effect on health and overall functionality, enhancing the body's ability to fight off diseases, maintain physical integrity, think clearly, and have the energy and motivation to engage in social activities.

As individuals age, numerous subtle changes occur that can gradually hinder their ability to maintain optimal nutritional status. These changes necessitate specialized nursing care, and the objective of this chapter is to outline an approach to nutritional assessment and management that considers the unique needs, limitations, and preferences of each older adult. Maintaining a well-balanced diet becomes increasingly challenging as people grow older.

This chapter examines the relationships between nutrition, physical activity, disease burden, and health outcomes. It then delves into age-related changes in body composition and appetite regulation that impact nutritional status and nutrient requirements. The chapter also covers malnutrition and obesity, as well as specific dietary considerations for optimal health. Nutritional disorders, inadequate dietary intake, and poor nutritional status can all affect the progression of various acute and chronic diseases, including coronary heart disease, cancer, stroke, diabetes, and osteoporosis, which are among the top 10 leading causes of death in the United States. Roughly two-thirds of all deaths in the United States are attributed to diseases linked to poor diet and eating habits.

Evaluating the diet quality of older adults is crucial for addressing health and nutritional issues. Such evaluations should be based on an understanding of what constitutes a balanced diet for each individual.

2.36 Changes in Appetite and Energy Expenditure

Maintaining a stable weight requires a steady balance between nutrient intake and energy expenditure. With age, the metabolic, neural, and humoral pathways that normally maintain this delicate balance by regulating appetite and hunger begin to lose their compensatory response to changes in energy needs. Psychological, socioeconomic, and cultural influences and multiple disease processes further contribute to the dysregulation. From the third to seventh decades of life, these factors combine to create an imbalance that typically leads to weight gain and increased fat deposition, at least in societies where food is abundant and the physical demands of life are light. However, after age 70, the risk of weight loss increases steadily with each year of survival. Body weight loss is associated with low dietary energy intake, which is common among healthy and frail older adults. Weight loss in late life is associated with many chronic diseases that increase the risk of death in old age, including Alzheimer's disease.

Pathophysiological changes lead to loss of taste, smell, and appetite with age. Several pathophysiological and age-related changes contribute to the difficulty older adults have in maintaining a balance between metabolic needs and nutrient intake. The appearance, smell, taste, and texture of food all contribute to the desirability of a meal and can stimulate or inhibit further food intake. Thus, the natural sensory systems are essential for the full enjoyment of food and are important regulators of nutrient intake. The ability to smell and taste food is of particular importance. The aroma of food can act as a powerful appetite stimulant. After food enters the mouth, aromatic substances released from the food reach the olfactory cleft through the nasopharynx and enhance flavor. The senses of smell and taste add to the enjoyment of food by stimulating secretions from the salivary gland, stomach, pancreas, and intestines as chemical signals for digestion. The texture, temperature, and quantity of food in the mouth also contribute to the pleasurable quality of a meal and contribute to increased consumption.

Therefore, deterioration in vision, olfactory function, taste, or the ability to sense the temperature and texture of food in the mouth can have a detrimental effect on eating habits and the likelihood of maintaining a healthy diet. This becomes a major concern as we age. Even healthy older adults experience a decline in their ability to detect odors and distinguish one odor from another. A similar pattern is seen for taste loss. Poor oral health and many diseases that reduce chewing, saliva flow, or the ability to swallow can also lead to a deterioration in taste and smell, negatively impacting appetite. Grinding and mixing food with saliva play an important role in releasing volatiles and in bringing the substances into contact with taste receptors, while swallowing movements are essential for pumping the released volatiles to the olfactory cleft where they are perceived.

2.37 Malnutrition in Older People

Malnutrition can manifest in various ways. A diet lacking essential components such as energy (calories), protein, minerals, fiber, or vitamins can result in nutritional deficiencies. The more severe and prolonged the food deprivation, and the more fragile the individual, the greater the likelihood of significant changes in body composition, functional impairment, or overt disease due to these deficiencies. Even mild dietary deficiencies can have notable health effects, such as subtle organ system dysfunction, decreased vitality, or increased susceptibility to illness. Protein and protein-energy malnutrition are common yet often overlooked forms of nutritional deficiency, with older adults with chronic diseases and individuals in institutional settings being particularly at risk. While the relationship between nutrition, disease, and clinical outcomes is complex, protein and protein-energy malnutrition seem to play a crucial role in disease-related morbidity and mortality in these populations.

At the other end of the spectrum, persistently consuming excessive amounts of one or more nutrients can have similar adverse consequences. Forms of malnutrition resulting from excessive consumption include high cholesterol, vitamin deficiencies, and obesity.

2.37.1 Obesity

Obesity is the most common nutritional disorder among older adults in Western societies, especially those living independently. Many obese older adults also suffer from other nutritional disorders. Protein deficiency is a serious and often overlooked issue among obese older adults with chronic diseases or poor functional status. This deficiency can be caused by various factors, such as an imbalanced diet, illness, and lack of physical activity (Table 2.2).

Table 2.2 Obesity-related disorders and conditions

Cardiovascular diseases	Hypertension (high blood pressure) Coronary artery disease Heart failure Stroke
Metabolic disorders	Type 2 diabetes Insulin resistance Metabolic syndrome
Respiratory problems	Obstructive sleep apnea Asthma Obesity hypoventilation syndrome
Musculoskeletal issues	Osteoarthritis Joint pain Gout
Gastrointestinal disorders	Gastroesophageal reflux disease (GERD) Fatty liver disease (non-alcoholic steatohepatitis) Gallbladder disease
Endocrine disorders	Hormonal imbalances Infertility (in both men and women)
Mental health issues	Depression Anxiety disorders Body image issues
Certain cancers	Breast cancer Colon cancer Endometrial cancer Kidney cancer
Skin conditions	Skin infections Intertrigo (inflammation of skin folds)

2.37.2 Weight-Related Complications

The impact of obesity on overall health, functional status, and quality of life is more pronounced in older people. Being overweight in old age is associated with similar risks for disease as in younger populations and also exacerbates many age-related conditions. The increased risk of disease associated with obesity may be due to the harmful metabolic effects of excess body fat and/or the adverse mechanical consequences of obesity. The latter effects include the relative excess of total body weight to muscle mass, which can contribute to osteoarthritis and other debilitating conditions while increasing the effort needed to perform daily activities. This leads to reduced functional reserve, chronic pain, and a higher risk of disability. Some heavier individuals have relatively less muscle mass than expected for their size, a condition known as sarcopenic obesity. For these individuals, the risk of disability is particularly elevated (Table 2.2).

2.38 Nutrients Needed to Maintain Health

2.38.1 Energy Requirements in Older People

Daily energy requirements per kilogram of body weight typically decline with age, decreasing by up to 33% between the third and ninth decades of life. Male gender and chronic disease are associated with greater rates of decline. However, energy requirements decrease with age even among individuals who remain healthy. The primary reason for this decline is the loss of muscle mass, which is almost universal with age. Muscle is much more metabolically active than adipose tissue. As muscle mass is lost, the ratio of fat to lean mass increases, leading to a greater decrease in resting metabolic rate or basal metabolic rate (BMR) than would be expected from a decrease in total body mass. Since BMR generally accounts for 60–75% of TEE, the net result of muscle loss is a significant decrease in total energy expenditure (TEE) and, consequently, energy requirements.

The second mechanism that contributes to the decline in energy requirements with age is a decrease in physical activity. Energy expenditure for physical activity (EEA) generally declines with age at the same rate as BMR, accounting for about 15–35% of TEE in most older adults. However, EEA can range from 5% in those who are bedridden to 50% in very active, fit older adults. Lifestyle plays a major role in determining the amount of energy expended in physical activity in older adults, just as it does in younger adults. Although the increasing prevalence of chronic debilitating diseases causes physical activity to decline with age, even healthy older adults are less active than younger adults. Some chronic conditions may lead to increased TEE, although this is controversial. People with Alzheimer's disease who are constantly moving at a rapid pace, such as those with persistent tremors, fall into this category. Even when a person appears sedentary, their EEA may be higher than expected, especially if they have certain disabilities such as a neurological disorder or amputation. This condition sometimes leads to a loss of neuromuscular energy efficiency and, as a result, exceptional levels of energy expenditure while completing even basic activities of daily living.

As people age, their energy requirements decrease, meaning that older people need to consume less food to maintain their weight and activity level. This puts older people at risk of protein and micronutrient deficiencies, as the need for these nutrients may not decrease as much as the energy requirement. Therefore, it is important for older people to increase their activity level and adjust their diet to include foods that are rich in protein and micronutrients.

The number of calories required by people as they age decreases for a variety of reasons and, therefore, care needs to be taken in food intake to avoid either too little or too much energy intake. The following can be mentioned as reasons for reducing the number of calories needed: With age, the amount of muscle in the body decreases and the amount of adipose tissue, which is made of fat, increases throughout the body. The rate and speed of metabolism in adipose tissue are much lower than in muscles. This process of replacing adipose tissue with muscle, which also increases, causes older people to have less energy than other age groups. Another factor is the reduction in the rate of basal metabolism. Basal metabolism is the lowest amount of energy that a person needs to survive. After the age of 25, this number decreases by 2% per year.

Decreased physical activity and mobility in old age are additional reasons for the reduction in the number of calories needed.

Taking into account the aforementioned factors and the significance of determining the energy needs of older individuals, a specific formula has been created. This formula calculates the number of calories required for older people based on their gender, age, and sex. The formula is as follows:

$$\text{Older men} : 66 + \left(\text{weight}^{*}13.7\right) + \left(\text{height}^{*}5\right) - \left(\text{age}^{*}6.67\right)$$

$$\text{Older women} : 65 + \left(\text{weight}^{*}9.6\right) + \left(\text{height}^{*}1.8\right) - \left(\text{age}^{*}4.7\right)$$

(In the formula above, weight is measured in kilograms, height in centimeters, and age in years.)

2.38.1.1 Protein

Due to the lack of high-quality nutritional studies with adequate representation of older age groups, current recommendations for protein intake do not differentiate between people over 65 years of age and younger age groups. The latest (2005) Dietary Guidelines for Americans, published by the Food and Nutrition Board and the Institute of Medicine, recommend 0.8 g/kg of body weight per day for men and women over 19 years of age. The question of whether protein needs change significantly with age remains controversial. Some experts believe that based on the available data, the recommended protein intake for older adults should be 1.0 to 1.25 g/kg per day. Due to the variability in estimates of protein needs in older adults, it may not be possible to resolve this discrepancy until better measurement techniques become available (Table 2.3).

Factors That Affect Protein Needs in Older Adults

A person's protein needs can change over time and are influenced by age, no protein content in the diet, activity level, medications, and health status. The energy content of the diet is of particular importance. The protein intake required to maintain nitrogen balance increases with reduced energy expenditure. Carefully conducted metabolic studies in healthy young men have shown that nitrogen balance cannot be achieved with any protein when total energy intake is less than 126 kJ/kg (30 kcal/kg). Although comparable data are not available for individuals over 65 years of age, the importance of energy intake in older people is well recognized. Negative energy balance often leads to negative nitrogen balance, particularly in individuals who are ill or have low activity levels. Whether progressive muscular resistance training, alone or in combination with a high-protein diet, can prevent the loss of lean body mass (LBM) in older people during periods of voluntary calorie restriction and weight loss is under investigation. As a general rule, protein requirements increase with higher levels of activity, such as sustained high-intensity exercise.

Table 2.3 (Amount of protein required (g/kg/day)

Age	Male	Female
General recommendation (>65 year)	1.1–1.2	1.1–1.2
Recommendation for acute and chronic disease (>65 year)	1.2–1.5	1.2–1.5

Many diseases and drugs can induce a catabolic state for protein by disrupt the normal balance between protein synthesis and degradation. Older adults who are both bedridden and have an injury, infection, or other acute inflammatory illness are particularly at risk for developing a profoundly negative nitrogen balance, which can lead to rapid loss of lean body mass, especially skeletal muscle mass. High doses of corticosteroids can have a similar effect. Determining the amount of protein that should be consumed to minimize loss of lean body mass and optimize recovery from such disease states is often difficult. In general, hospitalized older patients who are critically ill or recovering from surgery or trauma warrant a protein intake of 1.5 g/kg of body weight per day, unless they have a condition that requires protein restriction, such as renal or hepatic failure. Chronically ill and older residents of long-term care facilities are likely to have equally high protein requirements. Whether one source of protein is better than another in meeting the nutritional needs of older adults is controversial. Although it is generally recognized that all older adults should consume a diet that provides adequate amounts of all essential amino acids, there is little agreement on the importance of the source of protein in the diet. Several animal and human laboratory studies suggest that protein or amino acid supplements containing high concentrations of branched-chain amino acids such as leucine may be more effective than other dietary proteins in stimulating muscle protein synthesis, particularly in sedentary or chronically ill older adults. However, other studies have disputed these findings.

2.38.1.2 Fat and Cholesterol

Fat serves as a key source of energy and essential fatty acids, as well as a vehicle for transporting fat-soluble vitamins. Even when obesity and elevated cholesterol or triglycerides are a concern, fat intake should not be less than 10% of the total energy requirements to allow for adequate absorption of fat-soluble vitamins (A, D, E, K). Essential fatty acid requirements are met through two main types of essential fatty acids, the omega-6 series, derived from linoleic acid (e.g., arachidonic acid and γ-linoleic acid), and the omega-3 series, which can be obtained from α-linolenic acid (from plant sources) or found in certain cold-water fish (e.g., eicosapentaenoic acid [EPA] and docosahexaenoic acid [DHA]). Essential fatty acids are necessary for the synthesis of cell membrane phospholipids and eicosanoids, which include prostaglandins, leukotrienes, and hydroxy acids. Cell membrane phospholipids influence the biomechanical properties of membranes and their membrane-bound receptors. Eicosanoids, primarily derived from arachidonic acid and EPA, serve many functions, including modulation of inflammation and host defense. It is currently recommended that the intake of omega-6 linoleic acids be at least 1% of total dietary energy. Clinical deficiency of these essential fatty acids is rarely seen in adults because Western diets typically provide 8–15 g/day and adipose tissue stores 0.5–1 kg. Omega-6 fatty acids are abundant in many common foods in the average American diet, including most vegetable oils, nuts, grains, seeds, and legumes. When deficiency occurs, it is usually the result of profound cachexia or extensive disease or necrosis of the small intestine and inadequate provision of nutritional support. Although current recommendations for omega-3 derivatives of alpha-linolenic acid call for at least 0.2% of the total dietary energy, many nutritionists recommend higher intakes because of their beneficial effects on lipid metabolism. The oils of cold-water fish, including herring, mackerel, and salmon, are potentially rich in omega-3 fatty acids. Currently, nutrition labels do not list the amount of omega-3 fatty acids in fresh fish. Farm-raised fish may have more or less omega-3 fatty acids than wild-caught fish, depending on the food they are fed. Many omega-3 fatty acid supplements are available.

The optimal fat intake for older adults must be determined on an individual basis. Although congestive heart disease is the number one killer of older Americans, the importance of dietary fat after age 65 remains controversial. It is unclear whether diets that restrict fat and cholesterol have beneficial effects in reducing mortality from congestive heart disease in this age group. In fact, such diets may have harmful consequences, especially in those who have difficulty maintaining their weight. Therefore, it seems prudent to limit fat intake only in healthy older adults who would otherwise not be affected by such dietary restrictions. Increasing the ratio of monounsaturated and polyunsaturated fat to saturated fat, without changing total fat intake, may be beneficial in some circumstances. For this reason, some experts advocate the use of the Mediterranean diet, which promotes the use of olive oil, tree nuts and peanuts, fatty fish, seafood, and white meat while avoiding red and processed meats. There is concern about the use of partially hydrogenated fats rich in trans fatty acids, as these products may have a negative impact on lipid metabolism. Although more study is needed before a specific diet can be recommended, it is advisable to focus on consuming natural fats derived from vegetable oils (mainly monounsaturated), nuts, and fish, while reducing the intake of fats from animal products and avoiding foods containing trans fatty acids. However, these recommendations may not be suitable for frail older adults, especially those who are involuntarily losing weight, have a BMI less than 20, or have medical conditions that restrict their nutrient intake. Because fats provide twice as much energy per gram as carbohydrates and proteins, a high-fat diet may be necessary for these frail older adults to meet their energy needs or address for deficiencies. Restricting the types of foods these individuals consume may have negative consequences.

2.38.1.3 Carbohydrate and Mineral Requirements

Requirements for protein, vitamins, and minerals also change with age, as shown in Table 2.4, and gender.

Recommendations for the carbohydrate content of the diet are usually based on two considerations: the source of carbohydrates and the individual's energy needs. Ideally, food sources should be high in fiber (see the Dietary Fiber Content section later) and provide primarily complex carbohydrates rather than simple sugars. The amount of carbohydrate that should be included in the diet is usually determined by default. First, the individual's energy, proteins, and fat requirements are determined. The carbohydrate requirement is then determined by subtracting the amount of energy provided by protein and fat from the total energy requirements. Since protein is required to make up approximately 15% of the total energy content of the diet and fat should ideally be less than 30%, carbohydrates typically make up 55–70% of the total. When carbohydrates are completely eliminated from the diet, the body's energy needs are met in part by incomplete oxidation of fatty acids, which leads to ketosis, which may cause lethargy and depression. This ketosis also contributes to anorexia, which is part of the appeal of low-carb weight loss diets. At least 50–100 grams of carbohydrates per day should be consumed to avoid ketosis.

Many older adults, whether they are healthy and living independently or frail, ill, or hospitalized, are at risk of micronutrient deficiencies. Several population-based nutritional surveys have shown that community-dwelling older adults typically consume less than 50% of the recommended daily allowance (RDA) for many vitamins. These findings highlight the fact that even healthy adults do not consistently consume the recommended amounts of fortified dairy products, fruits, and vegetables. Risk factors for inadequate intake, adverse drug-nutrient interactions, and nutrition-related diseases all increase

Table 2.4 (Minerals required by men and women

Nutrient	Function	Recommended intake
Calcium	Bone health, muscle function, nerve transmission.	Men: 1000 mg/day (1200 mg/day for those over 70) Women: 1000 mg/day (1200 mg/day for those over 50)
Iron	Oxygen transport in blood, energy metabolism.	Men: 8 mg/day Women: 18 mg/day (8 mg/day after menopause)
Magnesium	Muscle and nerve function, blood sugar control, bone health.	Men: 400–420 mg/day Women: 310–320 mg/day
Potassium	Fluid balance, muscle contractions, nerve signals.	Both men and women: 2500–3000 mg/day
Zinc	Immune function, protein synthesis, wound healing.	Men: 11 mg/day Women: 8 mg/day
Phosphorus	Bone health, energy production, cell function.	Men: 700 mg/day Women: 700 mg/day
Selenium	Antioxidant function, thyroid hormone metabolism.	Both men and women: 55 mcg/day
Copper	Iron metabolism, nervous system function.	Iron metabolism, nervous system function
Manganese	Bone formation, metabolism of amino acids, cholesterol, and carbohydrates.	Men: 2.3 mg/day Women: 1.8 mg/day
Iodine	Thyroid function, metabolism regulation.	Both men and women: 150 mcg/day

with age, making clinical (and subclinical) deficiencies of vitamins and minerals more likely, especially in cases of frailty and the need for institutionalization. Commonly deficient micronutrients include vitamins C, D, E, B12, thiamine (B1), and folic acid, as well as the minerals calcium, magnesium, and zinc.

For this reason, many nutritionists recommend that older adults incorporate a daily, non-iron, general vitamin and mineral supplement that meets the Dietary Reference Intakes (DRI) for most micronutrients to their diet, although there is no evidence to support this recommendation. Studies of multivitamin supplements in noninstitutionalized individuals have found no benefit in reducing cardiovascular or cancer risk. It is also unclear whether intakes of individual micronutrients above the DRI are beneficial in selected populations. High intakes of certain micronutrients such as vitamins A, D, and pyridoxine are known to cause toxicity, which may manifest subtly and nonspecifically, making harmful effects difficult to detect. High supplementation of other vitamins or provitamins like vitamin E and beta-carotene, once considered safe, is now associated with adverse health outcomes. Older adults should be advised not to exceed the tolerable upper intake limit for vitamins and to disclose all vitamin and mineral supplement use when medications are reviewed by any healthcare professional. Vitamin and mineral supplements should not be used as a substitute for an overall healthy eating plan, which includes a high intake of fruits, vegetables, and whole grains and low intake of saturated and trans fats.

Vitamin B12 (Cobalamin)

Low serum vitamin B12 levels become more common with age, and approximately 10–15% of older adults are vitamin B12 deficient. Therefore, low levels do not reflect normal aging. Pernicious anemia, an autoimmune disorder that causes decreased production of intrinsic factor, is a rare cause of deficiency in older adults. Cobalamin deficiency in older adults is most often due to malabsorption of cobalamin from foods, usually due to atrophic gastritis. B12 supplements in crystalline form are not affected by atrophic gastritis and are poorly absorbed. Stomach acid helps remove the vitamin from food and makes it bioavailable. There may be other causes of deficiency in older people that are not yet known. Disorders that interfere with enterohepatic absorption (such as intestinal disease or surgery) lead to deficiency more quickly than low intake because the high efficiency of enterohepatic reabsorption of vitamin B12 is impaired and the vitamin is lost in the feces. Vitamin B12 deficiency can manifest clinically as two relatively independent disorders. There is a blood disorder that causes macrocytosis and anemia and a neurological disorder that can cause peripheral neuropathy, including paresthesia and numbness. Neurological symptom may include spinal lesions, loss of vibration and position sense, sensory ataxia, limb weakness, orthostatic hypotension, and plantar extensor responses. Additionally neuropsychiatric symptoms may occur. These signs and symptoms of vitamin B12 deficiency are nonspecific and in many older people there are associated disorders. When there are multiple possible causes for neurological signs and symptoms, vitamin B12 supplementation is usually associated with measurable but sometimes disappointing neurological or behavioral improvement. The older the patient and the more profound the signs and symptoms, the less likely it is that improvement will occur. However, some patients may respond, especially if the deficiency is relatively recent. Because patients with more severe hematologic symptoms often have less severe neurological impairment and vice versa, it is important to consider vitamin B12 deficiency, even if the patient does not have macrocytosis or anemia. Therefore, screening all older people for vitamin B12 deficiency should be considered, and supplementation is recommended for all patients with vitamin B12 deficiency.

Folate (Folic Acid)

Folate deficiency is often linked to general malnutrition, especially in cases of alcohol abuse, or exposure to specific folate antagonists such as methotrexate, phenytoin, sulfasalazine, primidone, phenobarbital, and triamterene.

Similar to vitamin B12 deficiency, folate deficiency can lead to macrocytic megaloblastic anemia. Supplementing with folate alone may improve the macrocytosis and anemia caused by vitamin B12 deficiency, but it will not address the persistent neurological issues associated with vitamin B12 deficiency and could even worsen neurocognitive function. However, individuals with normal B12 levels who consume high amounts of folate are less likely to experience cognitive impairment.

While tests for vitamin B12 and folate levels are typically part of the evaluation for macrocytosis, low folate levels are not a common cause of this condition. The fortification of cereals with folic acid in the United States since 1998 has led to a decrease in neural tube defects in developing fetuses. Concerns have been raised that this fortification, providing around 100 mcg of folate daily, could mask vitamin B12 deficiency, but this has not been conclusively proven. It is still recommended to consume a diet rich in fruits, vegetables, and fortified cereals as the best source of folic acid, although folate supplements are more easily absorbed by the body.

Folate status can be assessed by measuring serum folate if dietary intake (diet or vitamin supplements) has not changed recently, or by red blood cell (RBC) folate levels if there has been a recent change in diet (such as after hospitalization). Homocysteine levels may be elevated in folic acid deficiency, but they can also be elevated in cases of renal failure as well as with deficiencies in vitamin B12 or B6.

Vitamin D

Vitamin D plays a crucial role in maintaining normal bone health. Evidence suggests that vitamin D has various physiological functions beyond bone and calcium metabolism, although the clinical implications of these effects are debated. Vitamin D receptors are present on different cell types, allowing vitamin D to regulate various physiological processes such as insulin production, myocardial contraction, B and T lymphocyte function, thyroid-stimulating hormone (TSH) secretion, muscle contraction and growth, and central nervous system function. Vitamin D levels are directly linked to significant clinical indicators of health and well-being in older adults, including muscle strength and mass, physical function, and the risk of age-related macular degeneration, periodontal disease, and mortality. While research findings are conflicting, evidence suggests that vitamin D supplementation can reduce the risk of falls and fractures in high-risk populations like older women. Investigations are currently ongoing to determine whether vitamin D or its analogs, given through dietary supplementation, might reduce the risk of diseases such as diabetes mellitus, inflammatory bowel disease, congestive heart failure, colorectal and prostate cancers, multiple sclerosis, and rheumatoid arthritis.

The incidence of vitamin D deficiency increases with advancing age. Vitamin D can be obtained from the diet and synthesized endogenously in the skin following UV-B exposure, but both ways of acquiring this vitamin may be impaired in the elderly. Solar radiation is the main source of UV-B exposure; however, with age, the skin's ability to synthesize vitamin D decreases. Furthermore, older individuals generally remain in the sun for shorter durations and use protective measures such as clothing and sunscreen to protect against skin cancer. Sunscreen, which can reduce skin vitamin D production by as much as 95%, is particularly effective in preventing vitamin D synthesis. Melanin content also plays a role, whereby vitamin D synthesis decreases for people with darker pigmentation; hence, this effect may help explain the higher incidence of low vitamin D levels in dark-skinned individuals compared to light-skinned individuals. Seasonal variations may also affect vitamin D production; thus, many areas in the USA experience very low production in winter. Although many foods are sources of vitamin D, older adults may not be able to consume enough of these foods to meet their needs for this nutrient. A cup of fortified milk or fortified orange juice is supposed to contain about 100 international units of vitamin D, although the actual concentration can vary greatly depending on the manufacturer's quality standards. Fatty fish, especially salmon, also contain vitamin D, although the amount in

Box 2.2 Different Sources of Vitamin D

- Salmon
- Tuna and sardines
- Cod liver oil
- Mushrooms
- D3-fortified milk
- D3-fortified cereal

Calcium

From adolescence onward, both men and women should aim to consume between 1000 and 1200 mg of elemental calcium daily, unless there are specific nutritional needs. Many older adults do not meet this recommended amount. Additionally, calcium absorption decreases with age and varies depending on the food source. For example, a cup of milk or yogurt provides about 300 mg of calcium. While green vegetables also contain calcium, they also contain other phytochemicals that can interfere with calcium absorption, limiting the bioavailability of calcium from vegetables. Due to dietary restrictions or other factors, many older adults may struggle to consistently obtain the recommended amount of calcium from natural sources and may need to consider calcium supplements. Some brands of orange juice and candy now include added calcium, increasing the availability of this essential mineral in food sources. Calcium is also available in tablet form, with calcium carbonate being the most cost-effective option, although it should be taken with food (high-fiber foods may slightly reduce absorption). Other formulas, such as calcium citrate, are better absorbed but may be more expensive and contain less calcium per tablet. It is important to note that calcium supplements can lead to increased constipation in some individuals. Those with calcium oxalate kidney stones should not severely limit their dietary calcium intake, as dietary calcium can actually help reduce the absorption of dietary oxalate and lower the risk of stone formation. While some observational studies have suggested a potential link between calcium supplementation and an increased risk of cardiovascular disease, more research is needed to clarify this association. In the meantime, it is advisable to focus on maximizing calcium intake from dietary sources.

2.38.1.4 Fiber

Dietary fiber is obtained from the structural components of plant cell walls and is made up of plant polysaccharides and lignin that cannot be broken down by intestinal enzymes. Numerous health organizations recommend a daily intake of 20–35 grams of fiber, or 10–13 grams of dietary fiber per 1000 calories consumed. Despite the potential health benefits linked to dietary fiber, such as lower rates of certain cancers, diabetes, heart disease, and obesity, the average American diet is lacking in fiber, usually providing only 10–15 grams per day.

There are two general categories of dietary fiber: insoluble fiber, such as cellulose, hemicellulose, and lignin and soluble fiber, such as gums and pectin. Each category of fiber has a different range of beneficial effects. Both types reduce the energy density of the diet. The added bulk also has a short-term satiety effect, which helps control appetite and prevent overeating. Insoluble fiber has a greater effect on retaining water in the intestinal contents, which increases stool bulk, reduces intestinal transit time, and reduces pressure within the colon. These properties of insoluble fiber make it an important dietary component because it reduces constipation and may help prevent the formation of colonic diverticula. Sources of insoluble fiber include fruits, vegetables, dried beans, wheat bran, seeds, popcorn, brown rice, and whole grain products such as bread, cereal, and pasta. About two-thirds to three-quarters of the dietary fiber in typical mixed diets are insoluble.

Soluble fiber increases the concentration of intestinal contents, prolongs intestinal transit time, and slows the rate of absorption of carbohydrates and bile acids in the small intestine. These effects may have important physiological consequences that could be used to their advantage clinically. By slowing the rate of carbohydrate absorption, a diet very high in soluble fiber may be effective in reducing the postprandial rise in serum glucose, which may be useful in the treatment and prevention of diabetes. Soluble fiber, through its effects on bile acid absorption, can reduce total cholesterol and low-density lipoprotein (LDL) cholesterol by 3–10%. There is an inverse association between total dietary fiber intake and the incidence of fatal and nonfatal myocardial infarction. Several meta-analyses have shown that higher intakes are associated with reduced all-cause mortality. Most of these effects of soluble fiber were demonstrated using fiber concentrates. Comparable amounts of fiber can be obtained from food sources such as apples, oranges, pears, peaches, grapes, vegetables, seeds, barley and rice bran, dried beans, oatmeal, oats, and rye. Diets rich in fiber from food sources also provide essential micronutrients and non-nutrient compounds such as xenobiotics, antioxidants, and phytoestrogens that may have important health-promoting implications. As a general rule, a diet rich in fresh fruits, vegetables, legumes, and whole grain products is recommended. Since most fruits and vegetables contain less than 2 grams of total fiber per serving and most refined grain products contain less than 1 gram per serving, legumes, whole grains, and cereal bran should be substituted for other foods whenever possible to increase fiber intake. Supplementing the diet with any of the commercially available concentrated fiber sources may be necessary, especially in frail older adults. High-fiber sources of dietary fiber may also be helpful in treating chronic constipation when a limited variety of foods is available or the amount of food consumed is inadequate. A large increase in fiber in a short period of time may lead to bloating, diarrhea, gas, and general discomfort. To avoid abdominal problems, it is important to gradually increase fiber intake over several weeks. Fiber supplements should always be taken with plenty of fluids to avoid aggravating constipation. Carbohydrates are rich sources of energy and fiber, but due to the inability of the endocrine system in older people to achieve regular and stable blood sugar, it is best to limit this food group in older people. If carbohydrates are consumed in excess, blood sugar and subsequent insulin secretion in older people will increase sharply, and there will be a risk of hypoglycemia or hyperglycemia (Table 2.5).

2.39 Diet for Older Adults

The US Center for Geriatric Nutrition Research, in collaboration with Tufts University, has recommended a diet plan called MyPlate for individuals over 70 years of age. This plan categorizes food into five groups, represented by a glass and a plate. The glass signifies the importance of consuming enough water and dairy products, while the plate represents the main components of the diet for older adults.

According to the MyPlate plan, half of an older person's daily food intake should consist of fruits and vegetables. Grains should make up another quarter of the diet, with proteins comprising the remaining quarter. Additionally, regular exercise is emphasized in this diet plan for older adults.

Research has shown that modifying and improving diets can lead to reduced healthcare costs. One crucial change that should be made as individuals' age is reducing fat consumption. It is recommended to minimize fat intake and replace animal fats with vegetable fats whenever possible. Some experts even advocate for completely eliminating saturated fats from the diet.

A study conducted in the United States reduced fat intake in older adults' diets to one-third of their usual intake over an 8-year period. The results were surprising, showing a much lower rate of cardiovascular disease compared to their peers.

Table 2.5 Fiber required by men and women

Age	Male	Female
Under 50	31 to 34 grams per day	25 to 28 grams per day
51 and older	28 grams per day	22 grams per day

2.40 Use and Abuse of Dietary Supplements

Half of adults regularly use dietary supplements and vitamins. These individuals often continue using supplements into old age, and some even increase their dosage. Additionally, some older people begin using herbal medicines and teas, like green tea, without consulting their doctor, which can potentially interfere with their prescribed medications. It is advisable for older individuals to discuss their use of herbal medicines with their healthcare provider.

2.41 Special Nutritional Needs in Older Women

Heart disease, cancer, and osteoporosis are common diseases in older women that are related to nutritional status. Modification of nutritional risk factors may contribute to a reduction in the incidence of these diseases. In women, the risk of cardiovascular disease increases substantially between the ages of 64 and 74, approximating the risk observed in men. In older women, reducing fat intake to less than 30% of total daily energy intake can significantly reduce the incidence of cardiovascular disease. While a low-fat diet is believed to also reduce the incidence of cancer, research is still ongoing in this area and definitive results are not yet available.

There is a direct relationship between alcohol consumption and breast cancer in women. Reducing daily alcohol intake to less than 40 grams per day can significantly help prevent breast cancer. Nearly all women who reach the age of 70 experience some degree of osteoporosis. The causes of this osteoporosis include reduced estrogen levels, inactivity, obesity, smoking, and excessive alcohol and caffeine consumption. The risk of bone fractures and their consequences make prevention in this area essential. To help prevent osteoporosis calcium supplements up to 1000 mg per day can be used. Calcium carbonate and calcium citrate tribemates are available on the market for this purpose, with calcium carbonate being more affordable and easily accessible. It is important to note that if doses above 500 mg are used, it is best to take them with meals to prevent damage to the gastric mucosa.

2.42 Improving Oral Health

Maintaining proper oral hygiene, promoting easy swallowing, and ensuring a sore-free, pain-free oral cavity can help older people consume a variety of foods and aid in easier digestion. The health of one's teeth is also a crucial factor in determining the nutritional status of older individuals. Typically, teeth begin to fall out after the age of 30, and by age 70, most people have lost all their teeth. Educating individuals on oral hygiene is essential for achieving proper nutrition. This can be accomplished by raising awareness about the symptoms of oral diseases, such as chronic bad breath and bleeding gums after brushing. Numerous studies have indicated that brushing is more effective than using soft pads or mouthwash for cleaning teeth.

2.43 Water Needs in Older People

As individuals age, the amount of intercellular fluid decreases. This fluid typically makes up around 60% of the body weight in young people, but in older individuals, it decreases to less than 50%. Consequently, even minor changes and reductions in body fluids can be dangerous for older people, as issues that younger bodies can handle well can become life-threatening in old age. The American Medical Association recommends that men over 50 drink 3.7 liters of fluid daily, while women should aim for 2.7 liters. However, this recommendation applies only if the individual does not have any restrictions on fluid intake, as conditions like heart failure or kidney failure may require limitations.

Some older individuals may refuse to drink fluids for various reasons, whether consciously or unconsciously. Common reasons for avoiding fluids include fear of urinary incontinence, reluctance to use the bathroom, lack of access to suitable fluids, changes in thirst, lack of motivation, mood disorders, and nausea and vomiting. Dehydration not only puts older people at risk for various infections, but also significantly increases the likelihood of cognitive disorders, electrolyte imbalances, and issues with bladder muscle function. Dehydration is a serious condition that can be identified by symptoms such as dry skin with poor elasticity, a coated tongue, concentrated urine, a blood urea level over 60, and, in some cases, confusion.

Oder people are also very sensitive to changes in volume and fluid loss. Renal and cardiac function are among the causes of this sensitivity. Fluid overload should be considered when giving intravenous fluids to older people.

Although fluid needs in adults do not change significantly with age, people over 65 years of age have a reduced ability to regulate their fluid intake and are much more likely to become dehydrated than younger adults when their health status or environment changes. Aging is associated with a decreased thirst response to fluid deprivation, delayed correction of increased serum osmolality, and a decreased ability of the kidneys to concentrate urine despite increased serum vasopressin concentrations. Urine output increases two to threefold with age compared with younger adults because the ability to concentrate urine decreases. Chronic diseases and injuries that impair cognitive or physical function further increase the risk of dehydration by altering thirst perception, decreasing the ability to express a desire for water, or decreasing the ability to access and drink adequate amounts of fluids. When an acute febrile illness occurs in an older person who is already physically or cognitively impaired, dehydration can develop rapidly. This scenario occurs with alarming frequency in nursing homes. The failure of many health care providers, family members, and personal care assistants to recognize the risk factors and early warning signs of dehydration contributes to the risk that a frail older person will become severely dehydrated. Many older people themselves are unaware of their risks and may inappropriately restrict their fluid intake, sometimes as a way to control incontinence. Prevention of dehydration should be sought by identifying those at risk, especially older people with cognitive or physical impairments, swallowing difficulties, persistent weight loss, diarrhea, fever, or uncontrolled diabetes, or those receiving enteral feedings, diuretics, or laxatives. The minimum daily intake for inactive adults in temperate climates is estimated to be 1–3 liters per day. A reasonable goal is approximately 30 mL/kg/day for most healthy older adults. Requirements increase with fever, activity, or prolonged exposure to high ambient temperatures. Prolonged exposure to high ambient temperatures, such as exposure during heat waves, may cause profound dehydration. Individuals at risk of dehydration should be given specific fluid prescriptions and their fluid intake should be carefully monitored. Whenever hydration status is suspected, the subject should be weighed, orthostatic blood pressure recorded, and serum electrolytes, urea nitrogen, and creatinine checked. Blood pressure measurements should be compared with baseline values, as many frail older adults have significant orthostasis even when fully hydrated. In some settings, monitoring of urine output may also be appropriate. Skin turgor is not a reliable indicator of hydration status and should not be used in the care of older adults. Patients, families, and all healthcare workers, especially in nursing homes, should be educated to recognize the importance of adequate fluid intake at all times and to carefully monitor fluid intake if there is a change in mental status, activity level, or health status, or if fluid needs increase, as occurs during heat waves.

2.44 Threatening Obstacles to Healthy Eating in Older People

2.44.1 Indigestion and Food Intolerance

Indigestion and food intolerance are very common in older people due to decreased gastrointestinal motility, decreased secretion of digestive juices, and increased gastric emptying time. To address these conditions, older people often turn to using antacids or reducing the amount of food they eat, both of which can have more serious complications in the long run. The most appropriate way to overcome this problem is to use smaller meals in smaller volumes. This method not only helps control indigestion in older people but also helps maintain blood sugar at a constant level and prevents fluctuations in blood insulin levels. Fried and spicy foods can be difficult for the digestive system of older people, so it is recommended to avoid these foods. Sitting in an upright position for half an hour after eating and avoiding lying down for 1–2 hours after eating can reduce the likelihood of esophageal reflux and heartburn.

2.44.2 Anorexia

Anorexia can occur due to various causes, the most common of which are: side effects of medications, inactivity, physical illness, changes related to aging such as changes in the sense of taste and smell, decreased secretion of the hormone leptin, and changes in the structure of the stomach that cause a feeling of fullness with a smaller volume of food. To better manage anorexia, one should first try to identify its cause. For this purpose, it is better to seek help from an expert or nutritionist. Low-volume but energy-rich diets can be used for older people. If necessary, tube feeding can also be used. Some plants, such as ginger, have the property of stimulating appetite and can be used to increase the appetite of these individuals. In people with anorexia, weight should be carefully monitored and its changes controlled. Losing more than 5% of body weight in less than a month or losing 10% of body weight in six months is a very serious and dangerous sign of the presence of disease in older people.

2.44.3 Dysphagia (Painful Swallowing)

Dysphagia, or painful swallowing, is more common in older individuals and can present in various forms. This includes pain when food is moving from the mouth to the esophagus, pain in the esophagus while swallowing, and pain as food enters the stomach. The primary cause of dysphagia is stomach acid refluxing into the esophagus, but conditions like strokes can also contribute.

2.44.4 Constipation

Constipation is very common in older people due to reduced bowel movements, immobility, side effects of medications, and their reluctance to consume fiber and fluids. The difficulty and pain of defecation during constipation may lead some older individuals to avoid eating until they feel the need to defecate, which can be dangerous. To prevent constipation, older people should be encouraged to consume an adequate amount of fruits and vegetables in their diet. Increasing dietary fluids is the next step in controlling and treating this condition. Exercise and physical activity are effective strategies against constipation as they help speed up bowel movements and prevent stool from remaining in the intestine. If these methods do not work, the use of laxatives is recommended. It is important to note that laxatives should not be used in long term as they can create a dependency. If oil-based laxatives are used, attention should be paid to replacing fat-soluble vitamins. Older people should strive to consume 20–30 grams of fiber per day or include 10–13 grams of fiber in their diet for every 1000 kilocalories consumed.

Box 2.3 Recommendations for Preventing Constipation

- Including fruits, vegetables, whole grains, and legumes in the diet provides a good source of fiber.
- Advice increasing fluid intake, as a lack of fluids can contribute to constipation.
- Recommend drinking 6–8 glasses of water daily, taking into account individual medical conditions.
- Incorporate sources of healthy fats like avocado, olive oil, and nuts, as they can help lubricate the intestinal tract.
- Eating meals at regular times may also help stimulate bowel movements.
- Encourage light exercises, such as walking, to help stimulate digestion.

2.45 Sleep Health

Sleep and rest are active, dynamic physiological conditions and are among the primary levels of human needs that occur every day in each person's life. They are essential for human existence, and lack of them can put human life in jeopardy. Sleep is considered a suitable process for recovering, replenishing, and restoring the function of the nervous system and physiological systems of the body. It can also affect the body's internal clock which is considered to be the brain. The brain is a vital and harmonious factor in regulating the body's blood pressure, heart rate, hormones, and other activities.

Sleep deprivation causes neurological, autonomic, and biological changes. As individuals' age and transition from youth to adulthood, sleep problems tend to increase linearly. Sleep is considered one of the most crucial circadian cycles, and it is a complex biological pattern that is quantitatively and qualitatively related to human aging. Various factors, including gender, age, socioeconomic status (SES), place of residence, physical health, mental health, and nutritional status, can cause sleep disorders. However, age seems to be the most significant factor contributing to sleep problems.

The aging process is linked to both objective and subjective changes in the quantity and quality of sleep. Consequently, complaints about difficulties with falling asleep, staying asleep, and overall sleep are more prevalent in older individuals compared to other age groups. Research indicates that sleep ranks third in importance for overall health in healthy individuals, following headaches and digestive disorders. Behavioral sleep disorders, such as frequent awakenings, early awakening, snoring, and decreased sleep duration, are commonly reported in older adults.

Studies comparing the sleep patterns of healthy individuals with those of older adults have revealed that older individuals spend less time in slow-wave sleep (SWS) and deep sleep.

Various studies have shown that insomnia at night can have a significant impact on a person's life, potentially leading to depression, agitation, and increased stress levels. Additionally, research has indicated that cognitive performance and daily activities can be affected by poor sleep, with insomnia and sleep disorders affecting 50–70% of older individuals. Insomnia is the most common sleep disorder among older people, with 40% of those over 60 reporting difficulties falling asleep or staying asleep. These disorders can result in a range of issues, including fatigue, headaches, sensory impairment, mobility issues, memory problems, instability, heightened sensitivity, and decreased performance. These consequences increase the risk of cognitive and psychological disorders, reduced quality of life, dependency, vulnerability, and mortality among older individuals.

Typical alterations regarding sleep patterns associated with age may, at times, jeopardize health effects and affect well-being. Older people may also have increased sleep latency periods, decreased sleep maintenance, advanced sleep-phase type, and excessive daytime sleepiness. Associated symptoms may include fatigue, anxiety, headache, memory impairment, gastrointestinal disturbances, irritability, and low energy levels. During sleep, chemicals such as norepinephrine, serotonin, and growth hormone are released, leading to chemical changes that improve cellular nutrition for daily activities. The nervous system also recovers, memory is consolidated, and learning is facilitated. Additionally, sleep helps relax tension, anxiety, and stress, allowing a person to regain energy and focus on life.

Lack of sleep can impair both the body and mind, leading to mood disturbances and cognitive dysfunction. It is also associated with delusions, metabolic issues, immune system impairment, and reduced coping abilities. Individuals with insomnia have increased stress reactivity compared to individuals without insomnia and are more likely to use emotion-focused coping strategies. The pathophysiology of insomnia represents a state of psychophysiological arousal. Increased stress reactivity, characterized by increased hypothalamic-pituitary-adrenal axis activity, promotes the development of insomnia. Emotion-focused coping increases arousal through the suppression of emotional and physiological responses, leading to increased insomnia.

2.46 Sleep Physiology and Age-Related Changes in Sleep

The human 24-hour sleep/wake cycle is tightly regulated by the master circadian clock in the suprachiasmatic nuclei of the hypothalamus. This clock is synchronized by external factors such as light and food. It is well known that, after sleep deprivation, more sleep is needed to compensate for the lack of rest (sleep homeostatic pressure). Therefore, the homeostatic system increases the amount of sleep required, while the circadian system optimizes the best time for sleep. The suprachiasmatic nucleus also regulates the secretion of melatonin by the pineal gland. Melatonin plays a key role in changing the circadian rhythm and signaling the transition from day to night. Levels of melatonin in the pineal gland are low during the day, increase after darkness sets in (around 9–10 p.m.) and peak during the darkest hours (3–5 a.m.). With age, the pressure for sleep homeostasis declines and contributes to the reduction in the slow-wave sleep. In addition, the effects of reduced circadian signals in older adults are lower temperature in the core body and increased times for both waking and sleep.

Normal sleep is divided into different stages that cycle throughout the night. Sleep stages have been categorized as rapid eye movement (REM) and non-REM (NREM) sleep based on polysomnography studies.

REM sleep, also known as paradoxical asynchronous sleep, is a stage of sleep during which muscle tone is significantly reduced. This stage is associated with bursts of paired gaze and dreaming. The relative amount of REM sleep is maintained into old age, until it shows some decline and occurs periodically in cycles of approximately 90–120 minutes of sleep. Four age-related changes have been consistently found in polysomnography studies: declines in total sleep time, sleep efficiency, and slow-wave sleep, and increases in wakefulness after sleep onset. With aging in adults, total sleep time, sleep efficiency, percentage of slow-wave sleep, percentage of REM sleep, and REM latency all decrease, whereas sleep latency increases.

NREM sleep is divided into four stages. Stages 1 and 2 make up light sleep, while stages 3 and 4 are considered deep sleep or slow-wave sleep (SWS). As individuals age, the amount of stage 1 sleep increases, leading to more awakenings in stage 1. Stages 3 and 4 significantly decrease with age. And in individuals over 90 years old, stages 3 and 4 may disappear entirely. Some studies, have shown that older women may have normal or increased stage 3 sleep, while men may have normal or reduced stage 3 sleep.

2.46.1 Time in Bed

Many older people spend their nights either staying awake without trying to sleep, or lying awake after unsuccessfully attempting to fall asleep. They also use the bed to rest and nap throughout the day.

2.46.2 Total Sleep Duration

The total sleep duration, from sleep onset to the final wake-up from the major diurnal sleep period, increases with age due to a higher number of arousals.

2.46.2.1 Total Sleep Time

Total sleep time is the total sleep period minus the time spent awake during the sleep period. Most studies have found that total sleep time either decreases or remains unchanged in the older population.

2.46.3 Sleep Latency

Sleep latency refers to the time from the decision to fall asleep to the onset of sleep. Studies have shown considerable variation across individuals. In women, sleep latency is related to increasing age and the use of sleeping medications, which reduce sleep latency.

2.46.4 Awakening After Sleep Onset

Wakefulness after sleep onset is the time from arousal from sleep until the final wake-up. The duration of wakefulness after sleep onset increases with age. In one study, Webb attributed 38% of nocturnal arousals to physical discomfort such as bladder distention and urinary urgency. Pain, restless legs, and shortness of breath during sleep are also identified as arousal factors.

2.46.5 Sleep Efficiency

Sleep efficiency is the ratio of total sleep time to the total time spent in bed at night. Most studies have shown a decline in sleep efficiency among older people.

2.46.6 Factors Influencing the Incidence of Sleep Disorders

Basic Sleep Disorders

- Sleep apnea syndrome
- Restless legs syndrome (RLS), periodic limb movement disorder (PLMD)
- Rapid eye movement sleep behavior disorder (RSBD)
- Disorders of the circadian rhythm of sleep-wakefulness (advanced and delayed sleep-wake disorder)

2.46.6.1 Organic Causes

Chronic illnesses are other adverse individual factors affecting sleep quality in the elderly. Sleep disorders are more prevalent in the older population with chronic conditions such as diabetes. This is related to reduced glucose tolerance during the night due to decreased sensitivity to insulin and reduced insulin secretion response to increased blood glucose levels. Glucose metabolism during the first half of the night is affected by a decrease in cerebral glucose intake. Conversely, a drop in peripheral glucose consumption can also contribute to sleep disorders. Hormonal changes after menopause and increased physiological and psychological sensitivity make women more prone to sleep problems and poorer sleep quality. Other physical factors include allergies, pain, cardiovascular issues, pulmonary conditions, metabolic disorders, gastrointestinal problems, urinary issues, psychiatric illnesses, neurological disorders, and itching.

2.46.6.2 Psychological Factors

Other factors that negatively impact the quality and quantity of sleep is mental disorders. Studies have shown an association and bidirectional relationship between depression and insomnia. If the symptoms of depression are left untreated, the quality of sleep will deteriorate significantly over time. In general, insomnia is associated with depressed mood and low quality of life.

One reason for poor sleep quality in single people compared to married people may be related to psychological and social factors. Married people have a significant source of social support, in their families, while single and widowed people are deprived of this support.

2.46.6.3 Environmental Factors

Among the environmental factors that contribute to sleep problems, living in a nursing home is significant. This can be explained by the fact that older individuals who are moved to nursing homes lose the protective and emotional support provided by their families. This can lead to depression, feelings of worthlessness, physical issues, social impairments, and ultimately impact the quantity and quality of sleep. Other environmental factors that can affect sleep in older individuals include being single, having low economic status, living in unsuitable physical environments with extreme temperatures, unwanted noise, and excessive traffic, and lack of contact with loved ones. Since environmental factors are easier to control compared to other factors, addressing issues such as uncomfortable sleeping conditions, excessive noise, light, and inadequate bedding can greatly improve insomnia problems in older individuals.

Behavioral factors related to sleep habits, routines, and activities also play a significant role in sleep quality. Changes in sleeping patterns, such as staying overnight at a relative's house or being hospitalized, can disrupt sleep. Additionally, a lack of social interaction before bedtime can negatively impact an older person's ability to sleep well.

Other activities that are considered risk factors for insomnia and sleep disorders among older people include inactivity and prolonged periods of lying down during the day, unemployment, low quality of life, lack of aerobic exercise and dependence on others to perform daily and instrumental activities of daily living.

2.46.6.4 Social Factors

Retired and unemployed older people are at a higher risk of developing sleep problems. For some, retirement coincides with other stressful life events such as illness or the responsibility of caring for a sick family member. In these situations, retirement is more likely to lead to poorer physical and mental health due to the loss of work-related roles and social connections. As a result, retirement can turn a once-healthy adult into a vulnerable individual with declining physiological functions and an increased susceptibility to various diseases and mortality. This, combined with the development of mental health issues like depression, cognitive disorders, anxiety, and addiction, lays the foundation for insomnia problems.

2.46.6.5 Lack of Physical Activity

Multiple studies have found a strong relationship between lower activity levels and short and poor quality sleep. Increased energy expenditure and endocrine secretions have been proposed mechanisms by means of which exercise is posited to improve sleep quality.

According to the body repair theory, sleep boosts the secretion of anabolic hormones like growth hormone, testosterone, and prolactin, while reducing the levels of catabolic hormones such as cortisol. This results in anabolic activity during sleep following catabolic activity during wakefulness, leading to protein synthesis in most muscles of the body. Since exercise stimulates the body's metabolism and increases catabolic activity for energy production, research suggests that exercise can promote sleep and enhance anabolic activity.

On the other hand, regular physical activity improves physiological efficiency by reducing body fat, especially visceral fat, and plays a significant role in deepening sleep. Additionally, consistent physical activity increases the production of lactic acid in the body, heightening the body's natural need for rest and sleep.

2.46.6.6 Drug Use

Psychostimulants, antidepressants (selective serotonin reuptake inhibitors), antihypertensive drugs (beta blockers, alpha blockers), antiparkinsonian drugs (levodopa), bronchodilators (theophylline), steroids, antihistamines (H1 and H2 blockers), anticholinergics, alcohol, and interferons are all substances that may contribute to an increased risk of falls in older adults.

2.47 Diagnostic Criteria for Insomnia Disorder

Insomnia is defined as a subjective sleep problem characterized by difficulty in initiating, maintaining or achieving quality sleep, even when adequate opportunities and condition for sleep are present. On the other hand, "insomnia disorder" is used to refer to a syndrome characterized by complaints of insomnia. The most recent edition of the International Classification of Sleep Disorders (ICSD) categorizes insomnia as a "chronic insomnia disorder" when symptom occur at least three nights a week for minimum of three months. This diagnosis is applied when insomnia symptoms are not linked to other sleep disorders and medical or psychiatric conditions, or when symptoms persist despite treatment for these conditions. If treatment of other sleep disorders, medical issues, or psychiatric conditions successfully resolves the symptoms of insomnia, the diagnosis of chronic insomnia disorder is not appropriate.

2.48 Common Sleep Disorders in Older People

Common sleep disorders in older people are divided into several categories. These include chronic insomnia, circadian rhythm sleep-wake disorders (CRSWDs), sleep-related movement disorders, and sleep-disordered breathing (SDBs).

Approximately 50% of older adults experience symptoms resembling insomnia. Sleep disturbance or insomnia is the third most common patient complaint, following headaches and colds. About 15% of the adult population in the United States has insomnia severe enough to require medical attention. In the United States 1.7% of the population, receives a prescription for a sleeping pill annually, and another 0.8% purchase over-the-counter sleep medications. Approximately 50 million Americans take some form of sleep medication at some point. In a sample of 649 adults, prescription medication for sleep was reported in up to 19% of cases.

Among older people, older females report more insomnia symptoms than older males. This was demonstrated in an epidemiological study that found that moderate to severe insomnia occurred in 35% of women and 13% of men over the age of 70. Sleep disorders are estimated to affect over half of individuals over the age of 64 living in their own homes, and two-thirds of those over 64 who reside in long-term care settings. Additionally, disturbed sleep is considered contributing factor to long-term-care placement.

In general, sleep disorders are underdiagnosed and a significant concern in older adult populations.

2.48.1 Sleep Apnea

. The term for this phenomenon is Obstructive Sleep Apnea, which is characterized by repeated temporary resumption of breath during sleep. Its causes can either be upper airway obstruction, central states dysfunction, or a mixture of both. Individuals with OSA may wake up gasping for air, wander during the night, and snore loudly while sleeping.

Since awakenings relieve OSA, avoid sedatives and hypnotics in these patients because such agents can further relax the pharyngeal dilators, thereby worsening apnea. Martin and colleagues found that among healthy older people living in community settings, the prevalence of OSA (defined as more than 5 apneas per hour) was 28% in men and 20% in women. They also reported an OSA prevalence of 33% among a random sample of patients in a medical ward; this may relate to a high incidence of CHF in this study group. It is also noted that a large number of the older people who are inpatients are treated with hypnotics, which tend to adversely affect the severity of the OSA. OSA occurs among 42% of the demented inhabitants of nursing homes and further impairs cognitive function. In the general population, prevalence of OSA can go as high as 49% in advanced age.

A synergistic interaction between OSA and cognitive decline in dementia has been suggested. Sedative-hypnotic medications likely worsen sleep apnea and are contraindicated in patients with OSA. OSA may manifest as excessive daytime somnolence, systemic hypertension, cardiac arrhythmias, corpulmonale, and sudden nocturnal death. Coronary artery disease is also a risk. Nocturnal hypoxia secondary to OSAs promotes an increased incidence of cancer.

2.48.2 Chronic Insomnia

The International Classification of Sleep Disorders defines insomnia as difficulty initiating or maintaining sleep that results in daytime disturbance. Symptoms must occur at least three times a week and persist for at least 3 months.

It is estimated that about 50% of older adults report difficulty initiating or maintaining sleep. Sleep problems are more prevalent in women than men throughout the lifespan from 10% of young adults to 30% to 48% of older adults. Self-reported sleep problems are particularly high for older Black women, especially those who have chronic illnesses and major depression. The most common form is sleep-maintaining insomnia, occurring in 50–70%, followed by difficulty initiating sleep in 35–60%. About 25% of older adults complain of non-restorative sleep.

Insomnia in older patients is almost always chronic and is associated with a variety of medical and psychiatric disorders. The higher risk with age is related to the causes rather than the aging process itself, and increases the risk of sleep disturbance. Diagnosis requires a detailed sleep history of sleep-wake cycle patterns, daytime effects, pre-sleep conditions, and daytime napping. Questionnaires, interviews, or a two-week sleep log should also be utilized to ask about medications, sleep medications, and details of insomnia. Likewise, a comprehensive sleep evaluation should rule out the following potential diagnoses: organic conditions, psychiatric disorders, and substance use disorders. The American Academy of Sleep Medicine does not recommend routine polysomnography or daytime testing for chronic insomnia. The diagnosis of sleep-related breathing disorders, narcolepsy, abnormal sleep behaviors, or treatment resistance requires polysomnography.

Nonpharmacological methods are the first line of treatment, with medications being considered if nonpharmacological approaches fail or symptoms worsen. These methods include cognitive-behavioral therapy for insomnia (CBT-I), sleep hygiene education, relaxation therapy, imagery, sleep restriction, and stimulus control therapy. The choice of medication should be based on symptoms, considering any underlying issues, and decided upon collaboratively between the physician and patient, typically for prescriptions lasting up to 5 weeks.

If initial medications are ineffective, alternative options may include atypical antipsychotics like quetiapine (25–100 mg/day), tiagabine (4–6 mg/day), gabapentin (100–600 mg/day), and pregabalin (150–300 mg/day).

Treatments with benzodiazepines or other sedative-hypnotics are not recommended as a first-line therapy for insomnia, agitation, and delirium in older patients due to increased morbidity and mortality. According to the American Academy of Sleep Medicine, it is best to avoid using multiple medications in the elderly. Additionally, hypnotics like benzodiazepines and nonbenzodiazepines (Z drugs) should not be prescribed for insomnia in older adults as they can lead to tolerance, dependence, ataxia, falls, and cognitive impairment.

Polypharmacy, especially when more than 3 central nervous system-active drugs are prescribed, has been linked to falls, overdose, cognitive impairment, and death. It is important to consider the side effects and drug interactions of these medications when prescribing them, and be mindful of any interactions with other medications the patient may be taking.

Furthermore, some drugs commonly used to treat insomnia, such as diphenhydramine, are considered contraindicated by the American Geriatrics Society due to their anticholinergic side effects. When combined with other anticholinergics, they can increase the risk of dizziness and falls in older adults.

A point of caution is the use of melatonin. Melatonin is a supplement taken by individuals suffering from insomnia. The synthetic chemical produced in the pineal gland works to mimic the original and has proved effective for sleep quality and morning alertness in older adults above the age of 55.

Valerian root is another common complementary treatment for insomnia. Valerian root is effective for subjective, but not objective, sleep parameters and may also cause side effects including gastrointestinal upset, allergic reactions, headaches, and restlessness. In a meta-analysis of 10 studies involving over 1000 patients, valerian root showed mixed results, but demonstrated no side effects and was deemed safe for patients ages 7–80.

Finally, patients with mild insomnia and discomfort from pain may benefit from taking over-the-counter acetaminophen before bed.

2.48.3 Circadian Rhythm Sleep-Wake Disorders

Disruptions in the alignment of an individual's endogenous circadian rhythm by external environmental cues (e.g., social obligations or physical activity demands) can result in circadian rhythm sleep-wake disorders (CRSWD). Factors such as age, decreased light exposure, food intake, and reduced activity influence this rhythm. Early morning awakenings affect 20% of the older adult population.

Shift work disorder is often caused by a decrease in total sleep hours due to changes in work schedules. Extrinsic circadian rhythm sleep-wake disorders (CRSWDs) include jet lag disorder, where the body's internal clock does not align with the time zone. On the other hand, intrinsic CRSWDs result from changes in the body's internal circadian rhythm system. Examples include delayed sleep-wake phase disorder, where individuals sleep at least 2 hours later than the expected social time, advanced sleep-wake phase disorder, irregular sleep-wake rhythm disorder, irregular sleep-wake cycles, and non-24-hour sleep-wake phase disorder.

Advanced sleep-wake phase disorder is a common issue among older adults. It involves an involuntary onset of sleep at least 2 hours before the expected time, with spontaneous awakenings occurring in the early morning. Even with a late bedtime, older adults may still experience early morning awakenings. It is important to rule out comorbid conditions that could be causing these early awakenings, such as obstructive sleep apnea (OSA) and periodic limb movement disorder (PLMD), as well as depression and bipolar disorder.

Management of CRSWD is primarily nonpharmacological, involving light therapy and behavioral interventions. Patients are advised to spend time in bright light early in the evening and to avoid light exposure in the morning to help delay their circadian rhythm. Additionally, the bedtime should be gradually pushed back by 3 hours every 2 days until the desired sleep schedule is achieved.

In terms of pharmacological treatment, melatonin receptor agonists are commonly used to shift the circadian clock phase and improve sleep. Ramelteon and tasimelteon are two options available in the United States. Tasimelteon, specifically, has been approved for the treatment of

CRSWD and non-24-hour sleep-wake disorder. Ramelteon, on the other hand, is the only non-benzodiazepine receptor agonist approved by the FDA for managing sleep-onset insomnia.

Overall, a combination of non-pharmacological and pharmacological approaches can be effective in managing CRSWD and improving sleep patterns.

2.48.4 Sleep-Related Movement Disorders

Sleep-related movement disorders include restless legs syndrome (RLS), periodic limb movement disorder (PLMD), and REM sleep behavior disorder (RSBD).

2.48.4.1 Restless Legs Syndrome

It is a neurosensory-motor disorder characterized by an unpleasant sensation in the legs that causes an urge to move them, typically occurring at rest or in the evening/night. The sensation of crawling, tingling, or pain prompts movement of the limbs to alleviate discomfort. It can affect one or both legs, and as the condition progresses, it may also involve the arms or even phantom limb, making it difficult to fall asleep. Symptoms worsen at rest or during the night but improve during the day. RLS is often linked to other conditions such as depression, anxiety, attention deficit hyperactivity disorder, renal dialysis, iron deficiency, uremia, neuropathies, and cardiovascular disease, as well as dysfunction of the dopaminergic system. Iron deficiency is believed to play a role in the development of RLS. Drugs like antipsychotics, antiemetics, antidepressants, beta-blockers, anticonvulsants, and lithium can worsen RLS symptoms and are best avoided. Lifestyle changes and dietary adjustments are typically effective in managing RLS. The American Academy of Neurology recommends supplementation with ferrous fumarate and vitamin C for patients with RLS and low serum ferritin levels, with IV iron replacement for severe symptoms. It is important to investigate and treat iron deficiency and rule out other potential causes of RLS, such as neuropathies, cardiovascular disease, hypertension, depression, and diabetes. In terms of medication, the first-line treatments for RLS are dopamine agonists like ropinirole and pramipexole, which have been shown to be effective and safe. If these are not successful, dopamine precursors like levodopa and other dopamine agonists such as cabergoline can be considered.

2.48.4.2 Periodic Limb Movement Disorder or Nocturnal Myoclonus

PLMD is defined as a sleep-related periodic movement phenomenon characterized by repetitive, stereotyped involuntary movements of the limbs. The leg movements are repetitive, jerking motions that resemble the Babinski sign: extension of the big toe, dorsiflexion of the toes and ankles, and often flexion of the knee and hip. Moreover, PLMD is related to a high cardiovascular and cerebrovascular risk since it is a motor manifestation of increased sympathetic hyperactivity, thus responsible for the nocturnal elevation of blood pressure and heart rate. PLMD can also be present in the absence of concomitant sleep or medical disorders. The cardinal symptoms for patients with PLMD include restless sleep and daytime fatigue. The prevalence of PLMD among patients with RLS reaches up to 80% and between 4% and 11% among the older population. The prevalence of both disorders increases with age and is commonly associated with other sleep disorders and other medical conditions, including congestive heart failure, diabetes, liver and kidney disease, migraine, alcohol dependence, and several neurological and psychiatric disorders. Some medications, including antidepressants and lithium, can trigger PLMD.

The first step in treatment is to avoid certain medications that may aggravate PLMD, including antidepressants such as mirtazapine, venlafaxine, sertraline, fluoxetine, and amitriptyline. Caffeine-containing products should also be avoided. Treating underlying conditions, such as iron deficiency anemia, is also helpful in cases associated with RLS.

Dopaminergic drugs like pramipexole, ropinirole, and rotigotine, as well as other drugs like gabapentin and pregabalin, reduce periodic limb movements in patients with PLMD. A few small studies show that clonazepam 1 mg at bedtime, melatonin 3 mg 30 minutes before bedtime, and valproate 150–600 mg at bedtime may improve quality of sleep.

It is a repetitive, unilateral or bilateral jerking of the legs that awakens the patient from sleep. In a random sample of 427 older volunteers, 45% had periodic limb movements of sleep (PLMS). This is associated with sleep dissatisfaction, sleeping alone, and kicking at night. Other estimates of PLMS prevalence have been 28.6% in a sample of 2162 and 29.3% in a random sample of 696. Nocturnal myoclonus incidence increases with age, and the likelihood of sleep and wake complaints is related to age, absolute number, and severity.

2.48.4.3 REM Sleep Behavior Disorder

In RSBD, there is typically a loss of muscle atonia during normal REM sleep. This is often due to dysfunction in the brainstem circuits responsible for maintaining normal REM sleep atonia and suppressing behaviors during REM sleep. These abnormal behaviors that occur during REM sleep can lead to sleep impairment or disruption.

The prevalence of RSBD is relatively low, around 0.5% in the general population and up to 5–7% in older populations. Over 70% of patients with RSBD develop neurodegenerative diseases within 12 years of diagnosis. Clinical diagnosis relies on observing vigorous motor behaviors during violent dreams, such as talking, kicking, biting, and punching. These behaviors typically occur during periods of emotional stress or when withdrawing from sedatives and alcohol, but can also happen in healthy individuals. Additionally, the eyes remain closed, and the surrounding environment appears to be moving vigorously. It is crucial to inquire about the quality of sleep from patients as this can aid clinicians in diagnosing untreated RSBD early. Diagnosis requires polysomnography, which reveals a loss of normal skeletal muscle atonia during REM sleep.

Idiopathic RSBD is linked to neurodegenerative disorders like Parkinson's disease, Lewy body dementia, and multiple system atrophy. RSBD is often an early sign of neurodegeneration in the brainstem before spreading to other regions of the central nervous system.

The median time for transitioning from idiopathic RSBD to an underlying neurodegenerative disease that accumulates alpha-synuclein in nerve cells, known as synucleinopathy, is 4–9 years from the diagnosis of idiopathic RSBD and 11–16 years from the onset of symptoms.

Approximately 33–46% of Parkinson's disease patients also have RSBD. Risk factors for idiopathic RSBD include previous head trauma, agricultural work, pesticide exposure, low education level, smoking, ischemic heart disease, and use of inhaled corticosteroids. Patients with Parkinson's disease and RSBD often experience cognitive decline and are more likely to be diagnosed with mild cognitive impairment. Most commonly, insomnias in people with Parkinson's disease are found to correlate with a higher level of depression, balance impairment, and gait disturbance in this condition. Most importantly, they define themselves through progressive decrement of sleep maintenance. Therefore, individuals over 50 years with symptoms of mild cognitive impairment and sleep disturbances are at a higher risk of developing neurodegenerative diseases. For patients with these risk factors, adopting a healthy lifestyle by quitting smoking and avoiding alcohol is recommended. Additionally, managing comorbid conditions such as hypertension, diabetes, anxiety, and depression may be beneficial.

Prioritizing environmental modifications to prevent injury and trauma is crucial in managing this disorder. Using bedside alarms, adjusting positions, treating underlying causes, and discontinuing medications that worsen RSBD, such as certain antidepressants, are key strategies. Notably, medications that can exacerbate RSBD include SSRIs, SNRIs, tricyclic antidepressants, monoamine oxidase inhibitors, beta-blockers (like atenolol and bisoprolol), tramadol, and cholinesterase inhibitors. Low-dose clonazepam (0.5–1 mg/day) is the preferred treatment for

RSBD, taken 30 minutes before bedtime, but caution is advised in patients with sleep apnea. Zopiclone is another effective option with a shorter half-life compared to clonazepam. Melatonin at high doses (3–15 mg) before bedtime, with a median effective dose of 6 mg, can also be beneficial. Pramipexole (0.1–0.5 mg) and other dopaminergic agonists, in addition to acetylcholinesterase inhibitors (e.g., rivastigmine), can also be alternative treatments for patients who do not benefit sufficiently from frontline therapies.

2.48.5 Sleep-Breathing Disorders

Sleep breathing disorders (SBDs) encompass a variety of conditions, including obstructive sleep apnea (OSA), primary or secondary central sleep apnea (CSA), non-obstructive hypoventilation, and hypoxemic disorders related to pulmonary parenchyma and vascularity. Other potential causes of SBD include neuromuscular or chest wall disorders, periodic breathing at high altitudes, Cheyne-Stokes breathing, and more. The prevalence of SBD is high, with rates as high as 34% in men aged 30–70 years, 17% in women aged 30–70 years, and an overall prevalence of 23.9% in patients aged 65–100 years.

Sleep apnea is the most common SBD, characterized by intermittent partial or complete closure of the upper airway leading to sleep arousal and arterial hypoxia. Apnea refers to a complete cessation of breathing, while hypopnea involves a 30% reduction in airflow with more than 4% oxygen saturation.

The Apnea-Hypopnea Index (AHI) measures the total number of apnea and hypopnea episodes per hour of sleep, with a score greater than 5 indicating the presence of the disorder. OSA, a type of sleep apnea, is marked by more than five breathing pauses during sleep due to a loss of ventilator drive. This condition is often associated with anatomical or neuromuscular factors, such as a large neck circumference, high body mass index, and structural issues in the pharyngeal airway.

Untreated OSA can lead to cardiovascular diseases like coronary artery disease, stroke, and atrial fibrillation. CSA, on the other hand, is commonly seen in conditions like congestive heart failure and can increase mortality in patients with heart failure.

Treatment for OSA is crucial, particularly in older populations, due to its link to vascular disease and cardiovascular events. Weight loss, positional therapy, and the use of positive airway pressure devices are recommended for managing moderate to severe SBD. Avoiding sedatives and hypnotics is also important in SBD treatment. eXciteOSA is a recently FDA-approved rechargeable mouthpiece that is placed on the tongue and delivers neuromuscular electrical stimulation to the genioglossus muscle to increase muscle endurance to increase airway patency. If daytime sleepiness persists even with positive airway pressure, stimulants may be used. Optimizing heart failure therapy may improve CSA. Nocturnal oxygen supplementation and theophylline have been shown to reduce the severity of CSA.

2.48.6 Sundown Syndrome

Sundown syndrome is a behavioral phenomenon closely related to disturbance in the circadian rhythm with an incidence rate as high as 66% in patients with dementia and in nursing homes. The disruption of the circadian rhythm that causes sundown syndrome may be associated with seasonal pattern, such as during winter or in geographic locations with limited sunlight exposure. It is behaviorally manifested by restlessness, aggressiveness, confusion, disorientation, and mood changes. The name, "sundown," suggests that it is usually observed in the late afternoon or evening. Sundown behaviors are associated with functional impairment, rapid cognitive decline, financial burden, caregiver burden, and increased risk of institutionalization.

2.48.7 Mental Disorders

Psychiatric conditions include dementia, with anxiety and depression often being associated with insomnia. In fact, 50% of older patients with major depressive disorders report significant sleep disturbance. It is important to evaluate these disorders using clinical tools such as the MMSE and/or the GDS before considering sleep therapy.

In depressed patients, there may be a lengthened sleep latency, shortened REM latency, lengthened early REM sleep, more nocturnal awakenings, less SWS, and premature awakenings.

Patients with dementia often have poor sleep efficiency, prolonged stage 1 sleep, reduced stages 3 and 4, reduced REM sleep, sleep/wake disturbances, nocturnal wandering episodes, and daytime napping.

Older patients typically take between 5 and 9 medications daily, some of which can affect their sleep and wakefulness. Sedative antidepressants like amitriptyline and neuroleptics such as chlorpromazine and clozapine can lead to impaired performance and daytime sleepiness. It is advisable to avoid prescribing amitriptyline to older patients due to its anticholinergic effects and potential to cause confusion. Beta-blockers, especially lipophilic ones like metoprolol and propranolol, can cause issues with falling asleep, increased awakenings, and vivid dreams. Less lipophilic beta-blockers like bisoprolol and atenolol are preferred to minimize sleep disturbances.

Long-term use of sedative-hypnotic drugs can disrupt normal sleep-wake patterns either due to drug withdrawal or lingering daytime drowsiness. Many older patients in hospitals receive inappropriate prescriptions for sedative hypnotics. Stimulants like theophylline and caffeine can reduce slow-wave sleep and overall sleep duration while promoting wakefulness. The effects of caffeine can last up to 14 hours, and older patients may experience heightened sensitivity due to reduced liver function affecting caffeine clearance. Moreover, caffeine is present in various over-the-counter medications, including painkillers, cold remedies, allergy medications, and appetite suppressants.

Nicotine, a stimulant, disrupts sleep in ways similar to caffeine. Several studies have shown that smokers of all ages experience more sleep issues than nonsmokers, including trouble falling asleep and shorter sleep duration. Additionally, smokers may also experience excessive daytime sleepiness.

Personality and emotional disorders can also contribute to poor sleep or complaints of poor sleep quality. This often presents as early morning awakenings, a reduction in stage 4 sleep, and a short REM latency, which is particularly common in older adults. Conditions such as bipolar disorder, schizophrenia, PTSD, and anxiety disorders can make it challenging to both fall asleep and stay asleep.

2.49 Other Causes

- Other causes of disturbed sleep include chronic pain disorders such as osteoarthritis and metastatic diseases. Osteoarthritis can cause nocturnal joint stiffness and painful movement during sleep.
- Left ventricular failure with orthopnea and nocturnal dyspnea can result in disturbed awakenings.
- Cheyne-Stokes breathing pattern due to cardiac or cerebral causes can be treated with respiratory stimulants or nocturnal oxygen therapy to improve sleep
- Patients with COPD may experience nocturnal exacerbations of hypoxemia, particularly largely during REM sleep.
- Lower urinary tract symptoms (LUTS) like benign prostatic hypertrophy and detrusor instability can also contribute to poor sleep.
- Individuals with Parkinson's disease may have frequent urination and difficulty turning and getting out of bed, leading to fragmented sleep.
- Tachyarrhythmia.
- Gastroesophageal reflux disease (GERD).
- Constipation.
- Pruritic skin conditions.
- Socioeconomic factors include lack of adequate support from spouse and family.

2.50 Improved Quality of Sleep

2.50.1 Sleep Hygiene

Sleep hygiene is described as a set of behaviors that promote sleep while also avoiding behaviors that can disrupt sleep. It consists of a list of recommendations including behaviors, environmental conditions, and other factors related to sleep that can be used in treating insomnia through single or multiple interventions. Sleep hygiene education involves counseling on various lifestyle and behavioral factors, as well as environmental and physiological factors such as light, temperature, noise, bed quality, pain, and unresolved concerns that can impact a patient's sleep quality and quantity. A study conducted by Taheri et al. found that sleep hygiene education may improve the quality of sleep, severity of insomnia, and overall health in older women, making it a justifiable method of treatment in primary health care due to its affordability and accessibility.

2.50.2 Music Therapy

Another non-pharmacological treatment method is listening to music, which has recently become a common strategy. Music serves as a source of support to induce and enhance relaxation, and reduce or control stress in individuals. It is an effective intervention for stress management, establishing relaxation, and anxiety control through self-management techniques. Music also significantly improves sleep quality and perception of sleep quality, increases sleep duration, efficiency, reduces onset time and disturbance, and enhances daytime performance.

A meta-analysis study revealed that music has a moderating effect on sleep disorders and can be beneficial for people with sleep issues due to its accessibility and low cost. Music initiates the sleep process by reducing noradrenaline secretion in the blood flow. Soft music with a steady rhythm of fewer than 80 beats per minute can relax anxiety and stress, lowering cortisol levels. Music also enhances subjective sleep in adults, raises the pain threshold, and decreases heart rate, anxiety, and depression among older individuals.

While there are various drug treatments for sleep disorders, issues such as drug dependence, resistance, and costs are disadvantages of these methods. Therefore, incorporating non-drug methods, such as music therapy, in treating sleep disorders seems like a logical approach.

2.51 Sexual Health

The other crucial issue within the realm of health, especially concerning the aging community, is sexual health. This aspect of health pertains to the situation where couples engage in appropriate and normal sexual relations, showcasing desirable physical and psychological statuses that reflect intimacy, love, and harmony in married life. The sexuality of older individuals is a significant indicator of their quality of life, yet despite its importance, many sexual health needs of older adults go unmet. Sexual health is an important part of any individual's total well-being and quality of life. It has many interconnections with identity and character and affects the different relationships a person has with oneself, partners, and society. Hence, sexual health is a salient aspect of overall health and quality of life, covering physical, psychological, and social dimensions of wellness. The World Health Organization defines it as "a state of physical, emotional, mental, and social well-being in relation to sexuality," emphasizing that it is more than just the absence of disease, dysfunction, or disability. Sexual health involves a positive and respectful attitude towards sex and relationships, fostering the potential for pleasurable and safe sexual experiences free from coercion, discrimination, and violence. Despite evidence showing that many adults maintain sexual activity in later life, negative stereotypes about asexuality persist among older age groups. As the population of older individuals grows, outdated beliefs about their sexuality persist, despite the fact that the need and desire for sex do not diminish with age. Sexual health in older individuals directly impacts their quality of life, physical health, and overall well-being. Contrary to common misconceptions that sexual desire declines significantly with age, research indicates that many older individuals remain sexually active and interested well into their later years. Cultural factors also play a role in maintaining sexual activity among older adults. Additionally, age-related sexual behaviors and attitudes, levels of sexual interest and activity among couples, and their current sexual relationships are all factors at play in understanding sexual health among older individuals.

Physical changes associated with aging do not inevitably result in sexual dysfunction: good physical and mental health, a positive attitude towards sex in later life, and access to a healthy partner are associated with continued sexual activity and regular sexual expression. However, the most common assumption is that an older person is asexual, and the greatest problem is that older persons find it hard to open up about this issue to their doctor or health provider. There are many possibilities that can act as sexual desire at an older age: a lack of a healthy sexual partner, depression, monotony of a repetitive sexual relationship, lack of physical attraction to a partner or spouse, hormonal variations, and illness and/or unpleasant factors.

These changes encompass the factors previously mentioned: physiological changes that come with age, comorbidities that affect the physical and mental health of older individuals, the use of multiple medications, and various aging syndromes that collectively have a negative impact on maintaining sexual activity among the elderly. However, sexual desire, sexual behavior, and intimacy remain important in every stage of adulthood and serve as crucial indicators of quality of life. Engaging in sexual activity and achieving sexual satisfaction are associated with numerous physical and mental health benefits, including a reduced risk of cardiovascular disease.

For most healthy adults, pleasure and interest in sex endure with age. Aging itself should not prompt a change in the sexual behaviors that have always brought you enjoyment. It may be necessary to make minor adjustments to accommodate physical limitations or the effects of certain illnesses or medications.

2.51.1 Psychological Aspects of Aging and Gender

These changes are influenced by various factors, including physiological changes with age, comorbidities affecting the physical and mental health of older individuals, the use of multiple medications, and various aging syndromes that collectively have a negative impact on maintaining sexual activity among the elderly. However, sexual desire, behavior, and intimacy remain important in every stage of adulthood and serve as key indicators of the quality of life. Sexual activity and satisfaction are associated with numerous physical and mental health benefits, including a reduced risk of cardiovascular disease.

For most healthy adults, pleasure and interest in sex can persist as they age. Age itself should not be a deterrent to enjoying sexual behaviors that have always been pleasurable. It may be necessary to make minor adjustments to accommodate physical limitations or the effects of certain illnesses or medications. Although masturbation is an option, older adults may view masturbation as unnatural or even unhealthy. Education and permission by a health care professional may help to dispel such myths.

There are also some misconceptions about how sexual desire changes with age. Self-critical anxieties about sexual performance or physical appearance can be a distraction or even a hindrance to sexual pleasure and arousal.

This societal focus on associating sexual desire primarily with the young can lead to feelings of shame among older individuals when it comes to pursuing their sexual interests. As a result, these individuals may be hesitant or reluctant to seek help from sexual counselors. Providing information from physicians about the normal changes that come with age and how they can impact sexual desires could offer encouragement and guidance on finding continued meaning in pursuing sexual relationships.

2.51.2 Sexuality, Medication, and Illness in Older Adults

Physical illness can directly affect sexual function by interfering with the endocrine, neurological, and vascular processes that mediate sexual response. It can also indirectly impact sexual function by causing weakness or pain, as well as psychologically by inducing changes in body image and self-esteem. Due to the limitations of this article, a comprehensive discussion of the effects of medical illness on sexual desire is not possible.

2.51.3 Other Issues That Can Affect Sexual Relationships

In addition to physical changes, cultural and psychological factors can sometimes affect sexual desire in later life. For example, today's culture often associates sexual desire with youthfulness and vitality. However, there is no age limit when it comes to experiencing pleasure through sex. Our physical and emotional needs evolve over time and in different situations. Intimacy and sexual desire may hold varying levels of importance for each individual. It is possible to lead a fulfilling life with or without engaging in sexual activity.

2.51.4 Risk Factors for Sexual Dysfunction

Sexual dysfunction is influenced by numerous risk factors, which include physical, psychological, and neurological conditions.

2.51.4.1 Physical Factors

- Chronic pain: It can limit physical mobility, cause discomfort during sexual activity, and reduce overall sexual satisfaction. Pain can interfere with closeness and lead to fatigue and exhaustion, leaving you with little energy or interest in sex. Chronic pain is often treatable and does not have to be a part of aging. However, some pain medications can affect sexual function. Always talk to your healthcare provider if you experience side effects from any medication.
- Arthritis: Joint pain from arthritis can be uncomfortable during sexual intercourse. Treatment may involve exercise, medication, or joint replacement surgery to alleviate the pain. Additionally, rest, warm baths, and adjusting sexual relations may be beneficial.
- Diabetes: This condition can lead to erectile dysfunction and yeast infections if poorly managed. It can cause discomfort and make sexual intercourse undesirable. Proper management is crucial to prevent these issues.
- • Dementia: Individuals with dementia may experience changes in sexual behavior and desire. It can be confusing and challenging to deal with. Seeking advice from a healthcare professional trained in dementia care can be helpful.
- Neurological disorders: Conditions like Alzheimer's disease, Parkinson's disease, multiple sclerosis, and spinal cord injury can cause sexual problems due to nerve damage. This can lead to decreased arousal, sensation, or orgasm.
- Heart disease: Arterial narrowing can impact blood flow, making it difficult to become aroused or maintain an erection. It can also affect orgasm. Always follow your doctor's advice if you have concerns about sexual activity after a heart attack.
- Urinary incontinence: Age-related bladder control issues can lead to urine leakage during sex. Changing positions or emptying the bladder before and after sex can help. Treatment options include medical treatments, bladder control training, and lifestyle changes.
- Hormonal imbalances: Low testosterone or estrogen levels can cause low libido and sexual dysfunction in both men and women.
- Stroke. Having a stroke can sometimes make it difficult or impossible to have sex. Changes in position or use of a device can allow sexual relations for those with ongoing weakness or paralysis. Some people who experience paralysis from the waist down remain capable of having an orgasm and pleasure.

- Surgery can be worrisome, especially when it involves the genital area, such as hysterectomy, mastectomy, and prostatectomy. However, most people are able to return to their previous sex life after these surgeries, and for some, it may even open up new options for sexual activity.
- Depression can also impact sexual desire, as a lack of interest in intimacy and sexual activity can be a sign of this condition. If you suspect you are depressed, it's important to speak with your healthcare provider about potential treatments that won't interfere with your desire.
- Anxiety, chronic stress, and neurological conditions can all contribute to sexual dysfunction. However, the most critical factors in determining sexual desire and function are relationship security, emotional intimacy, and communication. People who have experienced past trauma or are currently in unhealthy relationships are more likely to experience sexual dysfunction, as these factors can have a significant impact on desire and function.

Addressing these underlying issues is crucial for effectively managing and treating sexual dys function. By recognizing and addressing these factors, individuals can work towards improving their sexual well-being.

2.51.5 Sexual Health Discussion

Many primary care physicians, especially those treating older patients, find it difficult or embarrassing to discuss sexual health. However, research indicates that patients struggle to bring up sexual issues with their doctors and would rather have their doctors broach the topic. This can result in insufficient attention being paid to sexual health concerns. In particular, men are less likely than women to always report sexual problems to their doctors. They may choose to ignore the issue, stop taking medications they believe are causing sexual dysfunction, or purchase medications online. These actions can lead to depression, social withdrawal, and delayed diagnosis of underlying conditions.

2.51.5.1 Sexual Activity Among Older Adults

Research indicates that the later years can still be filled with passion. In fact, according to the National Project on Social Living, Health, and Aging, a majority of older adults remain sexually active: 73% of adults aged 57–64 years, 53% of adults aged 65–74 years, and 26% of adults aged 75–85 years report being sexually active.

Sexual activity and sexual satisfaction are positively related to self-reported health and marital status.

2.51.5.2 Sexual Satisfaction in Older People

A satisfactory sexual life plays a crucial role in overall health and happiness, significantly impacting close relationships and adding quality to our lives. Sex is considered essential for maintaining happiness in a relationship. Studies have shown that both men and women over the age of 65 who reported engaging in sexual activity within the past year had higher life satisfaction scores compared to sexually inactive older adults. Sexual activity has been found to have an inverse relationship with feelings of happiness and overall well-being. The data suggests that satisfaction with one's sex life peaks in the mid- to late 30s and gradually declines after the age of 70. These findings emphasize the importance of addressing sexuality as a key component of health throughout our lives.

2.51.6 Physiological Changes Associated with Aging

Aging brings changes to the endocrine, vascular, and nervous systems, which have direct and indirect effects on sexual arousal and function.

Box 2.4

Age does not protect individuals from sexually transmitted diseases (STDs). Older individuals who are sexually active may be at risk for diseases such as syphilis, gonorrhea, chlamydia, genital herpes, hepatitis B, genital warts, and trichomoniasis. Sexually active individuals, regardless of age, may also be at risk for HIV, the virus that causes AIDS.

In fact, the number of older individuals living with HIV/AIDS is increasing. If you or your partner has multiple sexual partner, you are at risk for HIV/AIDS if you engage in unprotected sex. To protect yourself, always use a condom during vaginal or anal sex and use a dental dam or other barrier method during oral sex. It is important to learn more about using condoms, dental dams, and other methods of preventing STDs.

2.51.6.1 Physiological Aspects of Aging and Sexual Desire in Men

There is considerable individual variation in the actual physiological changes that occur with age and affect sexual function. It is estimated that 55% of men experience erectile dysfunction by age 75. Changes leading to a decline in sexual function, particularly erectile dysfunction (ED), are multifactorial. These factors may be organic, such as those from disease or medication effects, and psychological, such as anxiety and guilt. It is clear that all phases of the human sexual response cycle, as defined by Masters and Johnson, are affected by age-related factors. However, there is no evidence to suggest that erectile dysfunction is inevitable among older men who are psychologically and physiologically healthy.

2.51.6.2 Sexual Response Cycle

Normal age-related changes that accompany the emotional phase of sexual response in men include a decline or lack of increase in testosterone levels. Reduced scrotal vascular congestion, decreased scrotal sac tension, and delayed erection are common. While a young man may achieve a full erection within seconds, an older man may require several minutes to achieve a similar response.

These changes may be partly explained by age-related alterations in adrenergic and cholinergic mechanisms. The process of erection is a vascular event mediated by the autonomic nervous system, where the body's smooth muscle tone plays a major role in erectile ability. Gap junctions and ion channel mechanisms are largely responsible for determining the degree of smooth muscle tone.

There is evidence that, with aging, there is a reduction in the number of β-adrenergic and cholinergic receptors, potentially leading to an increased dominance of α-adrenergic activity. This increased smooth muscle tone could interfere with the relaxation of the body's smooth muscle necessary for the initiation and maintenance of the erectile response.

Age-related cellular changes may adversely affect the erectile response through increased deposition of connective tissue, resulting in reduced penile dilation.

Penile sensitivity also decreases with age, making achieving and maintaining an erection more reliant on direct physical stimulation and less responsive to visual, psychological, or non-genital stimuli.

As a result, the sexual partner may need to assist in stimulating the erectile response through manual or oral means before and during sexual activity to maintain an erection until orgasm. Penile rigidity typically decreases with age, starting in most men around age 60. While rigidity is usually sufficient for vaginal intercourse, couples may need to explore different sexual positions or incorporate manual stimulation to enhance the experience.

The plateau phase of sexual response lengthens with age, and pre-ejaculatory discharge and secretions decrease or disappear. Previous issues with premature ejaculation may improve in older men due to increased arousal and the time needed to reach orgasm. The duration of orgasm decreases with age, with less frequent and intense spastic contractions of the prostate and urethral muscles, as well as a decrease in the force of ejaculation. The time before ejaculation decreases from 2 to 4 seconds in young men to about 1 second in older men, and there is a gradual decrease in semen volume with each ejaculation. Occasionally, orgasm may occur without ejaculation. The final phase after orgasm, or resolution of sexual response, is marked by a faster loss of vasoconstriction and a longer refractory period.

For a 20-year-old male, the refractory period may be just a few minutes, while for an 80-year-old man, it could take several days, likely reflecting the time needed to restore normal levels of ions and neurotransmitter concentrations.

2.51.7 Physiological Aspects of Aging and Sexual Desire in Women

2.51.7.1 Effects of Menopause

Menopause, which typically occurs around age 50 for most women, is marked by a notable decrease in estrogen, progesterone, and androgen levels. After menopause, estrogen is primarily derived from the peripheral conversion of adrenal androgens. Around age 65, there is a further decrease in adrenal androgen production, known as adrenopause.

The decline in estrogen levels during menopause is the cause of many of the typical age-related changes in the genital tract. These changes include a reduction in pubic hair, a decrease in fat and subcutaneous tissue in the mons pubis, atrophy of the labia majora, and a shortening and loss of elasticity in the vaginal canal.

The amount of vaginal discharge decreases due to atrophy of the Bartholin glands and a decrease in the number and maturity of vaginal cells. The vaginal epithelium, which is highly estrogen-dependent, becomes thinner and loses glycogen. This results in a reduction in the numbers of Lactobacillus species and the subsequent production of lactic acid, leading to an increase in vaginal pH. These pH changes disrupt the balance of the vaginal microbial population, putting postmenopausal women at risk of bacterial infections. Decreased epithelial thickness, from about eight to ten cell layers to three to four layers, combined with a loss of vaginal lubrication, can cause postcoital bleeding, mild burning sensations during intercourse, and pain. Because of these factors, dyspareunia is the most common sexual complaint among older women seeking gynecological advice.

The size of the uterus reduces along with total collagen and elastic content that are reduced by 30–50% due to reduced stimulation of estrogen. Weight and stromal tissue of the ovary also become fibrotic and sclerotic. When systemic administration of estrogen is provided in high doses as a replacement therapy, beneficial effects occur in the urogenital tissues. However, increased doses carry a risk for the development of breast and endometrial cancers.

2.51.7.2 Sexual Response Cycle

A number of age-related changes influence the sexual response cycle of women. The arousal stage is characterized by less vigorous vaginal blood flow and genital engorgement, and it occurs more slowly than in younger women. This phenomenon appears to occur less frequently in women who remain sexually active than among virgins, although the mechanism is poorly understood. In Vaginal lubrication is delayed and reduced in quantity.

Whereas in younger women the arousal phase with lubrication may last only 10–15 seconds, in postmenopausal women it may last up to 5 minutes or more. Reduced vaginal vasoconstriction and lubrication may contribute to vaginal dryness and may cause painful intercourse. A variety of topical lubricants have been used successfully to compensate for inadequate vaginal lubrication. For women who do not like using lubricant during coitus, nonhormonal preparations like Replens or vitamin E oil capsules inserted vaginally every alternate day may significantly decrease vaginal dryness, as may oral zinc. Notwithstanding these age-related physiological changes, a number of studies have reported that postmenopausal women typically report little change in their subjective feelings of sexual arousal. In older women, the plateau phase of the sexual response tends to be prolonged. Additionally, the uterus descends to a lower position, and the labia majora do not elevate to the same extent as they did in earlier years. Breast tumescence is reduced, and the nipples exhibit less pronounced erection. While the orgasmic response itself does not appear to change significantly with age, there is a noticeable reduction in the number and intensity of vaginal and anal contractions. Younger women typically experience an average of 5–10 vaginal contractions during orgasm, whereas older women may only have approximately two or three.

2.51.8 Sexual Disorders in Men

2.51.8.1 Erectile Dysfunction (ED)

ED is defined as the consistent inability to achieve or maintain an erection sufficient for satisfactory sexual intercourse. The prevalence of ED increases with age; approximately 70% of men over the age of 70 experience some degree of ED, compared to 45% of men in their 60s and 15% in their 40s. While advancing age is a significant risk factor for ED, other contributing factors in older men include hypertension, diabetes mellitus, hypogonadism, medication side effects, metabolic syndrome, elevated body mass index (BMI), hypercholesterolemia, and decreased high-density lipoprotein (HDL) levels. Certain medications, such as beta-blockers, thiazide diuretics, and antidepressants, are also known to contribute to ED. Given the increased prevalence of cardiovascular disease in older populations, the relationship between cardiovascular health and sexual function is particularly relevant. Indeed, ED is increasingly recognized as a potential early indicator of concomitant cardiovascular disease and, in some instances, overall mortality. The underlying pathogenesis of ED in older men is largely attributed to systemic atherosclerosis, with symptomatic manifestations occurring in smaller blood vessels, including those supplying the penis. Long-term effects of hypertension and other peripheral arterial diseases lead to damage within these small vessels, resulting in reduced nutrient and oxygen delivery to the sexual organs. Furthermore, endothelial dysfunction, which is frequently secondary to metabolic syndrome conditions, contributes to the pathophysiology by impairing the production of nitric oxide in penile tissue, a critical factor in achieving erections. Management of ED typically includes lifestyle modifications such as smoking cessation, regular exercise, and an improved dietary plan, often yielding significant therapeutic results. Given the well-established association between hypogonadism and erectile function, testosterone replacement therapy aimed at normalizing hormone levels can also improve erectile quality.

According to the most recent guidelines issued by the American Urological Association (AUA), a morning serum testosterone level should be measured in all men presenting with ED. In men diagnosed with hypogonadism, a combination therapy involving phosphodiesterase type 5 inhibitors (PDE5i) and testosterone replacement therapy (TRT) may be considered as a viable treatment option.

More effective treatment measures include improvements in sexual satisfaction scores, erectile stiffness, and morning erection frequency with early testosterone supplementation. Concomitant to lifestyle modifications, TRT in symptomatic men with hypogonadism should be considered along with the use of PDE5i in those not currently using nitrates for chest pain. In those patients with high cardiovascular risk, consideration of nitrates may be an indication for counseling about sexual activity before any drug treatment for ED.

The AUA recommendations suggest that men who have appropriate counseling may be offered intracavitary injections, vacuum erectile devices, or penile prosthesis surgery. Testosterone supplementation is available in many formulations, including intramuscular injections, topical agents, subcutaneous implants, and intranasal sprays. In addition to these exogenous options, endogenous agents such as selective estrogen receptor modulators (e.g., clomiphene citrate) or aromatase inhibitors (e.g., anastrozole) may increase testosterone production in the body.

Other treatments include pulsatile GnRH administration delivered subcutaneously by pump. In this population, the role may be limited, as the primary benefit of this approach is in men seeking to preserve fertility.

2.51.8.2 Hypogonadism

Testosterone levels decrease with age. The AUA defines hypogonadism as testosterone deficiency with signs or symptoms associated with low serum total testosterone. These changes can be associated with dysregulation of the hypothalamic-pituitary-gonadal axis at all three levels. At the gonadal level, a decrease in Leydig cells reduces testosterone production. In the hypothalamus, rhythmic secretion of GnRH may be reduced. Finally, less luteinizing hormone and follicle-stimulating hormone are produced by the pituitary gland. Consequently, unlike women during menopause, men maintain sexual activity and fertility later in life because of these changes. These physiological changes result in reduced testosterone and symptoms of hypogonadism. Reduced testosterone also results in reduced bone mineral density and osteoporosis. About 30% of men experience hip fractures and demonstrate higher morbidity and mortality from these fractures compared to women. The cause of osteoporosis in aging women is clearly a direct effect of estrogen deficiency. In men, however, it is assumed that there is combined effect. Adequate aromatization of testosterone to estradiol helps prevent the decline in bone mineral density and, consequently, bone loss associated with aging.

Androgen decline is also associated with substantial changes as men age. The prevalence of symptomatic androgen deficiency in men between the ages of 30 and 79 was 5.6% and increased significantly with age to 18.4% among those 70 years of age. Various symptoms such as a significant decrease in libido, ED, osteoporosis/osteoporotic fractures, lethargy, sleep disturbance, depressed mood and poor physical performance are associated with low androgens.

Symptom Management

To counteract these effects, testosterone supplementation has been the standard treatment for male hypogonadism. It is important that testosterone supplementation is only given for symptomatic testosterone deficiency. Asymptomatic testosterone deficiency, or symptoms with normal testosterone, is not an indication for supplementation. Some of the benefits included preventing bone loss at the femoral neck, increasing bone mineral density, and increasing functional status, as well as improving upper and lower body strength, libido, ED and mood with testosterone supplementation. Testosterone supplementation is generally a safe treatment, but there are risks such as enlarged prostate, infertility, erythrocytosis, venous thromboembolism and worsening sleep apnea. The decision for hypogonadal men to take testosterone supplements should be evaluated on a case-by-case basis and should not be implemented in all men experiencing symptoms.

2.51.9 Female Sexual Dysfunction

2.51.9.1 Menopause

Menopause is defined as the cessation of hormone production by a woman's ovaries with the absence of menstrual periods for 12 months. The resulting changes in estrogen levels contribute to many of the potential pathologies of aging, such as osteoporosis, dyspareunia, and decreased libido. Loss of estrogen leads to uninhibited osteoclast activity and bone resorption, which leads to a weakening of the bone structure. Some of the unpleasant sexual health features experienced by older women are contributed to by low estrogen levels. The sensitivity to estrogen is decreased in the vaginal epithelial cells leading to vaginal dryness and reduced lubrication with sexual activity. Pain during intercourse, or dyspareunia, is another finding frequently reported to be associated with physiological aging in sexually active women. Despite these disadvantages, older women remain sexually active and consider it an important part of their lives. Also, the decline of estrogen in women due to menopause results in neuro- and psychosexual changes, including mood, irritability, anorgasmia, impaired sexual function, and decreased libido. In women, decreased libido is very likely a result of many sexual problems such as vaginal dryness, dyspareunia, decreased clitoral sensitivity, and decreased orgasmic intensity.

Management

One of the factors contributing to a decline in libido in a postmenopausal woman is reduced levels of androgens. Testosterone fluctuations have been linked with a decrease in libido. Evidence has revealed that women who received treatment with testosterone in addition to estrogen have enhanced libido. However, increased breast cancer, endometrial cancer, increased fractures, and cardiovascular disease have reduced the application of hormone replacement therapy (HRT) among women.

2.51.9.2 Vulvovaginal Atrophy/Orgasmic Changes (VVA)

Vulvovaginal atrophy is one of the common causes of immense physical and emotional distress for older women. Features of VVA primarily exist among postmenopausal females and its prevalence is around 4% in early postmenopausal women to about 47% in late postmenopause. The primary pathophysiology is a direct result of the effect of reduced activity on the vaginal epithelium. The thinning vaginal epithelium is thus lined with fewer cells that get shed in the vagina; this increases the pH, leading to disturbance of normal vaginal flora by Lactobacillus. A number of symptoms have been identified associated with the condition including labia minora, vagina dryness, irritation, postcoital bleeding, and dyspareunia. Associated complications of the conditions are incidence of recurrent urinary tract infections, as well as development of urinary and stress incontinence.

Management

The discomfort experienced by VVA among women drives many of them to seek either hormonal or non-hormonal treatment. Treatment is chosen based on a number of factors that include the severity of symptoms, preference, and safety and efficacy of the patient based on individual patient reports. Non-hormonal medications include topical agents such as vaginal lubricants, which are used during intercourse to prevent dyspareunia. Women are counseled about various lubricants, the most commonly used being water-based and silicone-based. Vaginal moisturizers are another form of non-hormonal treatment that is used daily to prevent vaginal dryness and provide longer-lasting relief. They are absorbed by the vaginal epithelium and lower the pH, thus mimicking the natural secretions of the vaginal mucosa.

The standard of care is estrogen therapy. Systemic or topical hormonal therapy can be administered. In the light of increased side effects associated with systemic use of estrogen for longer periods of time, topical estrogen would be more suitable for VVA. Either personal or familial history of malignancies of the breast and gynecologic organs needs counseling about the oncological risk of estrogen agents. These include creams of vaginal estradiol containing estradiol and conjugated estrogens, a sustained-release ring that delivers estradiol, and a vaginal tablet of micronized estradiol hemihydrate. Overall, most of these treatments have similar efficacy in relieving symptoms. However, there were more side effects associated with the pill related to uterine bleeding, perineal pain, and breast pain. Also, the ring was more prevalent because it was considered an easy method, highly convenient, and satisfactory in general.

New treatments for vulvovaginal atrophy are much more satisfying for postmenopausal women. A new treatment, with the use of a CO_2 laser, also called the Mona Lisa Touch, holds great promise. This may be an encouraging and promising life-changing sign for all women who cannot alleviate symptoms with mainstream treatments.

2.51.9.3 Hypoactive Sexual Desire Disorder (HSDD)

This is a very complex and multifaceted disorder that seriously affects women's sexual health. Otherwise known as hyposexuality or inhibited sexual desire, HSDD is characterized by a persistent lack of interest in sexual activity. To be clinically diagnosed, this lack of interest must cause significant personal or relationship distress, distinguishing it from normal fluctuations in sexual desire. This critical qualitative aspect helps in the identification of HSDD as a disorder that diminishes overall well-being and intimate relationships. Treating HSDD is crucial to enhancing the quality of life and emotional well-being of affected individuals.

Symptom Management

Bremelanotide (Vyleesi) and Flibanserin (Addyi) are two FDA-approved medications developed to treat HSDD in women. Bremelanotide (Vyleesi) has been found to notably improve sexual desire and reduce distress associated with HSDD in women. These medications relieve symptoms but do not cure the underlying condition. Addressing HSDD requires a comprehensive approach that includes psychological support and counseling to reduce its broader impact on personal and relationship well-being. Continued research and development in the field of sexual medicine is essential to improve the effectiveness of treatments and enhance the quality of life for affected women.

> **Box 2.5 Recommendation for Older People**
> - Get enough rest
> - Schedule sexual activity
> - Take painkillers 2 hours in advance
> - Encourage sporadic intimacy through touching and hugging, and also communicate openly
> - Utilize aids if necessary, and stress comfort, warmth, and delight

Lifestyle-Oriented Approach

Lifestyle medicine places the practice of healthy behaviors as the foundation of health and, as such, has great relevance to the sexuality of older adults. The six pillars of lifestyle medicine—nutrition, physical activity, stress management, avoidance of hazardous substances, restorative sleep, and social connection—are essential for improving disease prevention and management and enhancing sexual desire.

- Nutrition: The physician should stress the need for a high-fiber, plant-based diet with abundant fruits, vegetables, whole grains, and legumes. This diet is crucial for cardiovascular health and has a direct impact on sexual function. Such nutrition can also help increase energy levels and improve sexual vitality and stamina.
- Physical activity: It is important to encourage older patients to undertake regular physical exercise to maintain sexual function as well as overall health. Physical activity increases circulation, improves flexibility, and strengthens muscle tone, all important in maintaining sexual function. Improved blood flow supports erectile function and vaginal lubrication, while better flexibility and muscle strength improve comfort and endurance during sex. Besides, physical exercise releases endorphins that reduce anxiety and depression. This mental boost has a direct and positive effect on sexual desire and performance, making exercise a powerful tool for improving overall health.
- Stress management: Clinicians should strongly encourage older patients to incorporate stress-reduction techniques such as mindfulness, meditation, and yoga into their daily routine. These practices can actually help in reducing stress, a common factor known to reduce libido. Healthy social connectedness and encouraging open communications about sexual needs and preferences will go a long way in further reducing stress. Such an approach will enhance not only sexual satisfaction but also emotional intimacy, thus fostering better, more connected relationships.
- Abstaining from drugs: It is also the role of the health professional to advise older patients to avoid substances that may deter sexual function and desire, such as tobacco, excess alcohol, and recreational drugs. Regular counseling is also quite necessary for the control of medications in order not to have any adverse impact on sexual function.
- Improving sleep: Healthcare practitioners should prioritize the role of quality sleep in promoting overall health, especially in relation to hormonal balance and energy levels. Adequate, restful sleep is essential for regulating hormones such as testosterone and estrogen, which directly affect sexual desire and function. Encouraging patients to practice

good sleep hygiene—such as maintaining a consistent sleep schedule, creating a quiet sleep environment, and limiting screen time before bed—can improve sleep quality.

- Social connection: Good social relationships are fundamental to the emotional and physical health, including sexual well-being, of everyone. Social engagement among older adults brings a sense of belonging and emotional security that has a positive impact on sexual function and satisfaction. Loneliness and social isolation, in turn, are known to increase the risk for depression, anxiety, and low libido. Health professionals should encourage older adults to participate in social activities and social clubs and be close to friends and family.

2.52 Sexually Transmitted Infections (STIs)

High-risk sexual behaviors among older adults, especially STIs like HIV, have been a growing public health concern. This population often has a lack of knowledge about sexually transmitted infections and is less likely to engage in safe sexual practices compared to younger generations, putting them at greater risk. According to the Centers for Disease Control and Prevention, reported STI rates among American adults aged 65 and over have more than doubled between 2012 and 2020. Growing, it is still destined to increase further as this population is aging.

Health care providers require adequate education on the identification of at-risk individuals and appropriate screening to decrease morbidity and mortality from the disease. It has been reported that the majority of older adults do not have sufficient time to discuss their sexual health with a medical professional and, therefore, may be suffering from undiagnosed and untreated infections. By incorporating preventive screenings that assess patients' knowledge about sexually transmitted diseases, providers can encourage open and effective communication about sexual health with their older patients. This approach will not only prompt meaningful discussions but also ensure that seniors receive important educational resources and interventions that promote safer sexual practices and better overall health outcomes.

Box 2.6

- You are not immune to STDs just because you are getting older.
- If one or both of you have multiple sexual partners, you can get HIV/AIDS if you have unprotected sex.
- Always use a condom for vaginal or anal sex to protect yourself and your partner.
- Use a dental dam or another form of barrier during oral sex.
- Learn more about using condoms, dental dams, and other methods to prevent getting and giving STDs

2.53 Elder Abuse

Abuse of elders is intentional or unintentional injury, usually inflicted by persons in positions of trust or caretakers. The World Health Organization defines it as "Any sexual act that is performed against a person's will, by any person, regardless of their relationship to the victim, in any setting." An indicator of suspicion for elder sexual abuse is very vital since the older person might conceal such an issue out of shame or stigma, fear of retaliation, or dependence on the abuser. It is often challenging for the older person to balance the need for benevolence—choosing between the good of others and the right to autonomy. In the case of dealing with sexual issues in cognitively impaired older patients, one should be aware of elder abuse. Some of the older victims cannot report the harm due to health conditions such as dementia or Alzheimer's disease. Older women are much more likely to be abused than older men. Most reports of elder sexual abuse come from nursing homes or other care facilities. Perpetrators can be caregivers, staff, other residents, or anyone else who visits the facility.

Sexual abuse of older adults also occurs outside of nursing homes. Often, perpetrators are caregivers, family, spouses, or friends.

2.54 Comprehensive Sexual Assessment

Physicians, including health care physicians, providers, therapists, and counselors, are in a unique position to address sexual concerns and provide much-needed support to their older patients. By creating a comfortable and nonjudgmental atmosphere, physicians can put discussion about sexuality at the forefront and help patients receive the guidance and interventions necessary to enhance their overall health. Most older adults do not seek help for their sexual problems, even though sexual problems significantly affect the quality of life. The discussion about sexuality and sexual assessment is generally not included in clinical practice. This stands for one of the main gaps in sexual assessment among older adults. These results indicate a dire need to perform complete sexual assessment by physicians as part of comprehensive management. Such evaluations include a detailed sexual history, including sexually transmitted disease and HIV status, current medications, and sexual functioning. Clinicians should also evaluate sexual behavior and associated risk factors, such as relationship status, number of sexual partners, frequency of sexual relations, injection drug use, types of sexual activities, and sexual abuse history.

2.55 Disability in Elders

Old age is the tender age of human life that has to face more vulnerable threats, chronic diseases, loneliness, and isolation. Due to physical and mental disabilities, their individual independence is often threatened. Long-term adverse health-related consequences include increased risk for geriatric syndromes, dependency, disability, hospitalization in hospitals and nursing homes, and increased risk of mortality. According to the WHO, disability is formed from the interplay of health conditions, personal attributes, and environmental context. The environmental conditions act as contextual factors influencing all components of a disabling process, including body functions and structures, an individual's activities, and their participation in society. Disability can also be thought of as a kind of generalized disturbance of the physiological homeostasis with respect to different bodily systems. It considers the disability as a defect, a problem in function, or the structure of the body and acts like an umbrella that covers injuries, activity limitations, and participation limitations. Activity limitation is a problem that an individual faces in the performance of a task or action; participation limitation is a problem that an individual experiences in engaging in life situations.

Disability is a complex phenomenon that reflects the interaction between the characteristics of the individual's body and the characteristics of the society in which he or she lives. Disability presents as increased vulnerability, reduced resistance to internal and environmental stressors, and diminished ability to maintain physiological and psychosocial homeostasis. Frailty is present in 20–30% of the older population over 75 years of age and increases with age. As a person ages, physical and cognitive functioning decline, increasing the risk of disability in areas such as walking/mobility, self-care, and household management that may affect an older adult's ability to continue to live independently in the community.

Beliefs or attitudes about disability vary depending on age, culture, location, and many other factors. No two people experience the same disability in the same way. In fact, one may have very different experiences of a particular disability at different points in their lifetime. As soon as we begin thinking about disability in old age, stereotypes quickly come into mind. We immediately think of someone in a wheelchair or someone who has vision impairments. The reality is that disability varies not only in nature but also in extent to which it affects or limits people. In old age, disability might be caused by preexisting conditions or by biological changes and related factors. An example of this is vision loss common with age: decreased accommodation (the ability of the lens to focus), contrast sensitivity, and even sensitivity to bright light. Changes in the eye cause visual impairment. Approximately 70% of adults aged 80 or older have cataracts, with 20% and 7% of the same age group experiencing age-related maculopathy and glaucoma, respectively. Similarly, with age, there is a predictable breakdown of cells in the inner ear. This can result in hearing loss, and 35% of males and 22% of females in the age group of 70–74 years suffer from hearing impairments, and the rate further goes up to 58% males and 49% females who are 85 years or older. Taste, smell and touch sensitivities decrease. In the case of touch, this can be particularly problematic—as loss of sensitivity to touch and pain can lead to accidents and subsequent disability. Finally, loss of bone density and muscle mass, along with reduced circulation and respiratory efficiency, are also part of the natural aging process.

Currently, it is estimated that 15% of the population worldwide—approximately 1 billion people—live with one or more debilitating conditions. Among older people—people aged 60 and over—more than 46% have a disability, and over 250 million older people experience moderate to severe disability. With the global trend of population aging and an increased risk of disability among older adults, it is likely that the population affected by disability will increase further. In addition, a lifetime of illness, injury, and chronic disease accumulation add to the increase in the rates of disability among the older people.

2.55.1 Factors Contributing to Disability

Many factors contribute to disability, and all have the potential to prevent effective participation in many activities of daily living. While aging increases the risk of disease and disability, factors such as cumulative lifestyle choices and environmental exposures can further accelerate the onset of disability. One of the most consistent predictors of disability is socioeconomic disadvantage. Poor nutrition, as well as a lack of access to health care increase the risk of disability. Low-income countries have a higher prevalence of disability when compared to high-income countries, and among the general population, those of low SES also have higher rates of disability. The effects of poverty often become more pronounced with increasing age as it is a cumulative influence, and there is also increased poverty among older adults. Those born in poverty are more likely to develop a disability—and to carry it with them if they survive to old age. The prognosis and quality of life for people with disabilities experiencing poverty are worse than among people with disabilities who do not experience poverty. Thus, there appears to be a cycle of disability—wherein poverty both causes and exacerbates disability.

2.55.2 Impact of Disability in Older People

The most obvious impact of disability on older adults is in the area of self-care. Physical disability in older adults can prevent them from being able to independently get in and out of bed, leave the house, and perform home maintenance. Considering that many people with disabilities require visiting the hospital as well as taking pharmacy medicines, any disability that confines these people to the house exacerbates the challenges associated with managing disability in case people do not have access to assistance. Disability can affect people's basic activities.

. In the elderly, the impairment suffered in self-care capacity is often indicated by limitations in performance of activities of daily living (ADLs) that serve as common indicators of disability. ADLs refer to very basic self-care functions, including bathing, dressing, ambulating, and toileting with independence. ADLs may be partially alleviated by accessible accommodations: for example, difficulty with bathing and toileting may be facilitated by the installation of showerheads, grab bars, and raised toilet seats. However, individuals with disabilities related to ADLs most commonly require the support of personal assistance and caregivers. Approximately 15% of adults aged 65–74 years' experience difficulty walking, as compared to approximately 50% of adults aged 85 years and older. About 20% of adults aged 65 years and older use walking aids—such as canes, walkers, crutches—or require a wheelchair for mobility.

Based on the proposed definition, a disability is the limitation on an independent living skill affecting the management of the environment by the individual. These limitations encompass instrumental activities of daily living (IADLs). Typical IADLs include skills such as finances, grocery shopping, meal preparation, medication management, telephone use, and money management. Thus, data indicate that 40% of those between 60 and 75 years old and close to 75% of those aged 80 or older have some form of disability. Of the severely disabled, 20% are 60 years old or above, and the figure rises to 50% for elderly persons 80 years and older. In a lot of cases, disabilities concerning IADLs start with physical weakness; for instance, doing laundry and chores can be beyond the individual's physical capacity. Importantly, when an older adult is limited in some capacity, the individual's health status declines more rapidly and recovery takes longer, thus increasing the likelihood of further disability, further limiting their ability to live independently. Chronic disabilities are a strong predictor of falls in older adults. Falls are the most common cause of limitation in daily activities. The more chronic conditions an older adult reports, the more likely they are to fall and fall frequently. Thus, disability itself places individuals at risk for future disability.

2.55.3 Participation in Society

In many parts of the world, people with disabilities encounter multiple barriers: attitudinal, environmental, and institutional that hamper their complete equal participation in all spheres of life. Older people with disabilities are often amongst the most vulnerable and encounter even greater age-related barriers in society. Disability in older people often places limitations on their ability to lead happy and fulfilling lives. This is not just because of problems associated with activities of daily living, such as walking and dressing. Impairments can also create barriers to social and occupational interactions. For example, poor vision may prevent older people from driving. Mobility problems may prevent them from taking public transport, as may the availability or affordability of public transport. Disability can thus make older people retreat from social activities or stop going to functions that are not within their walking distance.

Physical and/or cognitive impairments can also hinder older persons' participation in work-related activities. There are several reasons for this. First, physical disability may prevent someone from doing the job they used to do-for example, walking problems may prevent a farmer from farming. But strong misconceptions about disabled older people—hopefully not by, but also for, the older people themselves—may as well prevent the older people who wish to work from seeking and obtaining work. Older persons with disabilities, for instance, are excluded from disability-related services promoting their rights and equal opportunities. As a result, older people with disabilities are often unable to benefit from programs designed to support them in seeking paid work. Older people with disabilities are also subject to discrimination. The emphasis on 'positive', 'successful' or 'healthy' ageing means that older people with disabilities are viewed as people who age 'badly' or 'unsuccessfully'. People with cognitive impairment and dementia are also sometimes seen as 'less than human' and are therefore not provided with time and companionship. Whether through the use of physical barriers, or through more subtle processes of social exclusion, isolation can have a profoundly negative impact on adults with disabilities. Principal predictors of longevity are the strength and quality of our social relationships. When these are limited by disability, whether through preventing social interaction or through increased incidents of discrimination, older people with disabilities are likely to experience reduced health and quality of life.

2.55.4 Social Impact and Management of Disability in Old Age

Given the increasing number of people with disabilities, there is a considerable global burden—both health-wise and financially. Financially, this cost is borne by the disabled themselves, governments and individual caregivers or families. In fact, most old people with a disability do not reside in an aged-care facility. The cost of caring about older people is not simply financial. It is emotional, too. Caregivers are often underpaid and overworked. Caregiving can be very stressful because it often involves negotiating and managing of both current impairment and future consequences of the impairment (palliative care and death) without acknowledgment by the public in general. In terms of the wider issue of disability, generally speaking, the World Health Organization suggests that several modifications of the environment can enhance the lives of those with a disability. For instance, access to education and health care policies should be designed in such a way that they consider the needs of people with disabilities. There is a need to increase funding and provision of services for people with disabilities. At a very basic level, built environments should be designed to be accessible to all. Negative attitudes and poor standards of care should be combated. In each case, extensive consultation of people with disabilities is desirable, and any programs should be carefully documented and evaluated (World Health Organization 2012). In terms of specific programs aimed at enabling older people with disabilities there are many examples of positive schemes. For instance, in Japan free community exercise classes, targeted at older people, can easily be accessed by the residents of major cities. In the United States, community-based programs have a purpose to prevent disability among older persons and also promotes self-management of illness, reduced functional decline, and also a reduction in length of hospital stay. On the individual level, managing disability in adulthood—for instance, disability itself—is rather complex. However, a variety of factors have been identified that dependably delay the onset of disability.

Most importantly, perhaps, exercise is a factor that has been shown to enhance both physical and mental health and is effective in delaying the onset of dementia and preventing physical disability. A second cognitive stimulation is considered important. Older adults who remain in the workforce late in life show better cognitive integration than those who retire early, and it is likely that cognitive challenge is protective. Finally, a strong social network is key. This does not mean that a large social group is the key to health for older adults; rather, they are much healthier when they report close, developed, and deep friendships. Reductions in smoking, drinking, and drug use also lower the risk of disability.

2.55.5 Risk Factors of Disability

Good physical functioning reduces cellular and molecular damage, delays the onset of disease and disability, and maximizes functioning throughout life. Social factors include gender, socioeconomic status, race, age, and culture. Individual well-being includes psychosocial and behavioral well-being. Biological processes include inflammatory responses, oxidative cellular damage, hormonal changes, and environmental factors of neighborhood characteristics and air quality.

- *Age*

Although the loss of physical function with age is inevitable, the effects of aging are quite variable among individuals, and age is a poor predictor of physical function. Many older adults age successfully without disability. However, age is associated with an increasing prevalence of diseases that strongly contribute to disability. Physical limitations in daily activities remain stable until age 45, then begin to rise: from 6.5% to 16.9% at younger ages, 26.9% at age 65, and 45.3% at age 75 and older. Among those over 85, 55% of women and 38% of men report being unable to perform basic motor tasks such as walking, bending, writing, or lifting 10 pounds. These physical limitations often are related to chronic disease conditions, making it difficult for scientists to separate biological processes from disease effects.

- *Disease*

The loss in physical function and rising disability within aging is closely related with the following diseases: hypertension, 53.3% for those 65 + years; osteoarthritis, 49%; cardiovascular disease (CVD), 30.9%; cancer, 21.1%; lung dysfunction, 20.6%; diabetes, 18%; and stroke, 9.3%. Cardiovascular disease and osteoarthritis are the major contributors to this burden, affecting roughly 80% of adults aged over 65. However, the overall prevalence of these conditions does not necessarily relate to their individual contribution to disability. Thus, conditions such as impairments in hearing and vision or osteoporosis, although less prevalent, substantially increase disability rates. Conversely, cardiovascular disease is both very prevalent and severely impacts both physical and cognitive function. Osteoarthritis, though prevalent, tends to have less of an impact on physical disability compared with CVD, sensory impairments, and diabetes. It disrupts cartilage integrity, increases perceived pain, and can lead to reduced muscle strength. However, people with osteoarthritis often require less personal assistance than those with other disabilities. The direct impact of disease on physical limitations can be evaluated through treatment outcomes. Such programs have been found to achieve positive results: surgical interventions, such as those for osteoarthritis, substantially enhance long-term physical function, whereas the SHEP trial significantly reduced cardiovascular events and incidents of physical disability using antihypertensive drugs. This evidences not only a strong reciprocal association but also one that can, through disease treatment, be readily reversed.

- *Obesity*

Recent estimates suggest that 35% of older adults are obese, and obesity in older adults is associated with a higher risk of physical disability. It was also determined that obesity raises the risk of physical disability in older adults, along with an earlier onset of severe disability. Moreover, obese older adults are two times more likely to be impaired in basic activities of daily living compared with normal-weight older adults. Obese older adults are deprived of basic activities of daily living for approximately 5 years less than normal-weight adults. Much of this excess disability is due to chronic conditions related to obesity. These conditions include diabetes, cardiovascular disease, osteoarthritis, chronic heart failure, hypertension, and cancers. Osteoarthritis is 2.6 times more likely in the obese than in the normal-weight persons, and physical disability also appears mainly affected by it in these obese persons. Moreover, among obese adults, the presence of comorbidities is also very common (2 or more), in 70–80% of cases compared with 40% in normal-weight adults. Such additional comorbidities with obesity may be a strong factor in the high rates of disability in older obese individuals.

- *Physical Functioning*

It mainly relates to functional limitations in the pathway to disability to conduct a physical activity. Probably the most widely used assessment of physical functioning is the Short Physical Performance Battery (SPPB) that the scientists from the National Institute on Aging created. Measures included walking speed, chair rising, and balance; scores on a national sample of the populations designated for epidemiological studies of the older people are included in this battery. Performance scores on the SPPB strongly predict health outcomes in the older people, including hospitalization, nursing home admission, mobility limitations, and dependence on primary care needs and mortality. For example, independent older adults who score in the lowest half of the functional scores are five times more likely to have a disability requiring primary care 4 years later. In addition, approximately 60% of those who score in the lowest third of the SPPB score will have a motor disability, while less than 10% will have the same condition 4 years later. The ability to successfully perform SPPB tasks is due in part to high levels of muscle strength.

- *Muscle Mass and Strength*

The neuromuscular system plays a key role in providing the backbone necessary for mobility and daily movements that are essential for maintaining physical independence. While disease conditions are a major factor in the occurrence of physical disability in older adults, the change in loss of physical function and the onset of activity limitations can be explained in part by characteristic changes in the neuromuscular system with age. Muscle tissue represents the major reservoir for free amino acids in the body and is linked to morbidity and mortality in states of HIV, cancer, and congestive heart failure. Greater quantities of muscle mass do not protect older adults from the onset of activity limitations; however, muscle strength is considered a major determinant of improved physical performance regardless of mass. Muscle strength is a strong predictor of severe mobility limitation, poor motor function, and mortality. Compared with older adults with high muscle strength, those with low levels are 2.6 times more likely to have severe mobility limitation, 4.3 times more likely to have slow gait speed, and 2.1 times more likely to die.

2.55.6 Types of Disabilities

There are a number of disabilities that seniors experience; however, the most common ones include mobility, agility, and pain disabilities.

- *Motor Disabilities*

Mobility disabilities are the most common type of disability among seniors and are more prevalent in women than men. A person experiencing a mobility disability may have difficulty going up and down the stairs, standing in one place for 20 minutes, or even moving from one room to another.

- *Agility Disabilities*

Agility disabilities are the second most common type of disability among seniors, and are more common in women than men. A person with an agility disability may have difficulty bending over, putting on or taking off clothes, getting in and out of bed, or picking up small objects.

- *Pain Disabilities*

Pain disabilities are the third most common type of disability among seniors, and are more common in women than men. A person with a pain disability may have persistent pain or frequent episodes of pain that significantly reduce the amount or type of activities a person can do.

- *Hearing Impairments*

As people age, hearing impairments become more common: About half of seniors aged 85 and older have a hearing impairment. Hearing impairments are more common among men. A person with a hearing impairment often has difficulty hearing when trying to talk to other people or on the telephone.

- *Visual Impairments*

As people age, vision impairments are much more likely to occur in older adults. Vision impairments are slightly more common among women. A person with a vision impairment may have difficulty seeing the face of someone across the room, even when wearing glasses.

- *Cognitive Impairments*

As people age, memory impairments become increasingly common. A person with memory impairment has difficulty performing daily activities because they become confused or forget things.

- *Communication Disabilities*

Most seniors with communication disabilities also have other types of disabilities, such as memory and mobility. A person with a communication disability often has a hard time understanding what others are saying.

- *Learning Disabilities*

Learning disabilities are not as prevalent among seniors as other types of disabilities. However, the rates for seniors 85 and older are higher. The rates are about equal between men and women. A person with a learning disability has difficulty learning new things and may have been diagnosed with conditions such as ADHD or dyslexia.

- *Emotional Disabilities*

While seniors generally have higher rates of all types of disabilities, seniors who live independently in their communities are less likely to have emotional disabilities than younger adults. A person with an emotional disability may have difficulty performing daily activities because of mental health problems, such as depression or anxiety.

2.55.7 Decline of Disability Over Time

In recent decades, disability rates have been declining rapidly and understanding the cause of the decline in disability is important as it can indicate a trend toward increasing or decreasing disability in the future.

The cause of the decline in disability depends on various factors.

- *Improved Medical Care*

One of the factors that have been effective in reducing disability is improved medical care. In the past, many older people were disabled by arthritis, which was treated with the advent of NSAIDs and COX-2 inhibitors and the invention of joint replacement surgery. The use of these technologies has expanded over time. The expansion of cataract surgery in people with visual impairments reduces disability related to visual impairment. The decline in cardiovascular disease mortality coincided with the implementation of Medicare, suggesting a possible link between improved access to healthcare and reduced mortality. Heart disease is a leading cause of chronic disability, making this connection particularly significant. Also, the role of certain medications in reducing high blood pressure, which was a major risk factor for stroke, has expanded.

- *Behavioral Changes*

Behavioral changes are also important in reducing disability. The effect of improved diets and reduced smoking on emphysema, heart disease, stroke, and chronic respiratory damage is increasing.

- *Expanded Assistive Devices*

Canes and walkers help frail older people stay out of nursing homes. Showers and grab bars prevent hip fractures and allow those with fractures to live independently. Microwave ovens make cooking easier for frail older people. And telephones with larger keypads allow people with low vision to communicate. Such assistive devices, which represent the growth of assisted living facilitics, may bc particularly important in reducing nursing home use.

- *Improved Socioeconomic Status*

An additional factor in reducing disability is improved socio-economic status. One key aspect of this is increased education among older people. Research has shown that the disability rate of more educated people is only about half that of less educated people. Added together, this finding and the great rise in the proportion of older people with high school and college degrees help explain the recent decades decline in disability. Education among older people is continuing to rise; in fact this is a trend that will probably continue for decades to come. Education can influence disability via several pathways: through increased availability of medical care resources, increased knowledge about appropriate health behaviors, and by the direct effect of mental stimulation on maintaining cognitive function. Educational attainment also has been shown to delay the onset of Alzheimer's disease.

Another dimension of occupational socioeconomic status involves the close association of job-related status with education. For the most part, today's older people tend to be healthier than older generations, due to differences in exposure to dust and smoke in past workplace environments compared to those today. The same applies to individuals who lived on farms, which were much more common a few decades ago than they are today.

Decreasing disability may reflect changes in the disease environment over time. There is growing evidence that infectious diseases encountered early in life affect health later in life. In particular, the link between rheumatic fever and rheumatic heart disease is well established. More tenuous links are also documented between heart disease and typhoid, measles, and malaria. Even pre-natal factors such as maternal malnutrition and failure to gain adequate weight may influence late life disease. Older generations were more exposed to these diseases and conditions during childhood than younger generations, which may partly explain the change in disability over time.

2.55.8 Preventing Disability Based on Prevention Levels

The occurrence of disability calls attention to the need for disability prevention, including rehabilitation.

WHO addresses this need by promoting a variety of prevention measures. The terms impairment, disability, and handicap are used as a reference for the primary, secondary, and tertiary prevention measures that are related to disability.

Primary prevention includes measures aimed at the prevention of diseases and injuries. Secondary prevention includes interventions that are used to treat diseases or injuries to prevent impairments. Tertiary prevention consists of a variety of measures aimed at eliminating or reducing impairments or disabilities. Since handicaps result from the interaction between people with disabilities and their societies, a change in society is also needed to reduce or eliminate handicaps.

- *Primary Prevention*

Positive beliefs and attitudes can reduce enormously the social handicap of disabled people. The measures promoted for the prevention of diseases that cause disabilities include immunization, particularly against poliomyelitis, measles, rubella and tuberculosis; prenatal care to ensure the healthy development and delivery of babies; appropriate nutrition, especially iron, iodine, and vitamin A, for mothers and children; and sanitary measures to prevent eye diseases, such as infections and trachoma.

Injuries may result from intentional or unintentional acts and injury prevention has several aspects. One is education regarding measures that can be taken to prevent acts that cause injuries. A second is protection, which uses environmental or technical devices such as seat belts, helmets and airbags to prevent injuries. A third aspect is the promotion of safety as part of general health promotion policies, and this is being developed under WHO leadership.

- *Secondary Prevention*

Medical interventions are thus necessary when diseases or injuries occur to prevent impairments, such as muscles that have been paralyzed, eyes and ears that are damaged, or a malfunctioning brain. These are medical treatments against infectious diseases of the eye, ear, spinal cord, and brain; proper nutrition against malnutrition; and treatment, both medical and other forms, for mental disorders.

- *Tertiary Prevention*

When impairments occur, they can be treated in order to prevent or to reduce disabilities, such as difficulty in seeing, hearing or walking. Eyeglasses can greatly reduce, or even eliminate, difficulty in seeing; a hearing aid can reduce difficulty in hearing; and leg braces can reduce difficulty in walking. When disabilities occur, measures aimed specifically at the limited function which a disabled person experiences can also be taken to reduce or to limit the progression of the disability. These are the measures commonly referred to as rehabilitation. Because they focus on the activities which people can or cannot do, they require their active participation. This rehabilitation process could include learning to dress or feed; a new method of communication; a different locomotion system, including probably using a wheelchair; and a new way of performing the activities of daily living.

Box 2.7 Recommendations Are Also Given for Family Caregivers and Older People

Physical Health

- Regular Check-Up: Encourage them with regular check-ups as needed to best manage a chronic condition or maintain general health.
- Screening: In addition to blood pressure and cholesterol testing, diabetes testing, and various types of cancer testing, other forms of screenings should also be done appropriate to one's age, to realize and intervene on problems earlier rather than later.
- Medication Management: The caregiver should help in managing medications by organizing them in pillboxes and taking them as scheduled to reduce the chances of missed doses and related health complications.
- Education on Common Health Conditions: Both the caregiver and the older adult should be educated on common health conditions affecting older people, such as heart disease, arthritis, and cancer, and ways of reducing the risk factors.

Physical activity

- Daily Movement: The guideline is to engage in at least 30 minutes of moderate physical activity on most days of the week, which can be broken down into shorter sessions to accommodate individual capabilities.
- Variety of Activities: Encourage a varied exercise program that includes aerobic activities such as walking and swimming, strength training with light weights or resistance bands, and flexibility and balance exercises such as yoga or tai chi.
- Safe Environments: Caregivers must ensure that exercise environments are safe and accessible, promoting physical activity in familiar settings to reduce the risk of falls.
- Motivational Strategies: Utilizing social engagement strategies, such as participating in group walks or fitness classes, can enhance adherence to physical activity routines.

Nutrition

- Dietary Balance: A diet that is balanced, with a variety of fruits, vegetables, lean proteins, whole grains, and healthy fats, is important for overall health.
- Nutrient-Dense Foods: Emphasize foods rich in essential nutrients, such as calcium and vitamin D for bone health and fiber for digestive health, to help manage age-related health conditions.
- Cooking Together: Involving older participants and caregivers in food preparation can make healthy eating more enjoyable and a social activity.
- Hydration: This is crucial to help avoid dehydration, especially when medication intake is high or when the level of physical activity is high.

Sleep Hygiene

- Sleep Routine: Engage in a regular bedtime schedule by having consistent timing of going to bed and rising, which would accordingly affect the body's ability to adjust the internal system related to sleep.
- Conduct a Sleep-Friendly Environment: Sleeping areas are designed to be quiet and dark, with cool surroundings; bedding should be appropriately appealing for comfort in getting sufficient rest.
- Avoid Stimulants: It is good to advise reducing the intake of caffeine and nicotine, especially before going to bed.
- Manage Screen Time: Electronic devices such as phones, computers, and televisions can be restricted for at least an hour before bedtime for better sleep quality.

Sexual Health

- Open Communications: An environment that allows talking openly about sexual health and intimacy can help alleviate confusions and reduce stigma pertaining to aging and sexuality.
- Education on Changes: One needs to be informed on the changes brought about in sexual health by aging; for example, a low libido and complications that can arise from it, as this will help in making informed decisions.
- Explore Options: Helping explore other aspects of intimacy and emotional closeness can foster interpersonal relationships.
- Health Factors: All caregivers and seniors should be encouraged to discuss any medications or health concerns that may impact sexual functioning with their healthcare providers.

Disability

- Enable Independence: Assisting older adults to utilize assistive devices, such as walkers and hearing aids, can greatly enhance both safety and independence in activities of daily living.
- Home Modifications: Recommendations toward modification of living spaces for better accessibility, such as the installation of ramps, widening of doorways, and addition of grab bars in bathrooms, are all important to support mobility and safety.
- Encourage Participation: Identifying community resources and programs tailored for seniors with disabilities can facilitate social connections and enhance the quality of life.

2.56 Summary

The aging process is complex and is a long phase of life that starts at birth. It is a phase of life that all of us will definitely experience at one point or another in our lifetime. As years go by, several changes occur naturally at the cellular level, and not just with individual cells, but also with all the organs of our body. These changes can set the stage for chronic diseases, making us generally more susceptible to a wide variety of health problems. Exercising regularly can go a long way in reducing the occurrence of such diseases and may even reduce the rate at which age-related diseases progress.

It is not only beneficial but absolutely essential and vitally important for the health of every individual to engage in physical activity, and this also includes the older people. Even though vulnerabilities may be more possible with older adults, this should not exempt them from the benefits of regular exercise. A safe and supportive environment along with regular, carefully designed exercise programs matched to the individual's capacity and limitations can go a long way in improving the overall health of the aged. This, in turn, can help in achieving better health parameters and at the same time reducing the chances of injury from falls or any other adverse incident.

Aging predictably brings about changes in many systems of the body, including the gastrointestinal tract. For older adults, these changes can predictably result in complications such as malnutrition or obesity, which are significant concerns in this age group. Therefore, it is absolutely critical for older people to adhere to a proper diet that is rich in essential nutrients and minerals, ensuring that their bodies receive the proper fuel necessary for optimal functioning and wellness.

Another area significantly impacted by the aging process is sleep patterns. Poor or insufficient sleep will further weaken cognition and impair mental clarity and mood.

Many people remain sexually active well into their old age; however, physical and hormonal changes due to the aging process will affect their sexual lives. While impotence can be regarded as a natural process of aging, it is, however, fair to mention that this particular disorder is more common among the older population due to the progressive deterioration in the functioning of different systems of the body with advancing age. Recognition of such changes is necessary for formulating adequate interventions and support mechanisms that will enhance the quality of life of the older people.

2.57 Summary of Research Studies

Abdul Hussein Al-Abidi, et al. conducted a cross-sectional study on 260 participants over 60 years of age entitled "Self-care of the older people and its related factors in primary health care centers" in 2024 with the aim of investigating the self-care abilities of older people and related factors in Iraq. In this cross-sectional study, older people were assessed through a questionnaire including demographic information and the self-care ability scale. According to the results of this study, 168 older people (64.6%) had satisfactory abilities and 19 (7.3%) had good ability for self-care. Married individuals (P = 0.003) demonstrated significantly greater self-care ability compared to those who were single, divorced, or widowed. Self-care capacity was also significantly lower among individuals with lower levels of education (P = 0.000). Therefore, the results showed that older people with diseases (0.000) have a low level of self-care. According to the study, the ability of older people with chronic diseases to take care of themselves is insufficient, which makes it necessary to plan and implement self-care improvement programs. The ability of older people to take care of themselves can be improved by organizing workshops based on identifying age-specific challenges and providing solutions to deal with them.

Amerzadeh et al. conducted a descriptive-analytical study on 374 older patients with type 2 diabetes in 2024 entitled "Self-care behaviors, medication adherence status and related factors among older patients with type 2 diabetes". The data collection tools included a demographic profile checklist, a summary of diabetes self-care activities questionnaire, and the Morisky medication adherence scale. In the self-care questionnaire, the highest score was related to adherence to the diet recommended by the treating physician and the lowest score was related to the frequency of checking inside shoes and foot examination, respectively. In addition, the results of self-care behaviors showed that self-monitoring of blood glucose (SMBG) decreased significantly with increasing education level. The level of self-care in physical activity, SMBG, and foot care among older people is below average. In addition, medication adherence in these patients is poor.

Casey et al. (2024) conducted a study titled "Self-care practices in the context of independent living of older adults" with the main goal of better understanding how older adults live independently and care for themselves and how assistive technology can be designed to support these practices. The study used semi-structured interviews with 12 participants living in and around a retirement village, focusing on studying the participants' self-care practices across physical, emotional and psychological, social, leisure, and spiritual dimensions. By extending Lee and Miller's self-care framework, this article provides rich insights into the everyday self-care practices of older adults, which go beyond the medical concepts of self-care. The main point of this study is that self-care assistive technology should be designed with the needs and preferences of older adults in mind, with a strong focus on enabling independence and supporting all aspects of self-care.

2.58 Critical Thinking (Scenarios Based)

Critical thinking in older people's self-care scenarios involves the analysis of different situations that older people may encounter concerning their health and well-being. Here are some scenarios with corresponding critical thinking questions and considerations:

- *Scenario 1: Medication Management*

Mrs. Thompson, an old lady, has recently been prescribed several medications for various health conditions. She often forgets to take her medications or takes them at inappropriate times.

Critical Thinking Questions:

1. What are some ways Mrs. Thompson could be encouraged to increase her compliance with her medication?
2. How might family members or caregivers help her with this?
3. What complications might arise due to medication noncompliance?

- *Case Scenario 2: Nutrition and Meal Preparation*

Mr. Johnson is an 80-year-old man who lives alone and often resorts to frozen meals or take-out because it is difficult for him to prepare nutritious meals.

Critical Thinking Questions:

1. What are the nutritional consequences of his current food selections?
2. What resources or social services would be helpful to Mr. Johnson in his preparation of meals?
3. How might the social components of eating, such as not eating alone, affect his mental status?

- *Case Scenario 3: Exercise*

Ms. Rodriguez was a walker but in recent months has become sedentary due to fear of falling and lack of motivation.

Critical Thinking Questions:

1. What are some low-impact activities in which Ms. Rodriguez can safely participate?
2. How might she overcome her fear of falling while exercising?
3. What is the role of social connections in her willingness to participate in physical activities?

- *Case Scenario 4: Cognitive Stimulation*

Mr. Lee has been withdrawn and disconnected from life over the past few months, with no particular interest in anything, including his usual hobbies of reading and playing chess.

Critical Thinking Questions:

1. What are some methods of cognitively stimulating Mr. Lee to reduce social isolation?
2. How might family or caregivers influence Mr. Lee to revisit prior interests?
3. What might be some consequences to Mr. Lee's overall health from being cognitively unengaged?

- *Case Scenario 5: Emergency Preparedness*

Mrs. Green is an older adult who resides alone in her home. She has never thought about what to do if she fell or experienced a power outage.

Critical Thinking Questions:

1. What steps can Mrs. Green take to prepare for an emergency?
2. How can technology help in an emergency?
3. What is the role of family and neighbors in making sure she is safe?

- *Scenario 6: Vision Changes*

Mr. Patel is a 75-year-old retiree who cannot see fine print and has difficulty reading labels and letters. This limits his ability to manage his medications and nutrition.

Critical Thinking Questions:

1. What are some environmental modifications that can be made to help Mr. Patel adapt to his vision change?
2. How might he best describe his problems to his eye doctor so he receives proper treatment?
3. What other resources are available for individuals experiencing age-related vision changes?

- *Scenario 7: Mental Health Concerns*

Mrs. Carter, an 82-year-old woman, has been feeling increasingly anxious and withdrawn since the death of her spouse. She has stopped attending her community events.

Critical Thinking Questions:

1. What steps can Mrs. Carter take to address her mental health needs?
2. How can her family help her reengage with her social circle?
3. What signs of depression or anxiety should family members watch for?

- *Scenario 8: Mobility Challenges*

Ms. Williams, a 78-year-old woman, has had knee surgery and is struggling with mobility. She is reluctant to use a walker, fearing it means she has become "too dependent."

Critical Thinking Questions:

1. What are the benefits of using mobility aids like walkers or canes for Ms. Williams?
2. How might her feelings about dependence be addressed in conversations with family or healthcare providers?
3. What alternative physical rehabilitation options can she explore?

These scenarios involve critical thinking and require the caregiver and the older people to consider solutions, resources, and decision-making strategies that support health, safety, and independence. They are multifaceted and call for comprehensive and thoughtful approaches toward older people self-care.

Bibliography

Adib-Hajbaghery M, Akbari H. The severity of old age disability and its related factors. Feyz Med Sci J. 2009;13(3):225–34.

Al-Abedi GA, Mansoor HI, Faris SH. Older adult self-care and related factors at primary health care centers. Bahrain Med Bull. 2024;46(1).

Amerzadeh M, Shafiei Kisomi Z, Senmar M, et al. Self-care behaviors, medication adherence status, and associated factors among older peoplewith type 2 diabetes. Science. 2024;14(1):19118.

Ancoli-Israel S, Ayalon L. Diagnosis and treatment of sleep disorders in older adults. Am J Geriatr Psychiatry. 2006;14(2):95–103.

Andrade M, Knight J. Anatomy and physiology of ageing 4: the renal system. Nurs Times. 2017;113(5):46–9.

apane KL, Resnik L. Obesity in nursing homes: an escalating problem. J Am Geriatr Soc. 2005;53(8):1386–91.

Barlow FK, Walker N. Disability and ageing. In: Encyclopedia of Geropsychology; 2015. p. 348.

Bauer J, Biolo G, Cederholm T, Cesari M, Cruz-Jentoft AJ, Morley JE, et al. Evidence-based recommendations for optimal dietary protein intake in older people: a position paper from the PROT-AGE study group. J Am Med Dir Assoc. 2013;14(8):542–59.

Brewster GS, Riegel B, Gehrman PR. Insomnia in the older adult. Sleep Med Clin. 2022;17(2):233–9. [QxMD MEDLINE Link].

Calder PC. n− 3 Polyunsaturated fatty acids, inflammation, and inflammatory diseases. Am J Clin Nutr. 2006;83(6):1505S–19S.

Casey B, Marston G, Vyas D. Self-care practices in the context of older adults living independently. arXiv preprint arXiv:2411.01815. 2024.

Daniels R, van Rossum E, de Witte L, et al. Interventions to prevent disability in frail community-dwelling older people: a systematic review. BMC Health Serv Res. 2008;8:278. https://doi.org/10.1186/1472-6963-8-278.

Deutz NE, Bauer JM, Barazzoni R, Biolo G, Boirie Y, Bosy-Westphal A, Cederholm T, Cruz-Jentoft A, Krznariç Z, Nair KS, Singer P. Protein intake and exercise for optimal muscle function with aging: recommendations from the ESPEN Expert Group. Clin Nutr. 2014;33(6):929–36.

DiPietro L. Physical activity in aging: changes in patterns and their relationship to health and function. J Gerontol: Ser A. 2001;56(suppl_2):13–22. https://doi.org/10.1093/gerona/56.suppl_2.13.

Escott-Stump S. Nutrition and diagnosis-related care. Lippincott Williams & Wilkins; 2008.

Fried LP, Guralnik JM. Disability in older adults: evidence regarding significance, etiology, and risk. J Am Geriatr Soc. 1997;45(1):92–100. https://doi.org/10.1111/j.1532-5415.1997.tb00986.x.

Fried LP, Ettinger WH, Lind B, Newman AB, Gardin J, Cardiovascular Health Study Research Group. Physical disability in older adults: a physiological approach. J Clin Epidemiol. 1994;47(7):747–60.

Gammack JK. Physical activity in older persons. Mo Med. 2017;114(2):105–9. PMID: 30228555; PMCID: PMC6140016.

Ghasemi S, Keshavarz Mohammadi N, Mohammadi Shahboulaghi F, Ramezankhani A, Mehrabi Y. Physical health status of the older people living at home in Tehran City, Iran. Salmand. Iran J Age. 2019;13(5):652.

Halter JB. Hazzard's geriatric medicine and gerontology. 2009.

https://patient.info/doctor/disability-in-older-people

Inelmen EM, Sergi G, Coin A, Miotto F, Peruzza S, Enzi G. Can obesity be a risk factor in older people people? Obesity Rev. 2003;4(3):14755.

Iranagh JA, Mohammadi F, Salem Safi P, Ayoughi V, Sedghiani A, Razi S. Non-pharmacological intervention to reduce sleep disturbance among older people: a randomized controlled trial study. Iranian J Ageing. 2023;18(2):162–77.

Jaqua EE, Hanna M, Labib W, Moore C, Matossian V. Common sleep disorders affecting older adults. Perm J. 2022;27(1):122.

Kim J-S, Wilson JM, Lee S-R. Dietary implications on mechanisms of sarcopenia: roles of protein, amino acids and antioxidants. J Nutr Biochem. 2010;21(1):113.

Knight J, Nigam Y. Anatomy and physiology of ageing 1: the cardiovascular system. Nurs Times. 2017a;113:22–4.

Knight J, Nigam Y. Anatomy and physiology of ageing 2: the respiratory system. Nurs Times. 2017b;113(3):53–5.

Knight J, Nigam Y. Anatomy and physiology of ageing 5: the nervous system. Nurs Times. 2017c;113(6):55–8.

Knight J, Nigam Y. Anatomy and physiology of ageing 7: the endocrine system. Nurs Times. 2017d;113(8):48–51.

Knight J, Nigam Y. Anatomy and physiology of ageing 8: the reproductive system. Nurs Times. 2017e;113(9):44–7.

Knight J, Wigham C, Nigam Y. Anatomy and physiology of ageing 6: the eyes and ears. Nurs Times. 2017a;113(7):39–42.

Knight J, Nigam Y, Hore N. Anatomy and physiology of ageing 10: the musculoskeletal system. Nurs Times. 2017b;113(11):60–3.

Langhammer B, Bergland A, Rydwik E. The importance of physical activity exercise among older people. Biomed Res Int. 2018;2018:7856823. https://doi.org/10.1155/2018/7856823. PMID: 30627571; PMCID: PMC6304477.

Lee SW, Patel R, Werner B, Yoo JW, Tiu T. The role of physical activity in older adults and practical intervention. HCA Healthc J Med. 2021;2(6):387–95. https://doi.org/10.36518/2689-0216.1352. PMID: 37427399; PMCID: PMC10324802.

Lorenzo-López L, Maseda A, de Labra C, Regueiro-Folgueira L, Rodríguez-Villamil JL, Millán-Calenti JC. Nutritional determinantsof frailty in older adults: a systematic review. BMC Geriatr. 2017;17(1):1–13.

Mahan L, Janice R. Krause and Mahans food & the nutrition care process. St Louis: Saunders; 2020.

Malafarina V, Uriz-Otano F, Gil-Guerrero L, Iniesta R. The anorexia of ageing: physiopathology, prevalence, associated comorbidity and mortality. A systematic review. Maturitas. 2013;74(4):293–302.

Manini T. Development of physical disability in older adults. Curr Aging Sci. 2011;4(3):184–91. https://doi.org/10.2174/1874609811104030184. PMID: 21529321; PMCID: PMC3868456.

Miller JM, Sabol VK, Pastva AM. Promoting older adult physical activity throughout care transitions using an interprofessional approach. J Nurse Pract. 2017;13(1):64–71.e2. https://doi.org/10.1016/j.nurpra.2016.08.006. Epub 2017 Jan 7. PMID: 34168522; PMCID: PMC8221589.

Nigam Y, Knight J. Anatomy and physiology of ageing 3: the digestive system. Nurs Times. 2017a;113(4):54–7.

Nigam Y, Knight J. Anatomy and physiology of ageing 9: the immune system. Nurs Times. 2017b;113:42–5.

Organization WH, University UN. Protein and amino acid requirements in human nutrition. World Health Organization; 2007.

Piercy KL, Troiano RP, Ballard RM, Carlson SA, Fulton JE, Galuska DA, George SM, Olson RD. The physical activity guidelines for Americans. JAMA. 2018;320(19):2020–8.

Popević M. Occupational sleep medicine: the sleep-related breathing disorders in high-risk occupations, protection and prevention approaches in occupational safety and occupational diseases [working title]. 2024. https://doi.org/10.5772/intechopen.1007579.

Pownall S, Taylor C. Use of thickening agents and nutritional supplements for patients with dysphagia following stroke. Br J Neurosci Nurs. 2017;13(6):260–8.

Raymond JL, Morrow K. Krause and Mahan's food and the nutrition care process E-book. Elsevier Health Sciences; 2020.

Riegel B, Barbaranelli C, Sethares KA, Daus M, Moser DK, Miller JL, Haedtke CA, Feinberg JL, Lee S, Stromberg A, et al. Development and initial testing of the self-care of chronic illness inventory. J Adv Nurs. 2018;74:2465–76. https://doi.org/10.1111/jan.13775.

Robinson S, Cooper C, Aihie SA. Nutrition and sarcopenia: a review of the evidence and implications for preventive strategies. J Aging Res. 2012;2012:510801.

Ross AC, Caballero B, Cousins RJ, Tucker KL, Ziegler TR. Modern nutrition in health and disease. Lippincott Williams & Wilkins; 2012.

Shahbazi MR, Foroughan M, Salman Roghani MR, Rahgozar M. The relationship between disability and depression, cognitive status and morale among older persons. Iran J Ageing. 2016;11(4):132–41.

Smith GI, Atherton P, Reeds DN, Mohammed BS, Rankin D, Rennie MJ, Mittendorfer B. Dietary omega-3 fatty acid supplementation increases the rate of muscle protein synthesis in older adults: a randomized controlled trial. Am J Clin Nutr. 2011;93(2):402–12.

Souza Júnior EV, Cruz DP, Silva CD, Rosa RS, Santos GD, Sawada NO. Association between sexuality and quality of life in older adults. Rev Esc Enferm USP. 2021;55:e20210066.

Soysal P, Smith L. Sexual activity and successful aging. Eur Geriatr Med. 2022;13:1235–8. https://doi.org/10.1007/s41999-022-00694-6.

Süderhamn O, Ek A-C, Pürn I. The self-care ability scale for the older people. Scand J Occup Ther. 1996;3(2):69–78.

Suzuki K, Miyamoto M, Hirata K. Sleep disorders in the older people: diagnosis and management. J Gen Fam Med. 2017;18(2):61–71. https://doi.org/10.1002/jgf2.27. PMID: 29263993; PMCID: PMC5689397.

Taghipour M, Hosseini SR, Pouraria S. The relationship between physical activity and balance control in the older people. Iran J Ageing. 2016;10(4):60–7.

Taheri M, Irandoust K. The relationship between sleep quality and lifestyle of the older people. Iranian J Ageing. 2020;15(2):188–99.

Villareal DT, Banks M, Sinacore DR, Siener C, Klein S. Effect of weight loss and exercise on frailty in obese older adults. Arch Intern Med. 2006;166(8):8606.

Volkert D, Chourdakis M, Faxen-Irving G, Frühwald T, Landi F, Suominen MH, et al. ESPEN guidelines on nutrition in dementia. Clin Nutr. 2015;34(6):1052–73.

Volkert D, Beck AM, Cederholm T, Cruz-Jentoft A, Goisser S, Hooper L, Kiesswetter E, Maggio M, Raynaud-Simon A, Sieber CC, Sobotka L. ESPEN guideline on clinical nutrition and hydration in geriatrics. Clin Nutr. 2019;38(1):10–47.

Weaver CM, Proulx WR, Heaney R. Choices for achieving adequate dietary calcium with a vegetarian diet. Am J Clin Nutr. 1999;70(3):543s–8s.

World Health Organization. United Nations University. Protein and amino acid requirements in human nutrition. World Health Organization; 2007.

3 Mental Self-Care

Fatemeh Bahramnezhad

In the end, the learner should be able to:

- Explain mental health and developmental tasks in older people
- Describe mental health and well-being
- Explain mental health and resilience
- Explain older people's psychological problems
- Identify older people's essential life skills
- Provide a mental self-care plan for older people

3.1 Mental Health and Developmental Tasks in Older People

The World Health Organization (2022) defined mental health as a state of mental well-being that enables people to cope with the stresses of life, realize their abilities, learn well and work well, and contribute to their community. Mental health is a complex and multifaceted concept with several key dimensions, experienced differently by each person, and it doesn't simply mean the absence of disorder. In the concept of mental health, individual factors, such as biological, emotional, behavioral, and interpersonal factors and cognitive status and, on the other hand, social, cultural, and economic factors, have a considerable impact on positive performance, emotional balance, and creating meaningful relationships.

Mental self-care includes purpose activities and practices to improve mental well-being, coping strategies, and resilience, and it directly affects psychological dimensions, such as emotions, thoughts, and relationships. In this chapter, we converse about older people's developmental tasks, well-being, resilience promotion, and the prevention of psychological problems and continue with social and spiritual self-care factors in the next chapters.

> **Box 3.1: Mental Self-Care: The Foundation**
> The first step in promoting mental health is having the right attitude toward the concept of mental health.

Older people's mental health is critical and can bring unique psychological challenges. One of the important issues in the mental health of older people is doing developmental tasks during aging. According to Robert J. Havighurst, developmental tasks for older people focus on adapting to several changes, and successful aging involves addressing key tasks that promote life satisfaction and well-being.

F. Bahramnezhad (✉)
Tehran University of Medical Sciences, Tehran, Iran
e-mail: bahramnezhad@tums.ac.ir

F. Bahramnezhad (ed.), *Self-Care in the Elderly*, https://doi.org/10.1007/978-981-96-9021-3_3

- Adjusting to decreasing physical strength and health
- Adjusting to retirement and reduced income
- Adjusting to the death of a spouse or close friends
- Establishing an affiliation with one's age group
- Adapting to social roles in a flexible way
- Establishing satisfactory physical living arrangements

3.2 Decreasing Physical Strength and Health

As aging often brings physical decline, individuals need to adapt to limitations and maintain health through proper care and lifestyle changes. Learning about natural physical changes of aging, common physical illnesses, easy access to medical services, and healthy lifestyle can play an important role in psychological adaptation to the reduction of physical strength and health in older people. Although no scientific method has been proven to prevent the aging process in humans, some strategies have been identified to manage the aging process and maintain physical health in older people.

1. *Daily exercise and physical activity:* Regular, low-impact exercises, like resistance training, balance exercises, and stretching, can help maintain muscle mass and reduce joint pain.
2. *Healthy diet:* Consuming adequate water, protein-rich nutrition, and calcium and vitamin D, which can help preserve muscle mass and strength, staying hydrated, and support bone density.
3. *Quality sleep:* Establishing a consistent sleep schedule, optimizing the sleep environment, and following a relaxing bedtime routine can help improve the quality of sleep.
4. *Management of physical health conditions:* Regular medical checkups, receiving medical treatments, and keeping chronic conditions, like diabetes, heart disease, or arthritis, under control can help track health changes, alleviate chronic pain, and improve mobility.
5. *Assistive devices:* Mobility aids, such as walking aids, grab bars, or chairs with arms and specially designed tools, like easy-grip utensils or jar openers, can enhance safety during movement and help maintain independence with daily tasks.
6. *Adapting to the environment:* Home and public areas' modifications, like installing handrails, improving lighting, removing tripping hazards, and providing suitable transportation, social activity plans, or home assistance for older people can make their homes safer and help them increase their individual independence.
7. *Positive thinking about aging:* Old age is associated with the loss of some abilities and reduced physical strength, but in most cases, it can bring about an increase in wisdom and awareness. Accepting physical changes instead of confronting them, recognizing small and big achievements, and giving meaning to life can play an important role in building self-esteem and coping with aging.

Box 3.2 Mental self-care recommendation
Adjust to decreasing physical strength and health, and love your valuable old body.

3.3 Retirement and Reduced Income

Adjusting to retirement and reducing financial resources is one of the big challenges in old age, which should be considered not only from the financial aspect but also from the emotional and social aspects. Loss or decrease of salary, increasing medical service and treatment costs, loss of social relationships with colleagues, and disruption of daily plans and life goals can have an important effect on the mental health of older people. The following activities are suggested to reduce the negative effects of retirement on mental health and increase adaptation in older people.

1. *Financial management:* Realistic budgeting and expense tracking, cutting down unnecessary expenses, estate planning, financial planning, and the use of medical insurance and available support services can reduce stress about money.
2. *Part-time or volunteer job:* The willingness and ability to do a part-time job can bring you extra income, and doing volunteer work will increase your social activities and make you feel useful.
3. *Creation of a new routine:* Replan your daily and weekly schedule, taking into consideration physical activities, fulfilling personal tasks, maintaining family and social connections, recreation, and entertainment. A routine can provide structure, which helps you stay engaged and feel a sense of purpose.
4. *Staying active in social networks:* Staying engaged with friends and family, finding new friends, and joining community groups can provide useful social connections. You can do daily or community group activities with them, travel, or stay in touch using video calls, social media, and messaging apps.
5. *Rediscovering purpose:* Determine short-term and long-term goals, including personal projects, learning new skills, family relationships, promotion of mental and psychological health, and charity work, or do anything that makes you feel better.
6. *Positive thinking about retirement:* Transitioning to retirement is a process, and adjusting expectations and gradually letting go of a previous lifestyle can make it easier to adapt. Without denying the unpleasant consequences of retirement, it offers the freedom to try things you did not have time for before, such as learning a new language, painting, gardening, or spending time with the people you love, and relax without feeling guilty.

Box 3.3 Mental self-care recommendation
Appreciate reaching your retirement age, and enjoy all of your free time.

3.4 Death of a Spouse or Close Friends

Learning to live with loss and coping with the death of spouse or close friends can be especially hard and is a deeply personal journey that has a profound impact on both emotional and physical health. In older people, we may lose those who played an important role in our daily lives, support networks, and shared history. Here are some approaches and insights that can be supportive when navigating this challenging experience.

1. *Accept your grief and your feelings:* Grieving involves a wide range of emotions, like sadness, anger, guilt, relief, or even numbness, and all of these are natural responses to loss. Allowing oneself to feel and express these emotions can be healing, even though it may take time to process the depth of the loss. It seems that facing the loss of loved ones shows some kind of attitude toward the concept and acceptance of death as the last stage of emotional maturity.
2. *The importance of physical health:* Grief is generally debilitating and can cause physical changes in people, such as sleep problems, disruption of eating habits, fatigue, negative thoughts, and self-blame. Physical activities, healthy eating habits, regular sleep, yoga, and meditation can help you in your physical self-care.
3. *Return to daily activities:* Try to focus on your daily activities, such as doing personal things, housework and taking care of your children, pets, and plants, or start doing volunteer activities, and create new goals for your life.
4. *Let others help you:* Strengthen the return to normal life and coping with loneliness by being with friends, family, and community. Let them accompany you in doing your daily activities, and share your feelings and experiences with others.
5. *Find a personal way to remember:* Praying, lighting a candle, planting a flower or tree, making a scrapbook, or engaging in the loved one's favorite hobbies can help keep the memory of the loved one alive.

6. *Professional support:* When symptoms of depression, anxiety, and insomnia are severe, talking to a therapist and seeking medical care can help you manage your emotions, cope with the death, and get back to normal life.

Box 3.4 Mental self-care recommendation
Accept the death of your loved ones because grief is part of the human experience, and you are not alone.

3.5 Affiliation with One's Age Group

One of the most important dimensions of mental health is communicating with peers, which plays an important role in coping with old age, which involves physical problems and moving away from work environments. Improving relationships with family, friends, and neighbors; maintaining relationships with colleagues; establishing new relationships with peers; and participating in social activities enrich the lives of older people and help increase satisfaction in life and have a successful old age. Considering the importance of relationships with others and social self-care in older people, a separate chapter has been dedicated to it in this book, where it will be fully investigated.

Box 3.5 Mental self-care recommendation
Participate in peer group activities, and enrich your life with a sense of belonging.

3.6 Social Roles in a Flexible Way

One of the other most important issues in mental health is accepting and adapting to social roles that people play as members of different groups, such as family, work, friendship circles, and social organizations. These roles come with certain expectations, responsibilities, and pressures that can have a positive or negative impact on one's mental health. Reaching old age can cause significant changes in social roles, and this role can be very different according to cultural, economic, and family structures. In most societies, the role of older people is highly respected, as it is one of the important components in maintaining social structures and intergenerational relationships. Although accepting new social roles in accordance with new developmental tasks, reducing the role of self-management, controlling individual life, and building a new identity in older people can be very challenging, they can increase self-esteem, self-confidence, and a feeling of usefulness in older people and improve their emotional and mental health. In the spiritual self-care chapter, we will talk more about these issues.

Box 3.6 Mental self-care recommendation
Create new social roles and goals, and search for the novel meaning of your life.

3.7 Satisfactory Physical Living Arrangements

Creating satisfactory living conditions by the time of reaching old age, which reduces physical capabilities and health, is one of the most important challenges for older people. Predicting, planning, envisioning, and providing a suitable, comfortable, dignified, and as independent a life as possible is essential and greatly helps improve coping skills and overall quality of life. As with other developmental tasks of aging, family, healthcare system, and society play a very important role in achieving this goal, and the following activities are recommended for older people to have a satisfying physical life.

1. *Safety and accessibility:* Aim to increase general self-help skills; it is better to make changes in their home and living environment individually, considering their physical capabilities and physical health. For example,

using mobility aids, wheelchairs, or walkers to help them move freely; installing grab bars, tall toilets, shower seats, and handrails in the bathroom; and using nonslip floors and good lighting throughout the home can reduce the risk of falls. Kitchen adaptations by making appliances available and providing pull-out shelves and lever taps for seniors who want to maintain their independence in preparing food can be very helpful.

2. *Comfort and personalization:* Considering older adults' sensitivity to temperature, noise, visual stimuli, smell, and touch, it is recommended to use efficient heating and cooling systems, reduce noise by providing a quiet environment, create a simple and pleasant setting with soothing scents, and offer comfortable, soft beds and chairs. Emphasis should also be placed on maintaining their current home environment while respecting personal preferences and choices.
3. *Healthcare and emergency preparedness:* Access to nearby clinics, pharmacies, and hospitals is essential, especially for seniors with chronic conditions. Regular health checkups, medication management, in-home care services, and the use of medical alert systems in an emergency situation play a very important role in creating a satisfactory physical life.
4. *Social connectivity:* Living close to family, friends or community centers, using shared spaces or gardens for social interaction, and having access to communication tools, such as by equipping homes with technology, phones with large buttons, smartphones, and virtual assistants, can help older people be in touch with others and reduce isolation.
5. *Cognitive support:* For older people with cognitive disorders, memory problems, and dementia, using cognitive aids, such as labeling and naming rooms, household items, tools, and food, and using digital clocks, speakers, large printed calendars, and voice reminders can help reduce confusion, support routines, and increase their independence.
6. *Caregiver support:* In cases of those who are in their old age or are suffering from chronic diseases, finding a caregiver and creating suitable environmental conditions, such as a private room or suite, and using monitoring tools, such as sensors, cameras, and remote monitoring tools, to provide privacy for both the older person and the caregiver can increase the quality of care and also reduce caregiver burnout.

Box 3.7 Mental self-care recommendation
According to your needs, create new satisfactory physical living arrangements.

3.8 Mental Health and Well-Being

Well-being is a broad concept that refers to the overall health, happiness, and life satisfaction, and it encompasses physical, mental, and social aspects. Well-being, like the mental health concept, is not just the absence of illness; it is feeling good about oneself, one's relationships, and one's environment and thriving and functioning well in various areas of life. Promotion of older people's well-being is a comprehensive approach that encompasses eight main components that focus on various aspects of our lives as follows.

- Physical well-being
- Emotional well-being
- Intellectual well-being
- Social well-being
- Environmental well-being
- Spiritual well-being
- Occupational well-being
- Financial well-being

3.9 Physical Well-Being

Considering the relationship between mental and physical health, the first dimension of general well-being is that physical factors directly influence one's mood and energy. Improving physical health by choosing a healthy lifestyle has a direct relationship with successful aging, while education and social supportive systems play an important role. Physical activity and exercise, a balanced nutritious diet, adequate sleep, regular medical checkups, and chronic disease management are scientific recommendations that are mentioned in various self-care sections.

> **Box 3.8 Mental self-care recommendation**
> Choose a healthy lifestyle that directly promotes your successful aging and physical well-being.

3.10 Emotional Well-Being

Emotional well-being refers to the ability to manage and express emotions in a healthy manner; cope with all aging-related developmental tasks; put on a positive outlook on ourselves, others, and life; and have pleasant feelings. Considering the overlap of the different dimensions of emotional well-being with the main issues of mental health, such as coping and resilience, and also the role of biological, emotional, behavioral, cognitive, social, environmental, cultural, and societal factors, learning the following techniques and general skills is recommended.

Emotional Regulation Technique Emotional management, or emotional regulation, as one of the essential life skills, shows a personal ability to understand, manage, and respond to emotions. It includes recognizing and accepting all the pleasant and unpleasant emotions, using emotional self-regulation and self-compassion skills, having emotional stability, and finally, expressing feelings to others through adaptive methods. The important point in teaching any skills to older people is the use of appropriate tools, concrete examples, and short behavioral and emotional techniques as personalized training, according to their demographic characteristics and cognitive abilities. The training instructions for emotion management will be given in the life skills section of this chapter.

Stress Management Technique Another essential life skill is stress management, which can have a significant impact on different aspects of mental health and significantly enhance the quality of life and life satisfaction. Due to the occurrence of various stressful events, such as the death of loved ones, reduction of physical and cognitive abilities, pain and chronic illness, economic problems, and a lack of control, the sense of insecurity and anxiety in older people has increased, and learning stress management skills seems vital. Correcting the right attitude toward the concept of stress, identifying resources and physical symptoms, practicing mindfulness and relaxation techniques, and learning thought control and problem-solving skills are the main topics of stress management that will be given in the life skills section of this chapter.

Adaptive Coping Strategies People use so many methods and techniques to manage stress and overcome crises or difficult situations, and these techniques are completely different in each person, like intelligence, personality traits, individual psychological factors, socioeconomic status, physical health, various life experiences, and resilience. Lazarus and Folkman developed a model of coping with stress, which emphasizes the appraisal and coping processes. In primary appraisal, an individual evaluates whether an event is a threat, a challenge, or a harm/loss, and secondary appraisal involves assessing the resources available to cope with it. According to these appraisals, we use different coping strategies, such as problem-, emotion-, and meaning-focused coping strategies.

1. Via problem-solving coping strategies, people focus on managing or changing a stressful

situation. It is like saying, "Okay, what can I actually do to fix this problem?" Defining the problem, generating solutions, weighing pros and cons, taking action, and assessing effectiveness are usually used in problem-focused coping strategies.

2. Per emotional coping strategies, people try to manage the emotional response to a stressful situation. It is like saying, "I can't change this, but I can change how I feel about it." Expressing emotions, relaxation techniques, positive reappraisal, distraction, and a sense of humor are usually used in emotion-focused coping strategies.
3. In meaningful coping strategies, people try to find positive meaning in a stressful event, often by focusing on personal values and beliefs. It is like saying, "How can I make sense of this, and how does it fit into the bigger picture of my life?" Reframing, finding purpose, spirituality, and personal growth are usually used in meaning-focused coping strategies.

The efficiency of each strategy is not certain, and it is not possible to accurately determine whether using this strategy by whom, how, and where is right or wrong. According to the evaluation of stressful situations and people's resilience, any of these strategies can be adaptive, incompatible, healthy, or harmful. In every stressful situation, the use of any healthy and adaptive problem-, emotion-, or meaning-focused coping method, which helps reduce unpleasant feelings, problem-solving or managing critical situations and increase resilience through creating new meaning or spirituality in painful, unavoidable situations, by people's own choice, is recommended.

Positive Thinking Technique Positive thinking is the ability to focus on the good and positive points in any given situation. Maintaining an optimistic outlook and reframing negative thoughts can significantly enhance your emotional well-being by fostering resilience and reducing stress, and it helps you see challenges as opportunities, appreciate the present moment, and feel better. Reframing thoughts, gratitude, self-affirmation, visualization, and surrounding yourself with positivity can genuinely alter your mindset and improve your emotional health. A very important point about positive thinking is having a logical attitude and belief toward the concept of positive thinking. You must have a realistic viewpoint of the situation, events, and opportunities; face it; and accept all facts, even hard or painful ones, while being able to stay positive. Positive thinking has no magical power to change or improve the surrounding situation, but it can help have a true view of situations, events, or life and help in emotional management, better problem-solving, and, ultimately, improving coping skills.

Effective Communication Skills Effective communication is an essential skill for building or maintaining relationships, requesting help and support, and improving your quality of life. It is the process of sharing information, ideas, or emotions in a way that is quite clear, concise, and understood by all parties involved while ensuring the message is both delivered and received accurately. Effective communication with older people needs special attention to their potential physical, cognitive, and emotional traits. Considering the two-way nature of the relationship concept, communication skills training is recommended for both older people and their families or caregivers. Effective communication skill training instructions will be given in the social self care chapter.

Finding the Meaning of Life The meaning of life is one of the coping strategies that is directly about creating a personal sense of purpose, embracing experiences, and finding what feels meaningful to each of us. There is no correct answer that suits everyone, and finding meaning in life can be a deeply personal journey. Helping older people rediscover meaning in life is about connecting them to what makes them feel valued, appreciated, and part of something larger. See the spiritual self-care chapter for more information.

Creating Joy and Happiness Happiness and joy are powerful emotional states of emotional well-being. They contribute to a positive mental state, promote resilience, foster connections, boost confidence, and offer protection against both physical and emotional stress. In general, creating joy for older people is about the appreciation of life that values their experiences, supports their needs, and uplifts their spirit. Here are some effective ways to bring happiness into their lives:

- Physical activities: gentle exercises, walking, dancing, swimming, or water aerobics
- Cognitive activities: puzzles and brain games, learning about new topics, and trivia competitions like 20-question competitions, pantomime, memoir writing, and storytelling sessions
- Artistic and creative activities: painting, crafting like knitting or pottery, gardening, listening to favorite songs, learning to play a simple instrument, and photography
- Mindfulness and relaxation: meditation and breathing exercises, aromatherapy, and spa
- Technology-based activities: visiting museums or going on historical virtual tours and travel, making video calls with family, and playing games on tablets or cellphones
- Outdoor activities: bird-watching, walk, fishing, gentle boating, and spending time with animals
- Social activities: book clubs, game nights, movie or documentary screenings, and social events, like tea parties, holiday celebrations, or themed dinner nights
- Volunteer and purposeful activities: mentoring or teaching younger generations; community service projects, like knitting for charities, creating cards for hospitals, or reading to children; and nursing pets

3.11 Intellectual Well-Being

Intellectual well-being is the aspect of health that keeps the mind active, curious, and continually engaged in growth and which can contribute to personal enrichment and build resilience. The intellectual well-being concept has two sides, emotional and mental factors. The emotional side is related to the motivating factors of enthusiasm, and the mental side is associated with abilities such as thinking, learning, and memorizing. Improving the intellectual well-being of older adults is essential to maintain cognitive function, boost their mood, and improve their quality of life.

1. Promote lifelong learning by participating in courses, workshops, or online training on new technologies or virtual reality.
2. Practice puzzles and brain games, and play brain teasers, games, and memory apps.
3. Introduce new hobbies, such as making art, gardening, photography, or playing music.

Box 3.9 Mental self-care recommendation
Promote lifelong learning, and introduce new hobbies to increase your cognitive abilities.

3.12 Occupational Well-Being

Occupational or career well-being means having work that aligns with personal values and allows for growth, and it refers to finding personal satisfaction, meaning, and balance through work or other meaningful activities. This dimension of well-being is not limited to paid employment; it applies to any productive or fulfilling activity that gives a sense of purpose and direction. Activities that engage everyone in tasks or roles, whether paid employment, volunteer work, creative pursuits, caregiving, or even hobbies, provide a sense of purpose, honor, identity, and social connection.

Retirement often marks the end of paid employment. Many older adults seek fulfilling activities that resemble or even extend their career roles, offering mental, emotional, and social benefits that contribute to their overall well-being. Here are some activities for occupational well-being for older people:

1. Part-time or flexible work, according to the level of knowledge, previous specialized

skills, cognitive capabilities, physical condition, and current energy level of older people
2. Mentorship opportunities to contribute by guiding the younger workforce
3. Community involvement to encourage older people to volunteer or participate in meaningful activities

> **Box 3.10 Mental self-care recommendation**
> Find your personal fulfillment through work or other meaningful activities.

3.13 Financial Well-Being

Financial well-being is a state where you feel secure and in control of your financial situation, allowing you to meet your current and future financial obligations comfortably. This includes managing money well, being free from financial stress, feeling prepared for both short- and long-term needs, and being able to plan for the future. Here are some specific tips to help seniors maintain or improve their financial well-being:

1. Optimize income sources by taking Social Security, managing your retirement accounts, and earning extra finances with part-time work or hobbies.
2. Create a sustainable budget by limiting debt, living within a fixed income, and prioritizing needs over wants.
3. Estate and legacy planning by power of attorney, current wishes directives, and gifting strategy can help reduce tax burdens and leave a legacy.
4. Minimize falling prey to financial fraud by getting educated on scams, adding a trusted contact to financial accounts, and maintaining a safety net.
5. Ensure lifestyle adjustments by downsizing the house, using free or low-cost services for seniors, optimizing medical plans, planning long-term care, and using health savings accounts.
6. Seek financial guidance on investment, budgeting, and estate planning, tailored to individual circumstances.

> **Box 3.11 Mental self-care recommendation**
> Control your financial situation, and have a plan for your future.

3.14 Environmental Well-Being

Environmental well-being refers to how the environment, such as the home, work, and surroundings, affects our quality of life. Environmental well-being is particularly important for people because a healthy environment can have a significant impact on their quality of life, physical health, well-being, and sense of independence. Promoting the environmental well-being of older people involves favorable, sustainable, and safe living conditions, with dignity and comfort. Here are some key aspects of the environmental well-being of older people.

1. Accessible and safe spaces
2. Clean air and water
3. Connection to nature
4. Community and social environment
5. Climate resilience and emergency preparedness
6. Accessible healthcare and amenities

> **Box 3.12 Mental self-care recommendation**
> Promote your quality of life by improving your environment and providing a desirable and safe life for yourself.

3.15 Social Well-Being

Social well-being is about how connected and supported a person feels by others, their sense of belonging, and their contribution to the community and supporting systems. Improving social well-being among older people is essential for enhancing their quality of life, promoting physical and mental health, and reducing isolation. All dimensions related to the social well-being of older people and self-care recommendations will be discussed in the next chapter.

> **Box 3.13 Mental self-care recommendation**
> Participate in social events, and create a sense of belonging.

3.16 Spiritual Well-Being

Spiritual well-being refers to a sense of peace, purpose, and connection that is often linked to beliefs, values, or experiences that give life a deeper meaning. It is not necessarily religious, though it can be for those who find spirituality through religious practices. At its core, spiritual well-being is about feeling aligned with something greater than oneself, which can involve personal growth, connection to others, or a relationship with the natural world or a higher power. Supporting the spiritual well-being of older people can be a meaningful way to help them find peace, purpose, and connection in their later years. Finding the meaning and connection of life, finding a connection to the universe, and achieving inner peace and personal values of life are the main subjects of spiritual well-being, which will be explained in the spiritual self-care chapter.

> **Box 3.14 Mental self-care recommendation**
> Connect to the universe, and find the meaning of your life.

3.17 Mental Health and Resilience

Resilience or resistance refers to recovering from difficulties and adapting to challenges and setbacks. It involves maintaining mental, emotional, and physical well-being during adversities and using these experiences for learning and personal development. It is noteworthy that the concept of resilience in psychology is used for various phenomena, such as the prevention of psychological disorders, successful coping, psychological growth, and recovery after life's adversities or trauma. Resilience is a multidimensional concept that involves psychological factors and adaptive strategies at the individual or community level, and it provides effective coping. The concepts of mental health and resilience are related. Strong mental health provides the foundation for resilience, and resilience supports mental well-being too. Mental well-being promotes emotional stability, self-esteem, and self-worth, and resilience also improves the use of healthy coping strategies. Resilience also helps reduce the risk of mental health problems, brings out positive relationships and support systems, encourages a growth mindset, and fosters self-compassion, and it can have a considerable impact over health, mental well-being, and quality of life. The most potentially causal resilience factors are related to meaning in life, physical activity, positive affect, and relationship satisfaction. Considering the factors affecting resilience, the following are recommended to improve resilience in older people.

1. Choose a healthy lifestyle.
2. Check your physical and mental health regularly.
3. Do daily and personal tasks yourself as possible.
4. Engage yourself in new learning and mental stimulation.
5. Have regular and structured care for yourself.
6. Be optimistic, and keep negative thoughts away.
7. Develop your emotional intelligence and stress management.
8. Learn life skills and coping strategies.
9. Increase your social connections with your family, friends, neighbors, and peer groups.
10. Be kind to yourself, and get help from others.

Box 3.15 Mental self-care recommendation
Strengthen your resilience by making healthy lifestyle choices and building enjoyable relationships.

3.18 Older People's Psychological Problems

Another important issue in mental self-care is the prevention and treatment of neuropsychological disorders, which can affect their cognitive abilities, mood, behavior, and performance. The prevalence of psychological disorders in older people is around 14%, which can be caused by normal brain changes associated with aging or neurological diseases. Early diagnosis and treatment interventions have an important role in reducing the progression of the disease and can have remarkable effects on quality of life, well-being, and independent functioning in older people. The common neuropsychological problems in older people are listed here.

- Dementia
- Delirium
- Parkinson's disease
- Huntington's disease
- Depression disorders
- Anxiety disorders
- Schizophrenia and late-onset psychosis
- Sleep disorders
- Substance-induced cognitive impairment

It is noteworthy that the screening, diagnosis, and pharmacological or non-pharmacological treatment management are performed by medical teams, such as family medicine, geriatrics, neurologists, psychiatrists, psychologists, rehabilitation specialists, social workers, and other medical professionals. Prevalent treatment interventions for older people's neuropsychological disorders are usually a comprehensive and multidisciplinary approach that includes the following:

- Medication management
- Physiotherapy and occupational therapy
- Cognitive rehabilitation
- Counseling and psychotherapy interventions
- Psychological and social support
- Lifestyle changes
- Teaching life skills
- Education of family and caregivers

Early diagnosis and treatment of neuropsychological disorders are very important, and they address all the physical and psychological sides of health. Considering the high prevalence of depression, anxiety, and dementia among other psychological disorders, we only introduce disorders and prevention methods. The following general activities to prevent mental disorders in older people are recommended.

1. Regularly visit the doctor, and get mental health screening done.
2. Follow your prescribed medical and nonmedical treatments.
3. Complete your treatment process and follow-up visits.
4. Plan your regular physical activities, sports training, and personal duties.
5. Maintain a balanced diet, and have healthy sleep.
6. Learn new skills, hobbies, and games.
7. Stay in touch with your children, relatives, and friends.
8. Participate in community or volunteer programs.
9. Create a new purpose and meaning for your life.

Box 3.16 Mental self-care recommendation
Follow your medical management programs and mental health screening.

3.19 Depression Disorder

Depression is one of the most common psychological disorders and presents a significant challenge in mental health. People with depression often experience low energy, loss of interest, sadness, boredom, disability, and hopelessness. Genetic factors, personality traits, environmental stressors, and unforgettable painful experiences can contribute to its development. In older adults, agitation, difficulty concentrating, sleep problems, loss of appetite, and physical complaints are common symptoms, which can sometimes worsen chronic pain and illness. Moreover, depression as a comorbid condition can occur alongside many physical illnesses such as cardiovascular disease, dementia, Parkinson's disease, and side effects from certain medications. Diagnosing depression in the presence of physical illness in older adults is important, as it can intensify physical symptoms, chronic pain, and anxiety. Therefore, simultaneous treatment of both the physical illness and depression is recommended.

Depression in older people can be seen as a depression disorder, late-life depression, and pseudo-dementia. Dysthymia or major depressive disorder in older people is usually seen before their 40s. Late-life depression can be caused by life changes in aging, such as retirement, death of loved ones, chronic illness, or loss of independence, and in both cases, common symptoms of depression, such as sadness, lack of interest, difficulty with sleep or appetite, fatigue, and feelings of hopelessness are seen. The diagnosis of pseudo-dementia depression in older people can cause dementia-like symptoms, such as memory problems, poor concentration, and confusion. These symptoms are temporary and improve with depression treatment but can sometimes increase the risk of dementia.

As mentioned, the treatment and prevention of depression in older people requires a comprehensive and multidisciplinary approach. After completion of diagnostic processes, medical management, and individual intervention planning, older people, their family members, and healthcare providers should work as a team with a compassionate and effective approach to promote personal activities and social relationships, encourage them to choose a healthy lifestyle, and provide opportunities for communication or social participation. The following are specific activities recommended to help prevent depression in older people.

1. Engage in enjoyable activities, and fill your surroundings with nature and beauty.
2. Control your negative thoughts and self-blame.
3. Talk to others, and share your feelings.
4. Promote your emotional management and problem-solving skills (Please read the section on older people's essential life skills in this chapter).
5. Use professional support.

Box 3.17 Mental self-care recommendation
Engage in enjoyable activities, and fill your surroundings with nature and beauty.

3.20 Anxiety Disorder

One of the most common psychological disorders is anxiety, which usually presents with the same symptoms in different age groups. People with anxiety usually report physical symptoms, such as headache, respiratory problems, sweating, nausea, and digestive problems, and also psychological symptoms, such as feeling too much stress or worry, agitation, irrational thoughts, forgetfulness, insomnia, and a desire to distance themselves from others. Like depression, a set of genetic factors, environmental stresses, and previous experiences can cause anxiety disorders. However, the common problems of old age, such as movement problems and physical diseases, inability to perform personal activities, financial problems, loneliness, loss of loved ones, and thinking about death, can cause extra anxiety in older people. One of the problems with diagnosing anxiety is that the symptoms of this disorder are common with other physical diseases, and early diagnosis is very important in the treatment of this disorder.

Types of anxiety disorders in older people include generalized anxiety disorder, phobia, panic disorder, and health anxiety. In generalized anxiety disorder (GAD), excessive worries about daily life events are seen with high intensity, but in phobias, people report high anxiety when being in certain situations and places. In panic disorder, people have frequent and sudden, severe panic attacks without any medical reasons, illnesses, or feeling of impending death, but older people with health anxiety disorder worry too much about contracting or spreading chronic diseases. In general, older people with anxiety disorders constitute a high percentage of clients in different medical systems, and their treatment requires more care and lowers their quality of life.

The treatment and prevention of anxiety in older people, like other mental disorders, is a comprehensive and multidisciplinary approach and includes a combination of medical treatments; psychological interventions, such as individual counseling and psychotherapy; emotional regulation techniques; and lifestyle modifications. The main goal of these interventions is to promote psychological well-being, strengthen coping skills, and create a supportive environment. The following are effective strategies recommended to help decrease anxiety in older people.

1. Limit exposure to stressors and bad news.
2. Practice relaxation techniques and deep breathing every day.
3. Control your negative thoughts.
4. Promote your stress management skills (Please read the section on older people's essential life skills in this chapter).
5. Use professional help.

> **Box 3.18 Mental self-care recommendation**
> Practice relaxation techniques and deep breathing every day.

3.21 Dementia and Cognitive Decline

The aging process can affect all physical skills as well as cognitive skills in everyone. Reduced speed of performing brain activities, increased distraction, concentration problems, and momentary forgetfulness are natural cognitive changes in old age. However, the process of cognitive aging is different in older people, and the recognition of natural cognitive changes or neuropsychological disorder diagnosis must be noted.

Dementia is a general term for a group of conditions resulting from a decline in cognitive function, such as memory, thinking, judgment, logic, and behavior, and it significantly affects the function, relationships, and daily life of older people. Alzheimer's disease, vascular dementia, frontotemporal dementia, and Lewy body dementia are the most common types of dementia.

Dementia prevention involves a multifaceted and proactive approach, but we still do not have a definitive cure or perfect prevention methods against dementia. However, by early diagnosis, medical interventions, and lifestyle changes, we can strengthen the cognitive function of older people and reduce the progression of dementia. The following are recommended to help cognitive function in older people.

1. Make your plans, and write down your daily activities.
2. As much as possible, do your own work.
3. Use stickers, note papers, and assistive technologies to do your daily tasks.
4. Follow the events and occasions in the daily calendar.
5. Concentrate on what you are doing, and follow the steps of the task.
6. Learn new skills, and challenge your mind.
7. Play mind games and memory exercises, or practice puzzles.
8. Participate in group activities and games.
9. Use professional help.

> **Box 3.19 Mental self-care recommendation**
> Learn new skills and challenge your mind every day.

3.22 Older People's Essential Life Skills

Life skills are a set of abilities and skills that help everyone have good and healthy relationships with others; solve their life problems in an effective way; manage mental stress and unpleasant emotions, such as anger, anxiety, and sadness; and make better decisions. As mentioned before, learning these skills helps us have better resilience and coping skills and have better mental health and quality of life. As individuals age, maintaining independence and quality of life becomes more important. Life skills for older people encompass a range of practical, social, and cognitive abilities that enable older adults to manage their daily lives effectively.

According to the content of this chapter, life skills related to the psychological domain, such as emotion management, stress management, and problem-solving, will be expressed in this chapter, and other life skills will be stated in the next chapters. It is noticed that the definition and effectiveness of essential life skills have already been stated, and here, we provide simple user-training instructions for older people. Life skills are learned and take time, and only practice and engaging with new experiences can guide you toward useful reactions and emotional balance.

Emotional Management Skill

- *Step 1:* Know your emotions, and tell yourself how you feel now.
- *Step 2:* Accept your emotions. All of your feelings, whether pleasant or unpleasant, are natural, and they are part of being human.
- *Step 3:* When you feel strong emotions, before doing anything, you should pause and take slow and deep breaths.
- *Step 4:* Analyze the situation, and think about possible reasons for your emotions.
- *Step 5:* After you have calmed down and assessed the situation, find helpful responses.
- *Step 6:* Now, according to your solutions, react to the situation. Remember, you can control your response, even if you could not control your emotions at first.
- *Step 7:* Reflect on what you learned from your emotional management. Think about what helped and what you could try next time.

Stress Management Skills

- *Step 1:* Know the physical signs and symptoms of your stress so that you can quickly identify your stress in different situations.
- *Step 2:* Practice deep breathing or relaxation techniques. Find a quiet, comfortable spot, if possible, where you can sit or lie down.
- *Step 3:* After you have calmed down, analyze the situation, and identify your current stress factors and sources.
- *Step 4:* Make a list of useful actions to deal with the source of stress or reduce your stress, and focus on helpful responses.
- *Step 5:* Considering the available resources and solutions, see if you can reduce or eliminate the stressor.
- *Step 6:* Considering the available resources and solutions, if you cannot control the source of stress, it is better to deal with your feelings, reduce your stress, and calm yourself by using emotion-oriented approaches.

Problem-Solving Skill

- *Step 1:* Identify your problem, and accept it.
- *Step 2:* Clearly define the current situation and problem, accurately identify the factors and components of the cause, and break the problem down into smaller items.
- *Step 3:* You should try to find different solutions. Consulting friends and relatives is also a good way to find useful and effective solutions.
- *Step 4:* Check your solutions, write down the advantages and disadvantages of each, and choose the best solution.
- *Step 5:* Plan your solution, and implement it.
- *Step 6:* If you solve your problem, say congratulations to yourself. If your solution is not effective, go back to the previous step, and choose another solution.

Box 3.20 Mental self-care recommendation

You can control your response, even if you could not control your emotions at first.

3.23 Mental Self-Care Plan for Older People

Self-care plan preparation for older people requires a comprehensive and multidisciplinary approach, focused on physical, mental, and social health. After the medical management process is completed, it will be planned as case formulation, and older people, their families, and caregivers will be educated on it. According to the goals of medical management, current problems, environmental and social factors, support systems, and older people's lifestyle, the self-care plans are individual, and they will be continuously monitored and updated until the end of life. The different areas of a case formula of self-care in older people are introduced here.

- *Current problems:* Describe the main problems or symptoms that older people, their families, and caregivers are experiencing.
- *Background information:* Review personal, medical, psychological, occupational, and family history and important life events of older people.
- *Current biological factors:* Include genetic predispositions, medical conditions, medications, and any physical limitations.
- *Current psychological factors:* Describe the client's personality traits, cognitive abilities, emotional responses, and any thought patterns that may impact their current mental state.
- *Current social factors:* Consider social relation ships, community engagement, family dynamics, cultural beliefs, and support systems.
- *Current strengths and resilience factors:* Identify any positive factors that could be leveraged in their care plan, such as personal skills, previous coping strategies, community resources, or family support.
- *Case formulation of the current situation of older people:* Describe all of an older person's biological, psychological, social, and environmental factors, and identify her/his coping strategy and current challenges.
- *Treatment goals and self-care plan:* According to the formulation, establish short-term and long-term goals and recommended interventions.
- *Adapting and updating the self-care plan:* Older people's health status and their needs can change over time, so review the self-care plan, provide feedback, identify results and challenges, and then, update the plan every 6–12 months.

Recommendations Are Also Given for Family, Caregivers, and Older People Aging is a natural and unavoidable stage of life that almost everyone will face, and each older person has their own care needs. The preparation of older people, family, caregivers, society, and the government through this stage is essential, and it maintains and improves their physical and mental health to have a healthy lifestyle. Considering the above, the following, regarding an older person's mental health, are recommended to families and caregivers of older people in three categories.

Box 3.21 Having a Positive Attitude Toward Older People

1. Old age is a natural stage of development.
2. Old age does not necessarily mean having illness and disability, and older people are only a population group with special needs.
3. The needs of older people are different at each stage and from person to person.
4. Although older people need our support, they are not our children.
5. Having a successful and dignified old age is one of the basic principles of human rights.
6. Helping promote the independence and empowerment of older people is one of the main duties of those around them, their caregivers, and society.
7. Showing a sense of respect, empathy, and kindness is of great importance in our communication with older people.
8. Caring for older people requires training and acquiring new skills.
9. Supporting older people can significantly help enrich their lives, and on the other hand, it can make your life incredibly purposeful and meaningful.

Having Essential Knowledge and Information Necessary for Older People

1. Increase your health literacy and basic medical knowledge.
2. Learn the necessary information about medical management plans, treatment methods, diet, and other care instructions for older people.
3. Access new technologies and educational resources.
4. Predict critical situations, and learn the necessary reactions and first aid methods.
5. Read older people's self-care instructions and, according to their abilities and needs, teach them how to follow the instructions.
6. Learn the psychological characteristics, developmental tasks, and special needs of older people.
7. Learn the concepts of mental health, resilience, and well-being, and help older people improve their mental health.
8. Provide the necessary conditions for older people to increase physical activity, strengthen cognitive abilities, and learn new things.
9. Create enjoyable hobbies, recreation, and social communication opportunities for older people.
10. According to older people's abilities, entrust them with the responsibility of housework and caring for children and pets.
11. Organize your support programs based on the severity of their problems and the amount of support they need.
12. Regularly assess and reassess needs.
13. Let older people take control of their lives.

Box 3.22 Having Your Own Self-Care Plan as an Older Person's Caregiver

1. Prioritize self-care.
2. Set realistic goals and perspectives for caring for older people.
3. Be positive, and accept the things you cannot change.
4. Strengthen your resilience, stress management, and communication skills.
5. You are not alone; build a support system for all family members, friends, and loved ones.

3.24 Summary of the Chapter

Mental health is a state of mental well-being that enables people to cope with the stresses of life, realize their abilities, learn well and work well, and contribute to their community. Mental self-care includes purpose activities and practices to improve mental well-being, coping strategies, and resilience, and it directly affects psychological dimensions, such as emotions, thoughts, and relationships. Some of the important issues concerning the mental health of older people are coping with developmental tasks of aging, well-being, and resilience. The most developmental tasks of older people are the following:

- Adjusting to decreasing physical strength and health
- Adjusting to retirement and reduced income
- Adjusting to the death of a spouse or close friends
- Establishing an affiliation with one's age group
- Adapting to social roles in a flexible way
- Establishing satisfactory physical living arrangements

Well-being is a broad concept that refers to the overall health, happiness, and life satisfaction, and it encompasses physical, mental, and social aspects. It is feeling good about oneself, one's relationships, and one's environment and thriving and functioning well in various areas of life; it encompasses eight main components, such as physical, emotional, intellectual, social, environmental, spiritual, occupational, and financial well-being. Learning life skills and some techniques can significantly help improve the emotional and psychological well-being of older people:

- Emotional regulation techniques
- Stress management techniques
- Adaptive coping strategies
- Positive thinking techniques
- Effective communication skills
- Finding the meaning of life
- Creating joy and happiness

Depression, anxiety, dementia, and neuropsychological disorders are common in older people, and early diagnosis and treatment of neuropsychological disorders are very important, as they address all the physical and psychological sides of health.

In general, mental self-care includes a set of targeted and learnable activities by strengthening various areas of well-being, coping skills, and resilience and managing neuropsychological problems in older people. The following general activities are recommended.

- Regularly visit the doctor and get mental health screening done.
- Follow your prescribed medical and nonmedical treatments.
- Complete your treatment process and follow-up visits.
- Maintain a balanced diet, and have healthy sleep.
- Plan your regular physical activities, sports training, and personal duties.
- Develop your emotional intelligence and stress management.
- Be optimistic, and keep negative thoughts away.
- Learn new skills, hobbies, or games, and engage yourself in mental stimulation.
- Learn life skills and coping strategies.
- Increase your social connections with your family, friends, neighbors, and peer groups.
- Participate in community or volunteer programs.
- Create a new purpose and meaning for your life.

3.25 Summary of Research Studies

Various studies have generally shown the effects of self-care training programs on the physical and psychological health of older people, a few examples of which we have provided here.

Gonzalez and Carman (2023) conducted a study titled "Self-care interventions of community-dwelling older adults: a systematic review and meta-analysis," with the aim of understanding and analyzing the efficacy of interventions in the physical and psychological self-care practices of healthy, community-dwelling older people. This systematic review shows that self-care interventions focus on physical health-related variables but not on psychological variables, and they significantly improve physical health-related variables, such as care visits, hospital admissions, medication, and gait speed.

Riegel et al. (2024) conducted a study titled "Does self-care improve coping or does coping improve self-care? A structural equation modeling study" to compare two models to determine whether self-care improves coping or coping improves self-care. The results show that the self-care model was the strongest. It decreases stress, promotes coping, and improves mental health. Also, promoting self-care may be more effective in improving mental health than interventions aimed at improving coping.

Esfahani et al. (2020) conducted a study titled "The Effectiveness of Behavioral Activation Intervention on Increasing Self-Care Behaviors and Life Expectancy in the Elderly", and it was aimed at investigating the effectiveness of behavioral activation intervention in increasing self-care behaviors and life expectancy. According to the findings of the study, behavioral activation intervention can be considered as one of the effective psychological interventions in increasing self-care behaviors and life expectancy in older people.

Mu et al. (2022) conducted a study titled "Association between self-care disability and depressive symptoms among middle-aged and elderly Chinese people." According to the results of the study, self-care disability is a risk factor for depressive symptoms among middle-aged and older Chinese people. A positive correlation between the number of self-care disabilities and the risk of depressive symptoms was found.

Miletic et al. (2021) conducted a study titled "Depression in Elderly with Different Comorbidities - Just a Small Problem or Something More?" and the aim of this study was to determine the incidence of depressive symptoms in patients hospitalized in the geriatric ward. The results obtained confirm the high incidence of depressive symptoms in patients hospitalized in the geriatric ward. Depression is not a normal part of aging and must be considered as a serious medical problem.

Maier et al. (2021) conducted a study titled "Risk factors and protective factors of depression in older people 65+. A systematic review." The results showed that chronic diseases and difficulty initiating sleep homogeneously increased the risk of depression, and findings hinted at a protective quality of physical activity.

The results of numerous studies have shown the effect of regular exercise, physical activity, dancing, walking, playing music, and pets on improving physical and mental health and cognitive function and reducing anxiety and depression in older people (Kazeminia et al. 2020; Nuzum et al. 2020; Huang et al. 2023; Wilson et al. 2019 and Giansanti et al. 2022).

3.26 Critical Thinking (Scenario Based)

3.26.1 Case Scenario: 1

- Sarah is a 71-year-old single woman who has recently retired, despite her inner desires. She has a PhD in economics and was a prominent executive in a large financial institution. She was diagnosed with breast cancer 10 years ago but has received successful treatment and is now free of physical illness. She lives alone in her large house in the suburbs and has few close friends or relatives. Since retiring, she has had trouble sleeping, has lost her appetite, and has a low energy level, and doctors have diagnosed a depressive disorder.

1. What do you think is Sarah's main problem?
2. Which factors would you consider in formulating a self-care plan for Sarah (based on the information provided or the need to obtain more information)?
3. Why does Sarah need to receive a self-care plan?
4. What are the primary and secondary goals of Sarah's self-care plan?
5. What are your suggestions for managing Sarah's mental health?
6. What activities would you suggest to reduce Sarah's depression?

3.26.2 Case Scenario: 2

- Jack is an 84-year-old man who lives with his 75-year-old wife, Rose, in a small apartment in the city center. They have four children and six grandchildren, two of them live nearby, and the entire family gathers for celebrations and occasions. Jack suffered a stroke 2 months ago and has just returned home after 45 days. He currently has speech problems, amnesia, and the inability to remember the names of people and places or perform simple tasks, such as turning off the lights when leaving the room or closing the door. Rose is the main caregiver for Jack, although she has a history of anxiety and digestive problems and worries a lot about taking care of her husband at home.

1. What is the main problem?
2. Which factors would you consider in formulating a self-care plan in this case (based on the information provided or the need to obtain more information)?
3. What are the primary and secondary goals in this case?
4. What are your suggestions for managing Jack and Rose's mental health?
5. What activities would you suggest to improve Jack's cognitive abilities?
6. What activities would you suggest to improve Rose's resilience?
7. What strategies can be implemented to empower all family members to take an active role in Jack and Rose's self-care plans?

Bibliography

Bandyopadhyay, G. (2018). Determinants of psychological well-being and its impact on mental health. In K. L. Banik (Ed.), Issues on health and healthcare in India: Focus on the North Eastern Region (pp. 53–95). Springer. https://doi.org/10.1007/978-981-10-6104-2_5

Brown Wilson C, Arendt L, Nguyen M, Scott TL, Neville CC, Pachana NA. Nonpharmacological interventions for anxiety and dementia in nursing homes: a systematic review. Gerontologist. 2019;59(6):e731–42.

Giansanti D, Siotto M, Parisi L, Aprile I. Pet presence can reduce anxiety in the older people: the Italian experience during COVID-19 lockdown assessed by an electronic survey. Int J Environ Res Public Health. 2022;19(10):6135.

González-González E, Requena C. Self-care interventions of community-dwelling older adults: a systematic review and meta-analysis. Front Public Health. 2023;11:1254172.

Havighurst RJ. (2018). Successful aging. In Process of aging (pp. 299–320). Routledge, Abingdon, UK.

Huang CS, Yan YJ, Luo YT, Lin R, Li H. Effects of dance therapy on cognitive and mental health in adults aged 55 years and older with mild cognitive impairment: a systematic review and meta-analysis. BMC Geriatr. 2023;23(1):695.

Kazeminia M, Salari N, Vaisi-Raygani A, Jalali R, Abdi A, Mohammadi M, Daneshkhah A, Hosseinian-Far M, Shohaimi S. The effect of exercise on anxiety in the older people worldwide: a systematic review and meta-analysis. Health Qual Life Outcomes. 2020;18(1):363.

Maier A, Riedel-Heller SG, Pabst A, Luppa M. Risk factors and protective factors of depression in older people 65+. A systematic review. PLoS One. 2021;16(5):e0251326.

Miletic B, Lekic A, Courteney U. Depression in older people with different comorbidities - just a small problem or something more. Psychiatr Danub. 2021;33(Suppl 4):471–4.

Ministry of Health and Medical Education. (2022). Active and healthy aging: Mental health in older people [Persian]. Tehran: Andishe Mandegar

Motamadi, A. (2020). Psychology of aging [Persian]. Tehran: The Organization for Researching and Composing University Textbooks in the Humanities

Mu TY, Xu RX, Xu JY, Dong D, Zhou ZN, Dai JN, Shen CZ. Association between self-care disability and depressive symptoms among middle-aged and older people Chinese people. PLoS One. 2022;17(4):e0266950.

Naji Esfahani F, Seirafi M, Kraskian Mujembari A. The effectiveness of behavioral activation intervention on increasing self-care behaviors and life expectancy in the older people. Aging Psychol. 2020;6(2):93–105.

Nuzum H, Stickel A, Corona M, Zeller M, Melrose RJ, Wilkins SS. Potential benefits of physical activity in MCI and dementia. Behav Neurol. 2020;2020:7807856.

Riegel B, Barbaranelli C, Stawnychy MA, Matus A, Hirschman KB. Does self-care improve coping or does coping improve self-care? A structural equation modeling study. Appl Nurs Res. 2024;78:151810.

Sisto A, Vicinanza F, Campanozzi LL, Ricci G, Tartaglini D, Tambone V. Towards a transversal definition of psychological resilience: a literature review. Medicina (Kaunas). 2019;55(11):745.

Stoewen DL. Dimensions of wellness: change your habits, change your life. Can Vet J. 2017;58(8):861–2.

Ungvari Z, Fazekas-Pongor V, Csiszar A, Kunutsor SK. The multifaceted benefits of walking for healthy aging: from Blue Zones to molecular mechanisms. GeroScience. 2023;45(6):3211–39.

World Health Organization. World mental health report: transforming mental health for all. World Health Organization; 2022.

Social Self-Care in Older People

4

Fatemeh Bahramnezhad and Banafsheh Ghorbani

In the end, the learner should be able to:

- Explain the definition and importance of social self-care
- Provide strategies for promoting social self-care
- Develop practical plans for social self-care
- Identify challenges to social self-care

4.1 Healthy Aging and Social Self-Care

4.1.1 The Foundations of Healthy Aging and Its Relationship with Social Self-Care

Longer lifespans can be considered a success for humanity. With this understanding, public policies have emphasized the positive meaning of aging and the contribution that older people can make with their knowledge, skills, and experiences in everyday life and work in society. For this positive sense of aging, different terms are used: successful aging, active aging, and, more recently, the resumption of the term healthy aging, proposed by the World Health Organization (WHO). The concept of an aging population is a relatively new problem from a historical point of view. An aging global population is the most important medical and social demographic problem worldwide. Older adults desire to stay healthy and active to engage fully in life. However, natural declines in biological, physiological, and cognitive systems due to aging may hinder their complete sociocultural and intellectual participation.

The number and proportion of people aged 60 and over are increasing. In 2019, the number of people aged 60 and over was 1 billion. This figure is expected to grow to 1.4 billion by 2030 and 2.1 billion by 2050.

This increase is occurring at an unprecedented rate and will accelerate in the coming decades, particularly in developing countries. Prioritizing healthy aging is essential not only in high-income countries today but also in low-income countries that are projected to have aging populations shortly.

According to the literature review, healthy aging is the process of maximizing opportunities for physical, social, and mental well-being that allows older people to participate actively in society without discrimination and to live independent and quality lives. In this regard, WHO defines healthy aging as "the process of developing and maintaining functional capacity that allows well-being into old age." Functional capacity, in turn, can be understood as a combi-

F. Bahramnezhad (✉)
Tehran University of Medical Sciences, Tehran, Iran
e-mail: bahramnezhad@tums.ac.ir

B. Ghorbani
University of Social Welfare and Rehabilitation Sciences, Tehran, Iran

F. Bahramnezhad (ed.), *Self-Care in the Elderly*, https://doi.org/10.1007/978-981-96-9021-3_4

nation of the inherent capacity of the individual, relevant environmental characteristics, and the interactions between the individual and these characteristics. Intrinsic capacity is the expression of physical and mental abilities (including psychosocial). Environmental characteristics are the context of life, including social relationships. Well-being is unique and permeated with subjective aspirations, including feelings of satisfaction, fulfillment, and happiness.

According to the WHO conceptual framework, there are four essential prerequisites for healthy aging:

(i) Changing our perspective on older people and aging,
(ii) Developing age-appropriate environments,
(iii) Reforming health systems to meet the needs of older people, and
(iv) Implementing long-term care systems.

These four conditions not only enhance the quality of life of older people but also provide benefits to society. In particular, changing our perspective on aging allows us to gain deeper insight into the abilities and experiences of older people and to utilize their skills in social, cultural, and economic contexts.

These four conditions enhance not just the quality of life for seniors but also provide advantages to society. Specifically, altering our perspective on aging allows us to gain a deeper insight into the abilities and experiences of older people and to leverage their skills in social, cultural, and economic areas.

Overcoming negative stereotypes about aging is also important. Ageism refers to the discrimination or bias against individuals due to their age, which is commonly found in society. It frequently results in negative stereotypes regarding aging and obstructs the happiness, social interactions, and overall well-being of older people.

A widespread misconception is that older individuals lose interest in the world beyond their surroundings as they get older. Indeed, older individuals often possess extensive life experience and have a strong desire to discover the surrounding world. A lot of them take pleasure in staying informed about current events, engaging in social events, and exploring new pastimes. An additional negative stereotype is that "older individuals do not desire or require intimate connections." Human relationships are a fundamental need throughout life and tend to gain significance as we grow older; older people individuals, like others, cherish close bonds with family and friends. These connections offer emotional backing, friendship, and a feeling of inclusion. Social isolation and loneliness can adversely affect both mental and physical health, making it crucial to develop meaningful connections for the well-being of older adults.

Some believe that as individuals grow older, they become entrenched in their habits and no longer require education or the pursuit of their interests, among other things. The belief that older individuals are more prone to encountering barriers is a stereotype that does not hold for everyone. Age does not imply inflexibility. Numerous seniors welcome change, acquire new skills, adopt new technologies, and pursue various interests. Their ability to adapt is commendable, as it enables them to keep growing and evolving.

Another notion that society has embraced is that "mental and physical transformations in old age are unavoidable." Although the aging process may cause physical and mental changes, this should not be a reason to hold back. Due to improvements in healthcare systems and a focus on healthy lifestyles, numerous older people are preserving their mental skills and physical health. Consistent physical activity, a nutritious diet, cognitive engagement, and proactive health practices can aid in minimizing the difficulties related to aging.

It is stated by some that "depression in older individuals is typical and expected."

Depression is not an inevitable aspect of growing older and must always be taken seriously. While mental health issues can impact individuals of all ages, it is essential to recognize that depression is a manageable condition. Older people showing signs of depression ought to pursue professional assistance and support. Tackling mental health issues is crucial for preserving a high quality of life in later life.

Age-friendly environments involve creating conditions that make older individuals feel safer and more at ease. The World Health Organization (WHO) released guidelines for creating age-friendly cities, highlighting multiple physical and social aspects of the community that are crucial for encouraging active aging: "outdoor spaces and structures," "transportation," "accommodation," "social involvement," "respect and societal acceptance," "citizen engagement," "communication and information," and "community assistance and health services."

Furthermore, the guidelines emphasize the significance of crafting public areas and services that offer enjoyable experiences for older people individuals. Locations like parks, communal areas, and cultural hubs can serve as venues for exercise and social engagement. These environments not only enhance quality of life but can also reinforce older individuals' sense of belonging to the community.

Transport is likewise a crucial element in establishing environments suitable for different ages. Offering secure and convenient transportation choices for seniors enables them to move from one location to another effortlessly and engage in social and cultural activities.

In terms of modification of health systems to cater to the requirements of older adults, rather than trying to manage a set of diseases and treat specific symptoms in a disjointed manner, the World Report on Ageing and Health suggests prioritizing interventions that optimize the physical and mental capacities of older people throughout their lives. This in turn requires changes in the way health and social services are organized; there needs to be greater integration within the health system and between health and social care services. As older adults age, health problems become more chronic and complex, and multiple chronic diseases become standard. Physical, sensory, and cognitive disabilities are more common, and older adults may experience complex health problems such as frailty, urinary incontinence, and an increased risk of falls. If not properly addressed through strong care coordination, these conditions can lead to polypharmacy, hospitalization, and death. Delivering care for older adults with multiple health problems is relatively complex. However, many existing health systems manage health issues in a disjointed and fragmented manner, with a lack of coordination between care providers and settings and in the timing of care provided.

Despite suffering from more health problems than younger adults, older adults use health services less frequently. Issues such as the cost of visits, lack of transport or inability to pay for transport, lack of accessible toilets, long queues, physical barriers to access, and communication barriers due to inadequate information provision for people with hearing or visual impairments affect older people. Access to health and medical services. Therefore, multi-sectoral measures that involve coordination between the health system, the transport sector, and social care are needed. Addressing these needs greatly facilitates social self-care. By overcoming these challenges, older people can interact more effectively with others, overcome loneliness and isolation, and experience happier lives.

Historically, families primarily took on the duty of caring for their parents and older relatives. Yet, currently, because of the one-child policy, swift urbanization, and heightened labor mobility, families are becoming smaller and more scattered, while multigenerational households are declining, leading to greater strain in caring for relatives.

The physical, mental, and financial difficulties encountered by family caregivers have attracted heightened attention from researchers, the public, and policymakers, leading to a shift in older people's care to long-term care settings. Providing services in these centers is highly important as it directly affects the physical, mental, and social health of older people individuals.

In this context, engaging social networks and social supports can significantly contribute to establishing an appropriate environment for older people's care and alleviating stress on families. The importance of policymakers' roles is also significant in this context. Offering financial aid to families caring for older people or to long-term care facilities will enhance the quality of life for seniors and support their social self-care.

Social support plays a crucial role in promoting healthy aging. Older people require a sense of belonging in society and chances to engage. This assistance can come from family, friends, and community organizations. Programs that link older adults and enable them to share their experiences can also promote a sense of belonging and fulfillment in their lives. These factors contribute to social self-care in older people, and the reciprocal effect of healthy aging and social self-care in older people is well-known. In general, healthy aging is a shared duty that necessitates teamwork among the government, nonprofit entities, and society as a whole. By prioritizing health, education, and initiatives to enhance social connections, we can create a community where older people not only live but also participate in social activities and enjoy a fulfilling life.

4.2 Understanding Social Self-Care

Social health is another critical component of human health and defines the ability of an individual to establish healthy and effective relationships with individuals, have social interactions, and belong to society. In older adults, this health component can play a major role in preventing depression, anxiety, loss of intellectual functions, etc.

Various studies have also identified that a considerable correlation between age and social health exists whereby increasing age has been observed to be correlated with decreasing social health. The more active the old are socially, the more incentives they possess and the ability to work for their welfare. Lonely old individuals might be deprived of motivation toward self-maintenance as well as achieving their physical, mental, and social deterioration at an earlier stage in life.

On this, social self-care is behaviors that get shaped to construct and strengthen relationships with other individuals. Literature review indicates that such care is aimed at social aspects and feelings of belongingness, which can prove very helpful in avoiding isolation and boosting self-esteem and happiness.

The worth of social self-care is to have positive social relationships by creating meaningful connections and forming a social identity. However, social self-care is not just passively enjoying others' presence. It also requires the active engagement of the individual with others. Passive communication refers to when the individual himself is around in a group but is not participating in social interaction, or their relations are casual and are devoid of emotional and intellectual sharing. Such a type of communication, despite looks, cannot meet the social and emotional needs of older adults and may even enhance the feeling of loneliness. In the elderly, it is necessary to remove passive communication and replace it with intentional, meaningful, and two-way communication; i.e., dialogue in which there is a feeling of being heard, respect for one another, and exchange of experiences. Such communication improves self-esteem, improves a sense of belonging, reduces loneliness, and improves mental well-being. Therefore, in social self-care, quality of communication is more important than being in a group.

For this reason, social self-care has been categorized as acts that are cultivated in order to promote and consolidate relationships with other people. When reviewing the literature, it shows that social care focuses on integration and sociality, which are very useful in preventing isolation and improving self-esteem and welfare.

The importance of social self-care is through positive social relationships by developing meaningful relationships and creating a social identity. However, social self-care does not necessarily mean simply enjoying other people's presence. It also requires the active involvement of the individual with others. Passive communication is where the individual is physically present in a group but fails to participate actively in social interaction or whose relationships are superficial and devoid of emotional and intellectual exchange. Such communication, as may seem to appear, cannot provide the elderly with their social and emotional needs and could even exacerbate feelings of loneliness. For older persons, passive communication must be eliminated and replaced by purposeful, meaningful, and two-way communication; i.e., conversations in which there is a feeling of being heard, respect for one another, and sharing. Such communication raises self-esteem, improves a sense of belonging, reduces loneliness, and improves mental well-being. In social self-care, therefore, quality of communication is more important than belonging to a group.

Some examples of these activities include interacting socially with family and friends, joining a group of people, or joining a cause such as volunteering. This care not only strengthens emotional and supportive bonds but also strengthens a sense of belonging.

Social support has been referred to as another method of social self-care, and they are presented as a complementary concept and play an essential role in the health of elderly people. Social support has been defined as what one receives from family, friends, neighbors, or social institutions in terms of assistance and provided resources. The elderly, with the ability of social self-care, can benefit more from existing social supports and even expand their supportive network.

Evidence has shown that social relations are one of the determinants of maintaining the self-care of the elderly.

When the elderly's social network comprises individuals who model, expect, and support the elderly in caring for themselves, there are increased chances of maintaining proper self-care activities.

These companions can also encourage the elderly to participate in social activities, interact with others, and express their feelings.

However, it can be observed that one of the requests of elderly people is the difficulty in maintaining themselves within their homes.

Most people would like to remain at home when they grow older, maintain their independence for as long as possible, and only seek assistance from family members or friends whenever the need arises. Living in their homes when older is known as "aging in place." However, some older adults, along with their families, feel concerned about security, transportation, or other routine practices. Living at home when older represents careful planning and prudence.

As a result, an in-depth program for social self-care in homebound elderly people is necessary, as will be explained in the subsequent pages.

4.3 Building and Maintaining Healthy Relationships in Older People

Healthy social relationships as a self-care practice must be fostered and sustained to increase the quality of life among elderly people and become more important as we age. Social contact is thought to increase the health of older people, and social isolation is a predictor of higher mortality.

Involvement in social relations greatly affects the physical and mental health of older persons. The lack of such relationships is associated with cardiovascular disease, hypertension, cancer, and slow recovery. Negative social relationships increase inflammation and immune dysfunctions, leading to poor health outcomes and increased risks of death. The quality of the relationships also matters; high-quality ones reduce stress levels, enhance the sense of belongingness, and improve quality of life and happiness, hardness, cognitive capacity, mental well-being, and overall physical health.

Larger social networks also go with improved mood, mental health, and the ability to cope with life's pressures. In contrast, social isolation can lead to depression, anxiety, and a poor quality of life.

Hence, teaching the elderly to plan and providing social programs that facilitate social relationships—such as those formed in parks, cinemas, and organized events—are particular concerns that must be taken into consideration by policymakers.

The following are some things that help social self-care in older people:

4.3.1 Stay Socially Connected

Research indicates that social isolation and loneliness substantially impact the physiological and psychological functioning of senior citizens. For example, aging individuals face higher risks of heart disease, obesity, cardiac arrest and strokes, Alzheimer's, and psychological disorders such as stress, anxiety, depression, and related conditions. Furthermore, physiological effects such as heightened inflammatory responses and weakened immune system function are also among the consequences of social isolation. Conversely, studies have demonstrated that sustaining social engagement offers numerous health benefits for senior citizens. Enhancing the body's immune response, resulting in reduced disease occurrence, strengthening emotional support and self-esteem, and ultimately elevating quality of life are among the positive effects of older people individuals' participation in social interactions. A key message and a piece of advice to older people is that they should make a habit of connecting with family and friends. This contact could be by means of physical contact, phone calls, video calls, etc. Membership in clubs like a book club, gardening and fitness club, and lunch club and in groups such as arts and crafts, painting, pottery, knitting, drawing, and photography helps lessen isolation and loneliness in seniors. By participating in these activities, seniors foster challenging of mind, physical strength, and emotional vigor. Groups and clubs are very enriching for seniors. Participating in these groups improves social self-care by providing social connections, sharing experiences, supporting each other, learning new skills, and increasing knowledge for seniors.

4.3.2 Wellness and Sports Clubs

As knowledge and medical studies advance and the population ages, the importance of exercise for all age groups, especially older people, is increasingly felt. As our awareness of aging and health and their relationship to exercise has increased, guidelines in this area have also changed. Between the 1970s and 1980s, it was thought that high-intensity exercise that put a lot of strain on the heart and lungs was appropriate. Since 1990, moderate-intensity aerobic exercise has been increasingly recommended. Physical activity and social participation are both critical components of healthy aging. However, many older adults are less physically active than adults younger than 65 years. Therefore, it is important to understand how physical activity promotes social self-care. Studies have shown that community-based interventions targeting older adults can increase their physical activity levels and are associated with significant benefits. Regular exercise has many benefits and releases endorphins. Improving mood and reducing stress, anxiety, and depression in older people are among the outcomes of exercise in this sensitive group. Older people may experience age-related challenges due to social withdrawal and loneliness, which regular group exercise helps to overcome. Engaging in physical activity with a peer group provides opportunities for conversation and social interaction, which are vital for combating loneliness and isolation. Participating in regular group exercise strengthens friendships and improves social connections. Also, developing communication skills is associated with social self-care through engaging in physical activity. Increased communication skills lead to better self-esteem, stronger relationships, and a greater sense of belonging. Group social activities for older people are also associated with cognitive benefits and improved performance in this area. Engaging in physical activity among older people is associated with a reduced risk of dementia. Participation in senior clubs has a positive impact on the functional status, quality of life, and physical activity levels of older adults. Studies have also shown that older adults who regularly participate in soccer clubs have lower body mass index, higher muscular endurance, and higher total body endurance, which have a positive impact on their physical health. This is because sports clubs provide an easy way for older adults to maintain social relationships, participate in physical activity, and feel fulfilled and happy. Older adults in sports clubs tend to stay active for longer and enjoy a higher quality of life and physical performance. In addition, they have lower body fat percentage and body mass index than those who do not participate. Given that physical activity levels decline with age, sports club membership can increase physical activity in older adults. Twenty to thirty minutes of daily exercise can improve physical performance in older men and women.

4.3.3 Walking Clubs

According to the WHO, one way to reduce healthcare costs and improve health is to encourage older people to be physically active. Group walking is a potentially attractive physical activity intervention that has particular potential to engage people who are interested in the outdoors, either for leisure or as a health intervention, and is cost-effective in increasing physical activity. Furthermore, the dynamism and social cohesion of walking groups have supportive effects on older people, encouraging and maintaining adherence and positive attitudes toward physical activity, companionship, and shared health experiences. If interventions are tailored to the needs of older people and target those who are inactive or more motivated to change, they will be encouraged to walk more. Health professionals and policymakers can also design walking routes that are helpful for older people. For example, access to drinking water, rest areas, and a place to sit, as well as planning a conversation with a specific theme, can provide more motivation for seniors to participate in group walks. Therefore, paying attention to this issue can help seniors' social self-care and a more active lifestyle.

4.3.4 Dancing Clubs

When engaging in physical activity, seniors can maintain an active level of physical, cognitive, social, and psychological functioning. Among the available forms of physical exercise, dance is popular among this population because it provides an environment of relaxation and fun where seniors can identify with people with similar cultural characteristics and interact socially with others, as well as express their emotions and relive life. Dancing also helps seniors maintain their balance because it requires coordination of movements. Every movement and rhythm of dancing can remind seniors of sweet memories. Improving coordination and balance of the body, the connection between the mind, and maintaining activity can reduce the risk of falls and physical injuries, which in turn increases the overall health of seniors. In addition, dance, as a group activity, provides an environment where seniors can distance themselves from loneliness and social isolation. Therefore, dancing can be beneficial for the quality of life of these people, as it eliminates many problems such as shyness, anxiety, and depression, and thus contributes to social self-care and a better quality of life. Therefore, professionals working with older people should seek to develop facilities or encourage greater participation by older people and consider ballroom dancing sessions as a way to promote physical and mental health and improve social self-care for older people. On the other hand, by providing suitable space and the necessary equipment for holding these sessions, it is possible to create more attraction for older people so that they are more motivated to participate in these sessions.

4.3.5 Swimming Club

Swimming can be an excellent form of exercise for older individuals due to its minimal injury risk. These activities can involve all the muscle groups in the body and serve as a thorough workout. In addition to the physical benefits, swimming facilitates social interaction and allows people to be part of a group. Evidence has shown that swimming lessons create a friendly environment of play and communication, in addition to providing swimmers with a sense of participation and also helping them to understand and accept their fellow human beings.

4.3.6 Golf Club

The main benefit of golf lies in its social aspect. Golf courses create a pleasant atmosphere that promotes interaction and networking among golfers. Golf is a beneficial leisure pursuit that provides physical, mental, and social advantages for older adults. Studies indicate that golf is a preferred pastime for seniors. This social interaction increases happiness, health, and a sense of belonging while reducing stress in older adults by engaging in activity in a pleasant environment. In addition, studies show that golf can enhance quality of life by increasing muscle strength, improving balance, and improving aerobic fitness (similar to weight training or yoga), along with promoting social self-care.

4.3.7 Pilates and Yoga Classes

Yoga and Pilates have gained notable popularity as exercise methods across various generations, including seniors. Both forms of exercise effectively enhance flexibility, strength, balance, posture awareness, mental well-being, breathing, and overall quality of life, while also fostering social connections. Yoga sessions are typically conducted in groups, offering seniors a special chance to gather and engage socially. Yoga and Pilates offer numerous advantages for older adults. They can enhance physical power and stability and extend the range of motion and flexibility. Certain seniors steer clear of physical activity and social engagement because of issues like osteoarthritis, limited range of motion for joints, and muscle discomfort. Nonetheless, doctors suggest yoga and Pilates as group activities that alleviate the symptoms of these conditions and enhance physical activity in older adults. The positions and stances in yoga and Pilates are excellent methods for helping seniors maintain balance. Alongside the previously mentioned benefits, these exercises enhance mood, memory, focus, and self-worth and diminish feelings of anxiety and depression, which ultimately results in a better quality of life and social self-care for older adults.

4.3.8 Tai Chi Exercise

Tai chi, an ancient Chinese martial art and healing art, combines martial art movements with chi (the circulation of vital energy), breathing, and stretching techniques. It offers many physiological and psychological benefits for older adults and improves the quality of life in their populations. A growing body of evidence suggests that tai chi improves balance, aerobic capacity, muscle strength, and flexibility and can relieve psychological problems such as depression, anxiety, stress, and mood disorders. In addition, this activity can provide a social opportunity where older adults can interact with each other and overcome feelings of loneliness and isolation, thus contributing to older adults' self-care.

4.4 Household Chores

These are the everyday activities individuals perform to keep their homes in order. Research indicates that engaging in housework correlates with favorable health outcomes, autonomy, well-being, social interaction, and personal self-care. As older adults have dedicated their lives to maintaining and managing their homes, they might find that as they age, they can no longer handle the same tasks as before, leading to feelings of incompetence and decreased self-esteem. Thus, it is important for children and caregivers of seniors to allocate tasks like dusting and vacuuming, assisting with kitchen duties, walking the dog, gardening, etc., which will provide older people with a sense of worth and increased productivity. This approach decreases isolation and loneliness among older people, leading to increased interaction with their surroundings and the community.

4.4.1 Technology and Aging: A Bridge to Social Self-Care

Technology is all around us, from the mobile phones that many of us have to the TVs we view, as well as how we search for details about eateries or holiday spots. Senior individuals are not excluded. They are progressively integrating different forms of technology into their daily routines.

The potential of technology to address the challenges of an aging population has been studied since the 1980s, and a wide range of major research topics has emerged, from the understanding, acceptance, and usability of technologies to the challenge of ensuring that older people are not technology-dependent. Given the positive impact of technology on all aspects of life and despite the limited current evidence on the effects of technology on the aging population, many studies have optimistically stated that technology can be an effective tool to improve the quality of life of older people. However, the concept of the nature and role of technology in aging is unclear. Studies have shown that the majority of the older people population prefers to age in their own homes. Aging in place, which can be defined as "living in the community, with a level of independence, rather than in residential care," is often seen by policymakers as a way to avoid the costly option of institutional care and as a means to address the expected shortage of healthcare professionals, and technology is often seen as a means to support aging in place. There are various types of technology specifically designed to support aging in place, and this technology is used in different parts of older people's lives. For example, assistive technologies are used in the homes of older people. These technologies create an environment in which devices are connected to home automation and enable communication with the outside world.

Technologies such as the Internet of Things (IoT), ambient/active assisted living (AAL) robots, and other artificial intelligence (AI) technologies have shown great potential to enhance independent living, improve mental and physical health, and enhance quality of life. At the same time, they can also reduce caregiver burden, which can lead to more targeted and better quality care. Also emergency assistance systems, vital signs monitoring, and fall detection systems. These technologies are sometimes referred to as smart home technology. A smart home is a comprehensive concept that refers to a complete system aimed at achieving health, safety, and well-being, usually with the possibility of remote monitoring of the individual's health status. Among the interventions intended to maintain and improve the active life of older adults as well as their health, interventions that involve e-health have received much attention due to their great potential to empower and inform older adults. These interactive interventions, such as telemedicine, electronic health records, virtual interventions, and personal health monitoring, can educate, engage, and empower older adults and are used to collect and share data through digital devices for early diagnosis and self-management of disease and self-care. However, despite playing an important role in successful interventions, the adoption of these technologies has been limited. One of the key barriers to wider adoption is that the process is based on preconceptions of technicians, or at best, geriatricians, about the needs of older adults, without taking into account the user's perspectives and preferences or their real-world limitations. These inconsistencies can hinder meaningful adoption and sustainable use and create the risk that the priority needs of end users are not met. By implementing these interventions, not only will their quality of life improve, but they will also be able to easily access their medical records, track their health status, and even communicate with health professionals. This creates a sense of independence, strengthens self-confidence and awareness of health conditions, creates greater security, and reduces stress and anxiety caused by health problems in older people. It will also serve as a tool for early identification of health problems. As a result, this process not only helps to improve their physical condition but also instills a culture of self-care and responsibility for health in them. Also, using technology as a bridge between older people and other people encourages them to interact with the world around them and ultimately contributes greatly to the social self-care dimension of older people. Also, studies have shown that the use of technological devices has a greater social benefit for older people and contributes significantly to the social self-care of older people rather than its technical dimension.

Studies have shown that technology adoption rates among older people are lower than those of younger people, as many technologies are not relevant to older people and are not adequately supported. Providing access and support to use technology, especially in the early weeks of its deployment, may be the most important step that needs to be taken to facilitate technology adoption. A promising way to address this issue is to integrate users into the innovation process following a participatory approach. Studies suggest that participatory design should follow a comprehensive strategy that starts with user needs and ends with evaluation to determine the effectiveness of the technology. Partnerships between researchers, designers, developers, and older people are also crucial throughout the innovation process, and attention to the diversity of the older people population (different cultural groups, geographical logic, attention to accessibility and technological literacy, etc.) is also required. This is how older people are encouraged to use technology and can benefit from its benefits, including the social dimension.

4.4.2 Game Club

Mathes (1978) stated that people have a set of basic needs that can be satisfied to some extent by participating in leisure activities. Playing may seem like a way to fill time or relax, but when playing, people can easily think, feel, and do something and be creative and innovative without fear of failure. When playing, seniors can gain new information and change their perspective on the world around them. Also, seniors have a lot of freedom of action when playing because they are not afraid of their independence being compromised or challenged, and they play with their peers free from prejudice or criticism. Games create a sense of excitement, enjoyment, focus, and freedom to experiment, explore, create, imagine, and bridge the gap between reality and dream. Seniors tend to participate in recreational activities that involve social interaction and are done in groups.

When a person plays in a group, it can increase the individual's connection with others, thereby increasing social connections and reducing feelings of loneliness. Many studies have been conducted on games in older people that have mentioned the positive results of games. For example, older people remember fun as a pleasant memory and define it as a release from commitment and a coping mechanism. Also, social participation in leisure and outdoor recreational activities is effective in the life satisfaction of older people. Studies show that the points and achievements older people earn while playing can be a good alternative to increasing self-confidence or job satisfaction. Also, preventing boredom, improving mental health, keeping the brain active, strengthening memory and concentration, cultivating imagination and creativity, relieving stress, improving mood, and encouraging socialization and bonding are other benefits of games for older people. Studies also suggest that to increase life satisfaction by involving seniors in fun activities, it is better to describe their interests, values, and culture before offering games and any fun activity to facilitate their motivation to participate. Studies also suggest that by using meaningful play as a tool to assess cognitive function, older adults can be assessed more in a natural context, without the additional effort of conducting tedious tests.

Based on studies, various games have been designed for older people that can help them with social self-care.

Puzzle Games (Puzzles, Ubongo, Cranium, Cluedo) are expected to stimulate the brain activity of older adults and promote the activation of their intellectual functioning, thereby delaying the development of dementia and providing more learning options for the education of older adults. Puzzle games are recommended for seniors in groups or pairs, and as a result, they increase interaction with the environment. *Board Games* (Chess and Checkers, Ticket to Ride, Dixit, Scrabble) and *Card Games* (Gin rummy, Old Maid, UNO, Solitaire) provide opportunities for lots of social interaction, which is vital for combating the feelings of loneliness and isolation common among seniors. Playing with friends or family strengthens relationships and builds bonds. Working with other team members to achieve a common goal increases trust and cooperation. *Dice Games* (liar's dice) have become popular among seniors today. The rules of the game are generally simple, allowing seniors to play without feeling harassed. Portable entertainment, stress reduction and relaxation, and group play are all benefits of dice games, which create a greater sense of belonging and lead seniors toward social self-care (58). Also, other types of games such as *Word Games* (Crossword puzzles, Hangman), *Number Games* (Sudoku, Battleships), *Memory Games* (Card Matching, Flag Game, The Tray Game, Pub Quiz), *Social Games* (Bingo, Name that Tune, Charades, Guess the Food), *Online Games* (Lumosity, Mahjong, Catan, Online Escape Rooms), and *Video Games* (Candy Crush, Civilization, Animal Crossing) that are recommended for older people are associated with increased social interaction and are recommended to be played with a group of older people or family members, which ultimately increases social self-care among older people.

4.4.3 Gamification for Older Adults

In recent years, we have seen an increase in the use of game-like elements and interactions in various non-gaming contexts. The use of gamification in older people is increasing as a new approach to improve the quality of life and increase their participation. These games, which are considered serious games, aim to transform daily activities into fun and engaging activities, help older people stay active, and familiarize themselves with new technologies, and thus increase their social interactions with other players such as family and friends. The use of gamification for older people is associated with many benefits. The increased motivation achieved by using game elements such as rewards and challenges makes older people more mobile. The use of applications that use game principles provides a platform for older people to communicate with each other, share their experiences, and improve their social connections. This reduces the feeling of isolation and loneliness in older people. Also, improving mental health, increasing motivation and morale of older people, and reducing stress are other benefits of using gamification for older people. Many older people may be afraid of using new technologies, which causes them to feel lonely and distance themselves from society. The goal of using this approach is to reduce this fear by performing simple yet attractive and purposeful tasks that are personalized based on their needs, making older people more active and their social interactions in line with technological advances.

The important point about using gamification is that because these games can be designed with a specific purpose and tailored to older people, they can play an important role in meeting the needs of older people. Another point is that to increase social self-care, gamification should be done in a group. Many gamified platforms strengthen social connections by allowing users to share achievements and compete with peers. This social aspect is very important for combating loneliness and improving the quality of life among older people.

4.4.4 From Words to Social Self-Care: Book Clubs

Book clubs are more than just study groups. They are dynamic communities where older adults can share insights and connect on a deeper intellectual level. Engaging with traditional literature and modern podcasts allows members to explore a wide range of topics and formats, from engaging storytelling to discussions of current events and specialized interests, thereby fostering friendships and reducing feelings of isolation. Studies have shown that participation in book clubs can improve cognitive abilities among older adults, potentially slowing cognitive decline. These discussions also encourage critical thinking and memory recall. These clubs include both older adults and younger participants, such as college students. Such settings have been shown to increase social interaction across generations while providing cognitive benefits through shared discussions, thereby fostering social self-care.

4.4.5 Volunteering in Support Groups

Living an active, disease-free life in old age can bring immense happiness. With aging recognized as a social issue, it is important to find ways to live a healthier, more active life as we age. Participating in volunteer work can increase a sense of purpose and social connectedness. Some studies have defined social connectedness as participation in various groups and organizations, including workplaces, churches, families, neighborhoods, and groups that engage in similar hobbies and volunteer activities. Volunteering allows seniors to interact with others while contributing to the community, which can improve mental health and well-being. Senior volunteer work increases quality years of life, reduces the risk of impairment in instrumental activities of daily living, improves cognitive decline, reduces symptoms of depression, and increases life satisfaction and well-being. Overall, seniors' participation in volunteer activities is effective in maintaining and improving their physical, mental, and social health. These activities are not only beneficial for seniors but also give them a sense of worth and are very important in social self-care.

Below are some volunteer activities that seniors can participate in:

4.4.5.1 Befriending Services

Befriending is a common type of initiative that is mainly implemented to build relationships and social contact with people experiencing loneliness and isolation in social and residential settings. These services are currently part of the social landscape in several countries, notably the UK, the United States, Canada, Australia, and Europe. Befriending is an internationally recognized low-cost way to increase social networks in older people and reduce their social isolation. Loneliness, which burdens both individuals and society, has risen globally. Befriending is described as "a connection among two or more individuals initiated, aided, and overseen by an organization that is expected to bring advantages to one or more of the involved parties." It is a "direct" form of formal, targeted intervention to reduce loneliness among older people. It is supported through socialization. Befriending can be carried out individually or in groups, over the phone or in person, at home or through "going out." Recent studies have pointed to the positive effects of befriending among older people, increasing empathy and social interactions.

4.4.5.2 Intergenerational Engagement

A major type of program involves intergenerational engagement, which often requires education, mentoring, and companionship. In this type of program, older adults usually share their experiences. The goal of this work is to provide meaningful intergenerational interaction and thus promote healthy aging in older adults. For example, visiting schools, kindergartens, and childcare settings, as well as reading books and stories to children and playing with them, is one of the volunteer activities of older adults. It allows older adults to connect with other people with a high enthusiasm for life and, in turn, increases social support for older adults and others. Examples of programs active in this field include Experience Corps® (EC) in the United States, a widely documented intergenerational training program and model. Also, the Research on Productivity through Intergenerational Empathy (REPRINTS) in Japan is an example of a program that is active in this field. In addition, there is an example of remote volunteering as part of Oasis, another nonprofit organization in the United States. One of Oasis's main goals is to promote healthier aging through intergenerational engagement. Also, to carry out this model of volunteer work, seniors are usually trained before the formal volunteering phase. Studies on these programs have shown that older people feel more meaningful and contribute to society. Improved quality of life and a sense of well-being were among the other benefits of this method. They also acknowledged that their social interactions had increased and they were better able to connect with the outside world, and the social dimension of self-care was more emphasized.

4.4.5.3 Support and Referral Hotline Services

The goal of these types of programs is to improve social interaction, psychological well-being, and volunteer skills (e.g., problem-solving) in volunteers to help service recipients. After training by professionals, volunteers provide counseling, referrals, and emotional support to clients regarding caregiving and family issues over the phone. According to these older volunteers, they reported feeling happier and empowered, having a sense of purpose, and improved communication skills while providing services. More than half also felt they were contributing to the community, improving their social interaction and relationships, and being able to understand their emotions and social self-care were other positive statements made by older volunteers. One example of a program that involves providing support and referral is the Phone Angel Program in the United States. In this program, Chinese American older volunteers work with fellow Chinese immigrants who are caring for a sick relative.

4.4.5.4 Home Visiting Services

Home visiting services, here, refer to structured social services in which volunteers visit older people living in the community who tend to be confined to their homes and socially isolated. Volunteer visitors in this program are accredited and accepted by the organizations that lead voluntary support groups. Both service recipients and visitors are usually older people. However, the program assumes that visitors are younger than the service recipients or, if older, are not housebound and active in the community. Volunteers regularly visit service recipients in their homes, engage in friendly conversations, and provide companionship. Studies conducted in this field showed that in this group, older people addressed challenges associated with aging (e.g., unfair treatment in society, how to adapt to their future aging), recognized strengths in the people they served, and developed appropriate social interaction between older people. The group reported that they learned from each other.

4.4.5.5 Dementia Care Services

Another volunteer program that seniors can participate in is dementia care services. In this volunteer program, which aims to promote activity participation in this group of seniors, seniors interact more with each other, and the senior volunteer actively facilitates the participation of people with dementia in appropriate group activities by creating a friendly and reassuring atmosphere and providing practical assistance to complete an activity. According to interviews conducted with senior volunteers in this group, it was concluded that the volunteers found their experience meaningful for themselves and the recipients of the services, enjoyed the teamwork, and gained more information about dementia and people with it. Overall, they experienced socio-emotional satisfaction from the interaction and connection they had with these people, their family members, and other volunteers of their age.

Other volunteer activities that seniors can participate in include volunteering in skill training classes, such as cooking, sewing, and gardening, and sharing their work experiences with others. Creating support groups for other seniors is another volunteer activity that can help each other with daily chores, shopping, or going to the doctor. Participating in environmental activities such as cleaning parks and recycling is also very useful. These activities give seniors a sense of pride, foster community interaction, and help them feel useful. They share valuable experiences gained over the years. Helping with food programs, such as cooking or distributing food to seniors in need through outreach programs, is especially valuable. Seniors can volunteer time in nursing homes and be active listeners or participate in senior group activities there. They can cooperate in libraries, museums, or cultural centers, where they can share their knowledge and experiences.

4.5 Empathy and Connection: Marriage as a Pillar of Social Self-Care to Combat Loneliness

Rising living standards, advances in medical care, and increased life expectancy have led to an increase in the older people population, and accordingly, studies focusing on older families have increased significantly in the past decade, driven by concerns about the capacity of families to care for their senior members and the adequacy of public pension systems to provide an adequate quality of life. Studies have shown that fewer adults are aging with their first and only partner, while increasing numbers are choosing to divorce, remarry, have romantic relationships, or live alone. Certain research has shown that more than a third of marriage dissolutions for people over 50 years of age occur through divorce. They have suggested that divorce may lead to greater loneliness in older people compared to widowhood. However, both divorce and widowhood are associated with increased loneliness in later life, as those who are divorced or widowed often feel lonelier and tend to have fewer social relationships with others than their married peers. Conversely, the children of older adults often tend to be independent and mobile, which may leave older widowed parents to fend for themselves. This scenario can lead to financial, social, and emotional problems such as loneliness. Support from others is crucial to reducing loneliness. This can come from a variety of sources, such as friends, family, and children. They found that support from friends reduced loneliness in old age. However, it should be noted that some believe that these friendships can provide a way to temporarily support older people during difficult times, which often reduces feelings of social isolation. However, spouses serve as an essential source of social support, and lack of support from spouses is a major factor in increasing loneliness among older people after the end of a marriage.

Since marriage is one of the most important institutions that affect the lives and well-being of individuals, improving the quality of life of older people and focusing on marital status as one of its concrete measures is of particular importance. Loneliness is a painful and distressing feeling that can have a variety of physical, health, and emotional consequences and can significantly increase the risk of mortality in older people. It may also be considered a factor affecting the mental health of older people. Older people use various strategies to cope with loneliness. Some older people remarry after losing their partner to eliminate the feeling of loneliness and increase their level of happiness in life. Feelings of loneliness, problems with not having a spouse, inability to express themselves, multidimensional fatigue, a feeling of aversion to dependence and lack of independence, and psychosocial vulnerability that is associated with a higher risk of mortality are all reasons that older people justify remarriage. At an older age, remarriage also creates a new sense of financial and emotional security and improves the person's physical health. The need for independence, sexual needs, and feelings of loneliness are among the reasons that older people cite for remarriage. Dissatisfaction and distress of children and interdependence of children and older people's parents, who think that remarriage leads to instability, are among the factors preventing the marriage of older people. Unpleasant experiences from a previous marriage are also important. Some older people do not have a good experience in their first marriage, which makes them reluctant to remarry. Older people believe that marriage at this age is not necessary and meaningful because of their inability to do the things they used to do in the past. Physical and sexual problems are also other obstacles resulting from inadequacy in marital relationships. Also, stereotypical beliefs, loss of honor and status in society, and fear of losing reputation prevent remarriage. Religious beliefs, reluctance, and a sense of need for marriage and independence were among the reasons for their unwillingness to marry.

4.6 Social Self-Care in Older People with Cognitive Impairments

As people age, many older adults develop mild cognitive impairment (MCI), a neurological disorder that is mild enough to not seriously interfere with daily activities and is usually considered a stage between normal aging and dementia, particularly Alzheimer's disease.

Older adults with cognitive impairments such as dementia or mild cognitive impairment face numerous challenges in maintaining social connections and self-care. Despite these challenges, however, social self-care—the ability to maintain and engage in meaningful human interactions—can significantly improve the quality of life of this group, helping to delay or even prevent the progression of MCI to dementia and leading to a sense of belonging, security, and peace of mind; reducing anxiety, depression, and confusion; maintaining mental and cognitive stimulation through conversation and interaction; maintaining self-esteem; and preventing isolation.

Participating in activities that promote cognitive training and stimulation, such as music therapy, dance therapy, art therapy, book therapy, and play therapy, can improve cognitive skills and overall health in older adults. Evidence suggests that online video games also have positive effects on cognitive function in older adults and can improve reaction time, memory, attention span, and the ability to multitask. When played in groups, multiplayer games such as World of Warcraft, League of Legends, Minecraft, and Ikariam can improve cognitive skills as well as increase a senior's sense of independence and social participation. Volunteer programs and intergenerational activities are also very beneficial for seniors with mild to moderate cognitive impairment. These programs involve seniors participating in activities such as reading to and tutoring children or volunteering in activities tailored to their interests and abilities. These measures not only help maintain and enhance cognitive abilities but also increase social interaction and improve the quality of life of the elderly. In this regard, we know that the elderly with cognitive problems may have challenges. For example, forgetting names, appointments, or relationships; inability to start or continue a conversation; confusion in crowded or unfamiliar environments; decreased self-confidence in communicating; and motor or language limitations. To overcome these challenges, it is important to observe several points. People who are in contact with this group of elderly people should create a safe and familiar social environment. Using quiet, low-stimulation, and predictable spaces and holding small group meetings with familiar faces is very helpful. Elderly people with cognitive disorders need support from family and caregivers, encouragement to be present in public and maintain old connections, and help to remember social appointments through a video calendar or phone.

The use of simple and understandable technologies also helps to create social relationships. Apps or tools with simple designs for video calling or using photos, music, or videos to remind people of relationships in this area are very important.

Engaging in purposeful social activities helps seniors with this problem not to be passive. Light activities such as group gardening, painting, or simple group games are voluntary activities appropriate to the individual's mental ability.

One of the important points is to teach those around them to communicate effectively with seniors with cognitive problems. Family and those around the elderly should know that speaking calmly, clearly, and in simple sentences and avoiding frequent corrections or pressuring the elderly greatly helps the elderly's self-care.

4.7 Social Self-Care in Older People with Disabilities

The increasing number of older adults with self-care disabilities is a major challenge for the aging population. It is estimated that more than 142 million older adults, approximately 14% of the global population aged 60 years and older, are currently unable to meet their basic daily needs, and this group of older adults with self-care disabilities places a significant burden on health care providers and other related services.

Disability is defined as an impairment in performing daily activities or the need for assistance with at least one daily activity. Disability is caused by a combination of social, individual, and environmental factors and is a growing public health problem, defined as a set of life barriers that affect an individual's physical, social, recreational, and occupational activities. The causes of disability are complex and multifaceted and include noncommunicable diseases, communicable diseases, and various injuries that older adults experience in their lives. In addition, factors such as gender, education, social networks, and disease status are influential in the development of disability. Social support and geographic characteristics of the area of residence also play a role in reducing or increasing disability in older people. According to some reports, the feeling of disability affects health status and quality of life more than actual disability, prevents older people from interacting with the environment, and makes them passive. Studies have shown that the prevalence of chronic disabling conditions significantly affects their ability to participate in daily activities, including social interactions, making older people highly vulnerable to psychological and social stress and forcing them to engage in social self-care. Social self-care is an essential aspect for seniors with disabilities, greatly influencing their mental well-being and overall life quality. By utilizing methods that encourage social interaction, including support groups, community participation, and technological resources, caregivers and healthcare professionals can improve the wellness of this demographic. Tackling the obstacles to social involvement is essential for enhancing self-care skills and creating a nurturing atmosphere for older people dealing with disabilities. The significance of social self-care is considerable. For instance, tackling isolation holds significant importance. Older adults with disabilities often experience loneliness and social isolation, and social gatherings are important for them, as they help them connect with others. Another is boosting self-efficacy. Studies indicate that self-efficacy—an individual's confidence in their capacity to achieve—is crucial in self-care. Increased self-efficacy correlates with improved self-care behaviors and lower disability rates in older adults. Social interactions can boost self-efficacy by offering support and motivation. Fostering social interactions can significantly contribute to social self-care by boosting self-efficacy through involvement in the community and bonding with family, friends, and others. Older people who are socially active tend to indicate improved health results and exhibit less worry about their health than those who are not engaged. Thus, enhancing the overall health aspect is also a vital part of encouraging social self-care among older people with disabilities. Thus, by employing various strategies to enhance social self-care for older people with disabilities, a meaningful difference can be achieved in their physical health, mental well-being, and overall life quality. Approaches to enhance social self-care consist of the following. Establishing or participating in support groups enables older people with disabilities to exchange experiences, difficulties, and methods of coping. These groups may concentrate on particular ailments or broader aging concerns, fostering a feeling of community. Promoting involvement in community events or volunteer activities can assist seniors in engaging with their neighborhood. The application of contemporary technology is quite beneficial and can enhance social interactions, particularly for individuals with mobility challenges. Video calls, internet forums, and social media networks can assist in preserving connections with family and friends. Exercise classes for groups or walking clubs specifically for seniors can enhance physical well-being and encourage social interaction. These activities offer chances for seniors to connect with others while engaging in advantageous physical exercise. Hosting workshops on engaging subjects (such as arts and crafts, gardening, or cooking) can foster involvement and cultivate new relationships among attendees, thereby enhancing self-care in seniors with disabilities.

4.8 Silent Isolation: How Social Self-Care Can Transform the Lives of Seniors in Nursing Homes

In a society with an aging population, concerns regarding loneliness and social isolation are gaining more significance. Research indicates that social isolation and loneliness have increasingly turned into a worldwide epidemic affecting older people. Loneliness and social isolation are recognized as risk factors for older adults, potentially resulting in heightened smoking, familial discord, loss of friends and loved ones, decreased mobility and income, mental health issues like depression and anxiety, poor overall health, increased chronic illnesses, extended average durations in nursing facilities, and an elevated risk of mortality. As reported by the World Health Organization, over 40% of seniors in nursing facilities experience feelings of loneliness. This may result from losing a partner, being far from family, or disinterest in interacting with others. Certain older people in nursing homes perceive themselves as a burden to others, leading to increased social isolation and loneliness and hindering their ability to interact and socialize with those around them. Furthermore, older individuals believe they have been cast aside by their relatives and companions, left to fend for themselves, which fills them with shame and leads them to avoid connections with Sarin, seeking to separate themselves from the community. Also, the lack of diverse and attractive programs in nursing homes reduces the participation of older people, and thus they are not willing to do social self-care. However, social self-care in older people living in nursing homes can be increased by providing solutions. Creating support networks, encouraging older people to create friendship groups, and holding group meetings for discussion and exchange of ideas with peers in nursing homes help to pay attention to social self-care. Holding workshops to teach conversation skills, express emotions, and share experiences through intergenerational activities is of great importance. Encouraging older people to participate in cultural programs, such as traditional celebrations and occasions, and holding art and craft workshops to enhance creativity and develop their skills so that they feel active and distance themselves from being passive. Given the availability of technology and the creation of appropriate platforms, training in the use of digital tools for video calls with family and creating online groups for discussion and social interaction is helpful. One of the most important issues that should be considered is training staff to establish positive and respectful communication with older people. Nursing home staff should establish effective and strong social communication with older people, especially those who are at risk of loneliness and social isolation and need more support. By involving them in self-care activities and considering additional programs and workshops, a sense of usefulness can be instilled in older people. It should be noted that the opinions of older people should be used to design programs and involve them at all stages. Considering counseling sessions and support sessions based on the problems that older people are facing and not ignoring them makes them feel that they are not abandoned and that they are still important to those around them. The role of policymaking in promoting social self-care for older people living in nursing homes is very important. Governments and responsible institutions should develop protective laws for older people living in nursing homes, allocate financial resources to improve social facilities and activities, involve older people in the discussion of social self-care, raise awareness through awareness campaigns for families and the general public, and encourage families to interact more with older people.

Recommendations Are Also Given for Family Caregivers and Older People

As mentioned, social self-care has many benefits for older people. However, despite its benefits, it also comes with challenges. Many older people feel lonely due to reasons such as the loss of loved ones, retirement, or reduced social relationships, and these things prevent them from doing social self-care, and they are not willing to participate in participatory activities at the community level. This challenge can be overcome by talking to older people, making them members of local support groups, encouraging them to participate in group activities, and establishing communication through technology (such as video calls).

Another issue is physical limitations, such as vision, hearing, and mobility problems, that make older people prefer to stay at home and prevent them from being present in the community. By designing flexible programs following the needs of older people, personalizing them, and providing transportation facilities, older people can be more actively involved.

One of the challenges that older people mention is financial barriers. Some older adults are unable to participate in paid social self-care activities, such as clubs, sports clubs, and groups, due to financial constraints. This challenge can be overcome by providing free or low-cost programs by governments and nongovernmental organizations and creating volunteer opportunities that do not require additional costs.

Older adults may not have enough confidence to make new connections and join groups due to a decrease in self-confidence following the aging process or past experiences. Holding psychological workshops to strengthen communication skills and self-confidence and encouraging older adults to do activities that lead to small successes are ways to increase self-confidence.

Older adults may also be unfamiliar with the benefits of self-care and may consider it unimportant. Some older adults consider this period to be lonely and isolated. However, by educating and informing older people about the importance of social self-care in mental and physical health and using media and public campaigns to raise awareness among them, they can be guided in this regard. Resistance to change and innovation is another challenge. It can be noted that some older people may feel dissatisfied with or afraid of new activities or new technologies. Providing simple and practical training in the use of technology and encouraging them to make small and gradual changes is an appropriate solution to this challenge.

Recommendations for Family Caregivers and Older Adults on Social Self-Care

1. Expand your connections:
   - Connect more with older people in your family, neighborhood, or community and try to meet their emotional and social needs.
   - Encourage seniors to participate in group or volunteer activities.
2. Implement innovative ideas:
   - Design and implement programs for seniors, such as reading groups, skill-building classes, or art activities.
   - Introduce technology as a tool to strengthen seniors' social relationships and help them use these tools.
3. Raise awareness:
   - Encourage seniors to participate in social activities by informing them about the importance of social self-care.
   - Use social media and networks to promote a culture of respect and support for seniors.

4. Strengthen your support role:
   - As an individual or family member, increase your support role in the lives of older people and help them overcome loneliness and isolation.
   - Collaborate with community or charitable organizations to provide better services for older people.
5. Explore and address challenges:
   - Identify barriers to older people maintaining social self-care (such as financial, physical, or mental health problems) and offer solutions.
   - Help older people overcome their fears or resistance to social participation.
6. Aim to improve quality of life:
   - Based on what you have learned, develop programs that focus on improving the mental, physical, and social health of older people.
   - Offer simple and actionable ways to encourage older people to engage in social activities.
7. Share your experiences:
   - Share your experiences and successes in working with seniors to inspire others.
   - Improve your approaches by studying more resources and using global experiences.
8. Think about the role of the community:
   - Provide suggestions to local organizations to improve infrastructure and social facilities.
   - Participate in or support local programs designed for seniors .

4.9 Summary of the Chapter

In this chapter, the concept of social self-care in older people, its importance for improving quality of life, and how it relates to physical, mental, and social health were identified. Social self-care provides an opportunity for older people to again feel valued and a part of something through strengthened social interrelations and moving away from isolation and loneliness.

Other different challenges exist in maintaining or improving the social self-care of an older adult, including physical and mental problems, financial aspects, or cultural issues. However, strategies such as creating groups, encouraging participation in different aspects, using technology, and further enlargement of public awareness can surmount these obstacles. This chapter also stressed the importance of family, community, and social organizations in the care of older people. Older people can be directed to a more active and meaningful life with appropriate programs and strengthened social skills.

Finally, readers are invited to use the material in this chapter in designing applications that improve the social well-being of older people and take practical steps to bring about positive changes in this respect. Social care for older people will not only help improve their lives but also lead to building a kinder and more supportive society.

4.10 Summary of Research Studies

A 2022 article titled "The Relationship Between Self-Care, Positive Family Environment, and Human Well-Being" tried to understand the impact of a positive family environment on self-care practices and overall well-being by Nisa Young-Torres. Soto et al. The results are as follows:

A good family environment increases the feeling of security and motivation of individuals, especially the older members, in self-care practices. Emotional support, shared responsibilities, and intergenerational bonding significantly enhance self-efficacy in health management.

This study highlighted family relationships in helping to combat social isolation among older people. Regular communication, involvement in family activities, and a feeling of belonging improve mental and emotional health. It also lists that positive family relationships support healthy behavior for older adults, including regular exercise, proper nutrition, and relaxation techniques that can be specifically adapted to deal with stress. All these preventive behaviors taken together reduce the respective risk factors for chronic diseases and depression. A stressful family environment, marked by conflict, ignorance, or no communication, negatively impacts self-care activity and promotes feelings of helplessness and poor health. This study supports interventions that strengthen family dynamics, such as counseling, educational programs, and structured family activities. It also highlights the need to integrate community resources to support older adults in dysfunctional families. It also suggests that by using the family unit as a primary source of social support, older adults can play an active role in their communities and improve their quality of life. Initiatives like family health workshops or caregiver support groups contribute to social self-care among older adults.

Another 2021 study, "Gamification for Older Adults: A Systematic Literature Review," by Jonna Koivisto et al., examines the use of gamification as a tool to increase engagement and well-being in older adults. The study shows how gamification can be used to improve social self-care among older adults by engaging them in meaningful and enjoyable activities.

Most gamified interventions also offer mechanisms for multi-person or group participation, thereby building communities and reducing social isolation in older adults. Activities involve team challenges or shared achievements that foster a sense of belonging and enhance social self-care.

Gamified platforms also encourage older users to engage in healthy behaviors such as exercise, cognitive training, or maintaining social routines. Positive feedback and rewards increase adherence to such practices.

Indeed, the study points to a number of challenges facing gamification among some older populations, including issues of technological literacy and accessibility. In such situations, the need for user-friendly design and appropriate training is suggested.

The study suggests that gamification can be integrated into social platforms, where it can become a useful tool for social self-care. Apps that balance simplicity and interactivity are likely to be successful in increasing social interaction and health behaviors in older adults. Gamified tools can also serve as a bridge to help older adults connect with their peers, caregivers, and family to make self-care a fun, collaborative experience. On the other hand, community-based games or apps for older adults ensure engagement, less loneliness, and emotional well-being.

A study titled "Managing Volunteer Activities Among Older Persons" was conducted in 2019 by Hiroe Yanahara et al. The study examines the importance of older people's involvement in volunteer work and the effective management strategies needed to support their participation. The findings of this paper include the following: The benefits of involving older volunteers include the diverse insights and experiences that are valuable in increasing organizational effectiveness. Older people have more responsibility because they have more time to devote to volunteer work, mentoring, and sharing their experiences with younger people. Older people prefer flexible roles that align with their interests and availability. Understanding these preferences is crucial for effective recruitment and retention. Technological approaches offer diverse volunteer opportunities that can be adapted to older people's schedules and enable them to participate in ways that best suit them. Digital tools also support older people in managing their volunteer activities and tracking their contributions, thus enhancing their sense of achievement. The article argues that organizations also need to identify and address the technological barriers that some older adults face to fully participate in volunteering activities. Empowering senior volunteers through thoughtful management and technology not only enriches volunteer programs but also enhances the quality of life of older adults. By creating inclusive environments and providing the necessary support, organizations can effectively harness the potential of senior volunteers.

Overall, research on social self-care provides valuable insights into how older adults can engage in their community. It also shows that with the social self-care of older adults, positive outcomes accrue to both older people themselves and their families and communities. Members of the community also benefit from their valuable experiences, and ultimately, we will have a healthier and happier society.

4.11 Critical Thinking (Scenario Based)

4.11.1 Case Scenario 1

In a small town called "New Life," the older people population is rapidly increasing. Many of the older people in the town feel isolated due to retirement, children being away, and the loss of old friends. In this regard, the municipality has decided to implement a project aimed at strengthening the social self-care of older people.

The project involves forming support groups, holding skills training classes, and providing access to communication technologies for older people. As part of the research team of this project, you must use critical and dynamic thinking approaches to identify and implement the best solutions.

Challenges in the scenario:

Resistance of some older people:
Some older people are distrustful of changes and new technologies and are reluctant to participate.

Lack of budget and resources:

The municipality is facing budget constraints, and it is not possible to implement all the programs simultaneously.
Differences in needs
Monitoring and review
Seniors with different conditions (in terms of physical, mental, and economic health) have different needs.

Critical thinking questions:

1. Which groups of seniors (based on physical, mental, or economic conditions) should be prioritized? Why?
2. What methods can be used to attract the participation of resilient seniors?
3. Is holding skills training classes more effective than providing access to technology?
4. How can you make the most impact in the senior community with a limited budget?
5. What types of group activities can provide the most motivation for seniors?
6. How can local resources (such as volunteers or donors) be used to strengthen programs?
7. What indicators can be defined to measure the success of the project?
8. If some seniors are unable to participate in the programs, how can alternative solutions be provided?

4.11.2 Case Scenario 2

Dayan, 72, lives alone in his apartment in a small town. He lost his wife years ago, and his children have moved to nearby cities for work.

Dayan is unable to perform many of his daily activities due to physical problems such as joint pain and poor eyesight. He spends most of his days at home due to his inability to move and a lack of regular social contact. Dayan used to ask his neighbors to help him with shopping or simple tasks, but he no longer asks for help due to shame and embarrassment. He is also unable to use communication technologies and has limited social interactions.

Given Dayan's condition, the need for social self-care is essential to maintaining his mental, physical, and social well-being. As a social worker, you have stepped in to help Dayan.

Critical Thinking Questions for Analyzing Dayan's Scenario:

1. Analyze the current situation:
   Why does Dayan feel uncomfortable asking others for help? Is this feeling caused by fear, shame, or social attitudes?

How has Dayan's social isolation affected his mental and physical health?
Have Dayan's physical problems directly affected his social abilities? If so, how?

2. Identify needs and priorities:
   What are Dayan's most important needs right now? Is his need for social connection more important than his physical needs?
   How can we prioritize the type of support Dayan should receive?
   Does Dayan need immediate help in specific areas (such as health care), or does he need more social connections and psychological support?
3. Assess available resources:
   Are Dayan's existing social and technological resources sufficient to strengthen his connections?
   What resources are available in the neighborhood or community that can help Dayan expand his social connections?
   How can technology be used to help Dayan connect with his children or friends?
4. Practical strategies to promote social self-care:
   How can Dayan be encouraged to participate in social activities (such as support groups or volunteer programs)?
   Is there a need for a counselor or coach to help Diane use technology?
   What types of social activities might be appealing to Dayan while also strengthening his social relationships?
5. Barriers and challenges:
   What factors might be preventing Dayan from participating in social activities? (such as physical problems, low self-esteem, or fear of being judged by others)
   How can these barriers be identified and addressed?
   Dayan may be reluctant to accept social support because of past experiences or feelings of shame. How can this be changed?
6. Sustainability and foresight:
   How can we design programs that will help Dayan live more independently and actively?
   Can we build a sustainable social network of neighbors, friends, and family for Dayan so that he does not feel alone?
   What steps can we take to ensure that Dayan can benefit from social self-care in the long term and continue to do so independently?

Bibliography

Abbott KM, Bettger JP, Hampton KN, Kohler H-P. The feasibility of measuring social networks among older adults in assisted living and dementia special care units. Dementia. 2015;14(2):199–219.

Anguera JA, Boccanfuso J, Rintoul JL, Al-Hashimi O, Faraji F, Janowich J, et al. Video game training enhances cognitive control in older adults. Nature. 2013;501(7465):97–101.

Araujo de Carvalho I, Epping-Jordan J, Pot AM, Kelley E, Toro N, Thiyagarajan JA, et al. Organizing integrated health-care services to meet older people's needs. Bull World Health Organ. 2017;95(11):756–63.

Asgari P, Navab E, Esmaeili M, Shali M, Bit-Lian Y, Bahramnezhad F. There is no fool like an old fool: the experiences of elderlies regarding remarriage in Iran. Iran J Psychiatry Behav Sci. 2021;15(2)

Ayala EE, Ellis MV, Grudev N, Cole J. Women in health service psychology programs: stress, self-care, and quality of life. Train Educ Prof Psychol. 2017;11(1):18.

Bacsu J, Jeffery B, Abonyi S, Johnson S, Novik N, Martz D, et al. Healthy aging in place: perceptions of rural older adults. Educ Gerontol. 2014;40(5):327–37.

Bastani F, Haghani H. Perceived stress and fear of COVID-19 among the older people referred to comprehensive health centers in Tehran, Iran. Iran J Nurs. 2022;35(136):134–49.

Bianco A, Patti A, Bellafiore M, Battaglia G, Sahin FN, Paoli A, et al. Group fitness activities for the older people: an innovative approach to reduce falls and injuries. Aging Clin Exp Res. 2014;26:147–52.

Boamah SA, Weldrick R, Lee TJ, Taylor N. Social isolation among older adults in long-term care: a scoping review. J Aging Health. 2021;33(7-8):618–32.

Breheny M, Pond R, Lilburn LE. "What am I going to be like when I'm that age?": how older volunteers anticipate ageing through home visiting. J Aging Stud. 2020;53:100848.

Buyl R, Beogo I, Fobelets M, Deletroz C, Van Landuyt P, Dequanter S, et al. e-Health interventions for healthy aging: a systematic review. Syst Rev. 2020;9:1–15.

Cacioppo JT, Cacioppo S. Social relationships and health: the toxic effects of perceived social isolation. Soc Personal Psychol Compass. 2014;8(2):58–72.

Caron A, Ayala A, Damián J, Rodriguez-Blazquez C, Almazán J, Castellote JM, et al. Physical activity, body functions and disability among middle-aged and older Spanish adults. BMC Geriatr. 2017;17:1–11.

Carter LA, Barnett JE. Self-care for clinicians in training: a guide to psychological wellness for graduate students in psychology. New York: Oxford University Press; 2014.
Casey A-NS, Low L-F, Jeon Y-H, Brodaty H. Residents perceptions of friendship and positive social networks within a nursing home. The Gerontologist. 2016;56(5):855–67.
Chan AW, Yu DS, Choi K. Effects of tai chi qigong on psychosocial well-being among hidden older people, using older people neighborhood volunteer approach: a pilot randomized controlled trial. Clin Interv Aging. 2017;12:85–96.
Claponea RM, Iorga M. The relationship between burnout and wellbeing using social support, organizational justice, and lifelong learning in healthcare specialists from Romania. Medicina (Kaunas). 2023;59(7):1352.
Cotten SR. Examining the roles of technology in aging and quality of life. J Gerontol B Psychol Sci Soc Sci. 2017;72(5):823–6.
Coyle CE, Dugan E. Social isolation, loneliness and health among older adults. J Aging Health. 2012;24(8):1346–63.
Dale B, Söderhamn U, Söderhamn O. Life situation and identity among single older home-living people: a phenomenological–hermeneutic study. Int J Qual Stud Health Well Being. 2012;7(1):18456.
de Oliveira DV, Muzolon LG, Antunes MD, do Nascimento Júnior JRA. Impact of swimming initiation on the physical fitness and mental health of older people women. Acta Sci Health Sci. 2019;41:43221.
Dehghankar L, Valinezhad S, Amerzadeh M, Zarabadi Poor F, Hosseinkhani Z, Motalebi SA. Relationship between perceived social support and disability with the mediating role of perceived stress among older adults. BMC Geriatr. 2024;24(1):276.
Dell'Osso L, Nardi B, Massoni L, Battaglini S, De Felice C, Bonelli C, et al. Video gaming in older people: what are the implications for cognitive functions? Brain Sci. 2024;14(7):731.
Dorociak KE, Rupert PA, Zahniser E. Work life, well-being, and self-care across the professional lifespan of psychologists. Prof Psychol Res Pract. 2017;48(6):429.
DSZAS M. Love hunger: contrasting dynamics of love and belongingness needs in the kite runner. PalArch's J Archaeol Egypt/Egyptol. 2020;17(1):458–69.
El-Ghoroury NH, Galper DI, Sawaqdeh A, Bufka LF. Stress, coping, and barriers to wellness among psychology graduate students. Train Educ Prof Psychol. 2012;6(2):122.
Fakoya OA, McCorry NK, Donnelly M. How do befriending interventions alleviate loneliness and social isolation among older people? A realist evaluation study. PLoS One. 2021;16(9):e0256900.
Feng Z, Glinskaya E, Chen H, Gong S, Qiu Y, Xu J, et al. Long-term care system for older adults in China: policy landscape, challenges, and future prospects. Lancet. 2020;396(10259):1362–72.
Ghaneh B, Saeed- Banadaky SH, Rahaei Z, Rezaeipandari H, Mohiti E. Disability and self-care among elders in Yazd. Elder. Health J. 2016;2(1):39–44.
González-González E, Requena C. Self-care interventions of community-dwelling older adults: a systematic review and meta-analysis. Front Public Health. 2023;11:1254172.
Guo Y, Wang T, Ge T, Jiang Q. Prevalence of self-care disability among older adults in China. BMC Geriatr. 2022;22(1):775.
Guy J, Norcross J. Leaving it at the office: a guide to psychotherapist self-care. New York: Guilford; 2007.
Hall AK, Stellefson M, Bernhardt JM. Healthy Aging 2.0: the potential of new media and technology. Prev Chronic Dis. 2012;9:E67.
Han A, Brown D, Richardson A. Older adults' perspectives on volunteering in an activity-based social program for people with dementia. Act Adapt Aging. 2019;43(2):145–63.
Hanson S, Jones A. Is there evidence that walking groups have health benefits? A systematic review and meta-analysis. Br J Sports Med. 2015;49(11):710–5.
Hemingway A, Jack E. Reducing social isolation and promoting well being in older people. Qual Ageing Older Adults. 2013;14(1):25–35.
Hong SI, Morrow-Howell N. Health outcomes of experience corps®: a high-commitment volunteer program. Soc Sci Med. 2010;71(2):414–20.
Indriana Y. Remarriage in older people: a qualitative research. J Mod Educ Rev. 2013;3(11):870–80.
Jin K, Simpkins JW, Ji X, Leis M, Stambler I. The critical need to promote research of aging and aging-related diseases to improve health and longevity of the older people population. Aging Dis. 2015;6(1):1.
Kappen, D., Mirza-Babaei, P., & Nacke, L. (2018). Gamification of older adults' physical activity: An eight-week study. In Proceedings of the 51st Hawaii International Conference on System Sciences (HICSS) (pp. 3907–3916). Hawaii. https://doi.org/10.24251/HICSS.2018.149.
Kim C-S, Choi S-I. The relations between participation motive and satisfaction level of the volunteer activities of the older people. J Korea Content Assoc. 2012;12(4):315–26.
Kim H, Kelly S, Lafortune L, Brayne C. A scoping review of the conceptual differentiation of technology for healthy aging. The Gerontologist. 2021;61(7):e345–69.
Koivisto J, Malik A. Gamification for older adults: a systematic literature review. The Gerontologist. 2021;61(7):e360–72.
Kotter-Grühn, D. (2015). Changing negative views of aging: Implications for intervention and translational research. In M. Diehl & H.-W. Wahl (Eds.), Annual review of gerontology and geriatrics, Vol. 35, 2015: Subjective aging: New developments and future directions (pp. 167–186). Springer Publishing Company.

Kyriazis M, Kiourti E. Video games and other online activities may improve health in ageing. Front Med (Lausanne). 2018;5:8.

Lai C, Leung D, Kwong E, Lee R. Factors associated with the quality of life of nursing home residents in Hong Kong. Int Nurs Rev. 2015;62(1):120–9.

Lee JJ, Miller SE. A self-care framework for social workers: building a strong foundation for practice. Fam Soc. 2013;94(2):96–103.

Lee CC, Czaja SJ, Moxley JH, Sharit J, Boot WR, Charness N, et al. Attitudes toward computers across adulthood from 1994 to 2013. The Gerontologist. 2019;59(1):22–33.

Liu Y, Tamura R, editors. Application of game therapy in the health of future older people: an experience design perspective. HCI International 2020–Late Breaking Papers: Universal Access and Inclusive Design: 22nd HCI International Conference, HCII 2020, Copenhagen, Denmark, July 19–24, 2020, Proceedings 22. Springer; 2020.

Macera CA, Cavanaugh A, Bellettiere J. State of the art review: physical activity and older adults. Am J Lifestyle Med. 2017;11(1):42–57.

Malmedal W, Steinsheim G, Nordtug B, Blindheim K, Alnes RE, Moe A. How volunteers contribute to persons with dementia coping in everyday life. J Multidiscip Healthc. 2020;13:309–19.

Mathes EW, Edwards LL. An empirical test of Maslow's theory of motivation. Journal of Humanistic Psychology. 1978;18(1):75–7.

McKenzie SH, Harris MF. Understanding the relationship between stress, distress and healthy lifestyle behaviour: a qualitative study of patients and general practitioners. BMC Fam Pract. 2013;14:1–8.

Middleton KR, Ward MM, Haaz S, Velummylum S, Fike A, Acevedo AT, et al. A pilot study of yoga as self-care for arthritis in minority communities. Health Qual Life Outcomes. 2013;11:1–14.

Mitzner TL, Savla J, Boot WR, Sharit J, Charness N, Czaja SJ, et al. Technology adoption by older adults: findings from the PRISM trial. The Gerontologist. 2019;59(1):34–44.

Mizobuchi, S., & Suzuki, H. (Eds.). (2023). Research and development of a bingo game using dice to prevent dementia. In HCI International 2023 Posters. Springer Nature Switzerland

Moffatt, F. (2017). The individual physical health benefits of swimming: A literature review. In The health & wellbeing benefits of swimming (pp. 8–25). The University of Nottingham

Mohsin NF, Jali SK, Bandan MI, Jali N, Jupit AJR, editors. Older adults and digital game trends, challenges and benefits. In: 2021 IEEE Asia-pacific conference on computer science and data engineering (CSDE). IEEE; 2021.

Mooventhan A, Nivethitha L. Evidence based effects of yoga practice on various health related problems of older people: a review. J Bodyw Mov Ther. 2017;21(4):1028–32.

Motaharinezhad F, Madani P, Seyed S, Avaz KA, Rasolzadeh M. The impact of the six-week walking on the older people's happiness and mental health. Middle East J Rehabil Health Stud. 2016;3(3):e60290.

Mu T-Y, Xu R-X, Xu J-Y, Dong D, Zhou Z-N, Dai J-N, et al. Association between self-care disability and depressive symptoms among middle-aged and older people Chinese people. PLoS One. 2022;17(4):e0266950.

Mui AC, Glajchen M, Chen H, Sun J. Developing an older adult volunteer program in a New York Chinese community: an evidence-based approach. Ageing Int. 2013;38:108–21.

Murayama Y, Ohba H, Yasunaga M, Nonaka K, Takeuchi R, Nishi M, et al. The effect of intergenerational programs on the mental health of older people adults. Aging Ment Health. 2015;19(4):306–14.

Nations U. Department of Economic and Social Affairs, population division world population prospects: the 2015 revision, methodology of the United Nations population estimates and projections. 2015.

Oliveira DV, Favero PF, Codonhato R, Moreira CR, Antunes MD, Nascimento JRA. Investigation of the emotional and psychological factors of older people persons frequenting ballroom dancing clubs. Rev Bras Geriatr Gerontol. 2017;20:797–804.

Onunkwor OF, Al-Dubai SAR, George PP, Arokiasamy J, Yadav H, Barua A, et al. A cross-sectional study on quality of life among the older people in non-governmental organizations' older people homes in Kuala Lumpur. Health Qual Life Outcomes. 2016;14:1–10.

Osmani N, Matlabi H, Rezaei M. Barriers to remarriage among older people: viewpoints of widows and widowers. J Divorce Remarriage. 2018;59(1):51–68.

Peek ST, Luijkx KG, Rijnaard MD, Nieboer ME, Van Der Voort CS, Aarts S, et al. Older adults' reasons for using technology while aging in place. Gerontology. 2016;62(2):226–37.

Peine A, Neven L. From intervention to co-constitution: new directions in theorizing about aging and technology. The Gerontologist. 2019;59(1):15–21.

Plummer J, Nguyen K, Everly J, Kiesow A, Leith K, Aging CoGSi, et al. How an intergenerational book club can prevent cognitive decline in older adults: a pilot study. Gerontol Geriatr Med. 2023;9:23337214221150061.

Pursley, E. (2024). The house of healing for the soul: Bibliotherapy and book clubs within geriatric care (Honors thesis, Baylor University). Baylor University Digital Collections. https://hdl.handle.net/2104/12711

Rico-Uribe LA, Caballero FF, Olaya B, Tobiasz-Adamczyk B, Koskinen S, Leonardi M, et al. Loneliness, social networks, and health: a cross-sectional study in three countries. PLoS One. 2016;11(1):e0145264.

Roh SY. Effect of a 16-week Pilates exercise program on the ego resiliency and depression in older people women. J Exerc Rehabil. 2016;12(5):494.

Schneider CE, Hunter EG, Bardach SH. Potential cognitive benefits from playing music among cognitively intact older adults: a scoping review. J Appl Gerontol. 2019;38(12):1763–83.

Scult M, Haime V, Jacquart J, Takahashi J, Moscowitz B, Webster A, et al. A healthy aging program for older adults: effects on self-efficacy and morale. Adv Mind Body Med. 2015;29(1):26.

Sharifi S, Khorzoughi KB, Rahmati M. The relationship between volunteering and cognitive performance in older adults: a systematic review. Geriatr Nurs. 2024;55:89–96.

Siette J, Cassidy M, Priebe S. Effectiveness of befriending interventions: a systematic review and meta-analysis. BMJ Open. 2017;7(4):e014304.

Sim M, Park J-M. A comparative study on factors influencing successful aging between elders attending senior citizen clubs and elders not attending senior citizen clubs. J Korean Gerontol Nurs. 2015;17(3):196–206.

Sleeman KE, De Brito M, Etkind S, Nkhoma K, Guo P, Higginson IJ, et al. The escalating global burden of serious health-related suffering: projections to 2060 by world regions, age groups, and health conditions. Lancet Glob Health. 2019;7(7):e883–92.

Stenner BJ, Mosewich AD, Buckley JD. An exploratory investigation into the reasons why older people play golf. Qual Res Sport, Exerc Health. 2016;8(3):257–72.

Sun XS. The situation, demand and obstacle of remarriage of rural older people-based on the survey of two villages in Hubei and Jiangxi Provinces. Sci Res Aging. 2014;2(9):20–7.

Thinley S. Health and care of an ageing population: alignment of health and social systems to address the need. J Health Manag. 2021;23(1):109–18.

Tong Y, Chai L, Lei S, Liu M, Yang L. Effects of tai chi on self-efficacy: a systematic review. Evid Based Complement Alternat Med. 2018;2018(1):1701372.

Toril P, Reales JM, Ballesteros S. Video game training enhances cognition of older adults: a meta-analytic study. Psychol Aging. 2014;29(3):706.

Torres-Soto NY, Corral-Verdugo V, Corral-Frías NS. The relationship between self-care, positive family environment, and human wellbeing. Wellbeing Space Soc. 2022;3:100076.

Tu J-C, Yang C-H, Liang C-Y, Chen H-Y. Exploring the impact of puzzle games for the older people from experiential learning. Think Skills Creat. 2022;45:101107.

Uchino BN. Social support and health: a review of physiological processes potentially underlying links to disease outcomes. J Behav Med. 2006;29:377–87.

Umberson D, Karas J. Social relationships and health: a flashpoint for health policy. J Health Soc Behav. 2010;51(1_suppl):S54–66.

Umberson D, Montez JK. Social relationships and health: a flashpoint for health policy. J Health Soc Behav. 2010;51 Suppl(Suppl):S54–66.

Upton RK III. The effects of golf on the mental health of older adults: a content analysis of the literature and a proposed future study. 2020.

Villavicencio MEF, Díaz MR, Julián González Pérez G, Barbosae MAV. Declive cognitivo de atenciÃ³n y memoria en adultos mayores sanos. Cuadernos de Neuropsicología/Panamerican. J Neuropsychol. 2020;14(1)

Voigt, M. (2019). Health inequalities in Spain: Analysis of structural inequalities and the effects on health and mortality (Doctoral dissertation, Universitat Autònoma de Barcelona). https://ddd.uab.cat/record/240743

Walsh R. Lifestyle and mental health. Am Psychol. 2011;66(7):579.

Weening-Verbree L, Huisman-de Waal G, Van Dusseldorp L, van Achterberg T, Schoonhoven L. Oral health care in older people in long term care facilities: a systematic review of implementation strategies. Int J Nurs Stud. 2013;50(4):569–82.

Wiles J, Morgan T, Moeke-Maxwell T, Black S, Park H-J, Dewes O, et al. Befriending services for culturally diverse older people. J Gerontol Soc Work. 2019;62(7):776–93.

Wright MR, Hammersmith AM, Brown SL, Lin I-F. The roles of marital dissolution and subsequent repartnering on loneliness in later life. J Gerontol B Psychol Sci Soc Sci. 2019;75(8):1796–807.

Yanahara H, Machida T, Nakazawa S, Suzuki E, Matsuo M. Management of volunteer activities among older people persons. GSTF J Nurs Health Care (JNHC). 2020;4(1). https://dl6.globalstf.org/index.php/jnhc/article/view/1994?utm_source=chatgpt.com

Yang Y, Li W, Guo Y, Liu Y, Li Q, Yang K, Wang S, Zeng N, Duan W, Chen Z, Chen H, Li X, Zhao W, Chen R, Kang Y. Early COPD Risk Decision for Adults Aged From 40 to 79 Years Based on Lung Radiomics Features. Front Med (Lausanne). 2022;9:845286. https://doi.org/10.3389/fmed.2022.845286. PMID: 35530043; PMCID: PMC9069013.

Yasunaga M, Murayama Y, Takahashi T, Ohba H, Suzuki H, Nonaka K, et al. Multiple impacts of an intergenerational program in Japan: evidence from the Research on Productivity through Intergenerational Sympathy Project. Geriatr Gerontol Int. 2016;16:98–109.

Zahniser E, Rupert PA, Dorociak KE. Self-care in clinical psychology graduate training. Train Educ Prof Psychol. 2017;11(4):283.

Zhu X, Dong Z, Wu Y, Xu DW. A review of different types of volunteer programs for older adults with and without cognitive impairment. Front Public Health. 2023;11:1164952.

Spiritual Self-Care in Older People

5

Fatemeh Bahramnezhad and Banafsheh Ghorbani

In the end, the learner should be able to:

- Understand spiritual self-care in older people
- Identify the spiritual needs of older people
- Explain the impact of spiritual self-care on various physical, psychological, and social aspects of older people
- Describe daily practices for cultivating spiritual self-care in older people

5.1 What Is Spiritual Self-Care in Older People?

Population aging is not a phenomenon limited to a country or region but a global issue, as the number of older people in the world continues to rise. Given this trend, it is essential to address the needs of older individuals.

According to the World Health Organization (WHO), health encompasses physical, mental, social, and spiritual dimensions. Spiritual health is interconnected with and influences other aspects of health at all stages of life. This dimension is crucial for creating a harmonious connection between internal forces, leading to stability, peace, harmony, and a strong sense of connection with oneself, God, society, and the environment.

Traditionally, health was defined solely in terms of physical, mental, and social well-being. However, recent studies have shown that without spiritual health, the other dimensions of an individual's well-being cannot function optimally, leading to a diminished quality of life. Therefore, it is vital to recognize spirituality as an essential aspect of human existence, as all individuals have varying spiritual needs that contribute to their overall well-being.

A review of the literature has shown that there is no universally accepted definition of spiritual health. However, several definitions of spiritual health have been proposed, which we will discuss below. The words, themes, and characteristics often used to describe spirituality in studies include journey, experience, life force, identity, self-awareness, wholeness, feelings, purpose, faith movement, certainty, connection, transcendence, and meaning in life, which researchers sometimes use in their studies on spirituality.

According to numerous studies conducted in this area, spiritual health has two dimensions. One is the vertical dimension, which includes the connection with the supernatural, and the other is the horizontal dimension, which involves the connection with the surrounding environment and others. Therefore, spiritual health is the spiritual experience of a person from two different perspectives: the religious health perspective, which focuses on how people perceive health in

F. Bahramnezhad (✉)
Tehran University of Medical Sciences, Tehran, Iran
e-mail: bahramnezhad@tums.ac.ir

B. Ghorbani
University of Social Welfare and Rehabilitation Sciences, Tehran, Iran

F. Bahramnezhad (ed.), *Self-Care in the Elderly*, https://doi.org/10.1007/978-981-96-9021-3_5

their spiritual life when they are connected to a higher power, and the existential health perspective, which focuses on social aspects and discusses the psychological concerns of individuals and how they adapt to themselves, society, or the environment.

In this regard, both religious and nonreligious researchers have defined spiritual health from two theoretical perspectives. From a religious standpoint, spiritual health is determined based on a monotheistic worldview. In contrast, from a nonreligious perspective, it is defined as a focus on beliefs, relationships, values, and goal choices rather than a belief in God. The results obtained showed that nonreligious spirituality is the achievement of the potential abilities of the human psyche, not dependence on a sacred or higher power. These researchers point out that it is very difficult to define spiritual health from a nonreligious perspective. Their view is that the use of spirituality is simply a tool to treat illness and cope with it better.

Fisher describes spiritual health as a fundamental dimension of health and well-being that acts as a coordinating and complementary force for other dimensions of human health (physical, mental, and social). The journal, citing Miller, defines spiritual health as an inherent and fundamental quality of an individual that includes a belief in something higher than oneself and a belief that life is affirmed and valued. Spiritual health can create conditions in society that promote social self-care and ultimately contribute to the well-being of older people. Some believe that spiritual health is an organized system of beliefs, practices, and rituals in a society to which its people adhere. Review studies have consistently shown that spirituality involves a personal and universal quest for answers to life's ultimate questions and their meaning, which may or may not involve religious beliefs, rituals, or ceremonies. It can also be entirely separate from religion.

Spirituality is a complex concept that is understood as both a religious and nonreligious construct. It is a concept that is ideologically linked to an individual's religious affiliation. Some believe that spirituality is closely tied to religion, leading to variations in the definition of spiritual health across different religions. Spirituality is influenced by various factors such as life events, belief background, religious practices, gender, culture, temperament, and the stage of life an individual is in.

In some studies, spirituality and religion are used interchangeably, with religion aiming to foster a connection to the sacred or transcendent, such as God or a higher power. However, spirituality provides a broader and somewhat vaguer definition. It is important to differentiate between spirituality and religion as a first step, as a spiritual person may not necessarily be religious and vice versa. For example, an older nonreligious individual may not prioritize spiritual self-care, while a nonreligious elder may also engage in spiritual self-care practices.

Spiritual care differs from religious care in its focus and approach. Spiritual care is personalized, centered on the individual, and does not make assumptions about a person's beliefs or lifestyle. On the other hand, religious care operates within the framework of shared beliefs, values, and practices of a faith community. It is important to note that spiritual care should not aim to convert individuals, should not be limited to religious settings, and should not solely rely on clergy or professionals.

Considering the increase in the older population, it is necessary to pay attention to issues related to this age group. While the likelihood of developing chronic diseases increases with age, old age does not necessarily mean disability. Changes that occur during aging can lead to a severe decrease in the ability of various body systems, resulting in diseases and, ultimately, a decrease in the efficiency and quality of life of older people. These complications can cause feelings of emptiness and burden in older individuals. On the other hand, studies have shown that spiritual beliefs in older people lead to indescribable peace, strength, and joy. Older individuals with strong religious and spiritual beliefs tend to face fewer cognitive problems. Religious beliefs, attitudes, and practices play important roles in adapting to the consequences of aging and ensuring the mental health of older people.

This can help reduce stress caused by life's challenges, including diseases.

Older adults need to find new ways to develop their spiritual self-care because numerous studies show that spirituality has a strong relationship with overall health. Recently, gerontological literature has focused on the influential role of existential factors like religiosity, spirituality, and personal meaning in the psychological well-being of older adults. It has been suggested that spirituality be examined as an independent component of "successful aging" in various cultural contexts. Spirituality or religious commitment is a complex and multidimensional part of the human experience that positively impacts health and well-being outcomes in older adults. Studies indicate that older adults are willing to use spirituality in old age and during struggles with diseases, suggesting that considering spiritual self-care in the aging process can lead to accelerated recovery. Research findings indicate that the religious beliefs of older adults significantly affect their quality of life, mental and physical health, and successful aging. Some researchers believe that spirituality includes hope, discovering purpose in life, making allowances for others' shortcomings, moral beliefs and principles, spiritual support, healthy relationships, faith in God, ethical behavior, and creativity. Similarly, self-expression, religious beliefs, and spiritual well-being increase with age. Following religious beliefs and precepts increases motivation to develop and strengthen self-care practices. Therefore, the deeper an older person's faith in God, the more effectively they can manage life's challenges. It appears that people with more spiritual inclinations have higher levels of hope and satisfaction.

Given the increasing prevalence of the older population and rising life expectancy, promoting health in old age is now a priority for health professionals, researchers, and policymakers worldwide. The aging process involves a dynamic interplay of biological, psychological, social, and economic changes that collectively impact later life outcomes. Some major challenges that often come with aging include physical limitations, social isolation, and economic difficulties due to reduced earning capacity. Older adults who lack the resources to cope with these challenges are at risk for depression and other negative mental health outcomes.

Spirituality is a complex and multilayered concept with diverse definitions and practices for spiritual self-care. The different layers of spirituality include faith, core experiences, related attitudes, and subsequent behaviors.

Therefore, to assess an individual's spirituality, it is necessary to consider a complex set of "indicators," each of which may have different significance in that individual's life. These are influenced by the individual's religious upbringing, cultural factors, specific life experiences, personality traits, etc. In general, spirituality involves awareness of a higher power and a relationship of harmony, peace, and tranquility, a way of understanding oneself and expressing personal satisfaction. It should be noted that spirituality cannot be offered as a cure, but it can act as a complement to specific treatments and contribute to the spiritual dimension of self-care in older people.

In addition, a growing body of research suggests that participation in religious activities influences spiritual well-being and may improve the general psychological well-being of older people. Their judgments of life satisfaction show that they are willing to participate in many spiritual activities to improve this dimension of self-care. Interestingly, the trend of increased spiritual growth and religious activity in older people continues in modern society, despite the significant secularization compared to 50 years ago. Given the issues of loss, physical illness, disability, and mortality that we face in old age, understanding an individual's spiritual perspective is increasingly important.

5.2 Spiritual Needs in Older People

The assessment of spiritual needs in older people has significantly advanced in recent years. Research has shown that spiritual or religious considerations and needs increase with life-threatening illness and old age. Additionally, research has argued that spirituality is a crucial source of coping with these conditions, and quality of life improves when spiritual needs are met and spiritual care is provided in appropriate ways for older individuals, thereby enhancing spiritual self-care.

When a need is fulfilled, joy, gratitude, satisfaction, and inner peace may result. However, when spiritual needs remain unmet for an extended period, feelings of giving up can lead to depression or emotional detachment. Therefore, assessing the spiritual needs of older people is essential to prevent such negative outcomes. Understanding the unmet spiritual needs of older individuals and the reasons behind them is necessary to prioritize and support the implementation of spiritual self-care.

Comprehensive biographical interviews have revealed that a person's spirituality is not a fixed state but an ongoing process that evolves at different stages of life. Some aspects may change in importance, as well as the significance of specific beliefs. The spiritual needs of older people are, therefore, defined differently at each stage of life. In general, a need indicates that something is missing, even if it cannot be precisely defined. Such needs can be physical, emotional, cognitive, psychosocial, behavioral, and spiritual. Therefore, spiritual needs suggest that there is a deficiency that may be felt and that compels the individual to seek meaning, cognitive, emotional, psychosocial, and behavioral satisfaction in their life, relationships, and experiences.

Spiritual needs and related issues are generally considered for older people, and these vary from person to person and in different circumstances. Addressing these needs helps to strengthen faith, peace of mind, and a sense of satisfaction with life.

Older people usually seek to strengthen their relationship with God and thus become closer to spirituality. For example, religious needs include praying, attending religious rituals, participating in religious ceremonies, and turning to a higher source. Older people need to be present in religious social environments, such as participating in religious gatherings and charitable activities. They are usually interested in passing on their religious and cultural values to future generations, which is pleasant for them. Older people may face problems such as illness, loss of loved ones, or feelings of loneliness. Religion can give them hope and strength to cope. Religious teachings can provide them with peace and reduce anxiety, fear of death, and worries related to aging. Attention to the existential needs of older people is related to deeper and more spiritual issues, including questions about the meaning of life, death, relationships with others, and identity, and is important for achieving spiritual self-care. These needs often become more important in old age, especially as one approaches the end of life. Finding and maintaining meaning in life, especially in the face of changes caused by retirement, the loss of loved ones, or a decrease in abilities, falls into this category of needs. Facing the reality of death and trying to accept it and find peace about the end of life and leaving the world are other spiritual needs that older people should be aware of. The need to have meaningful and deep relationships with others, especially family and friends, and a sense of belonging to a community or group that shares common values are important aspects of spiritual self-care. Having freedom in personal decision-making is very important. In this way, older people feel that they have the right to freedom and choice. Another important issue in examining the spiritual needs of older people, which should be given special attention, is participation in activities that give them a sense of purpose and usefulness, thus increasing their motivation in life and enhancing their quality of life. Inner peace is another spiritual need of older people that should be paid attention to. It refers to a mental and spiritual state in which a person feels calm, balanced, and accepting of themselves, life, and existing circumstances. Reviewing life and accepting decisions, successes, and failures, as well as feeling satisfied with the past life and coping with regrets, are necessary for inner peace in older people. Creating a positive perspective on old age and life after retirement, emotional peace, soothing conversations, focusing on the present moment and appreciating the small and beautiful things in life, creating social connections with others, and experiencing a connection with nature are among the needs that lead older people toward inner peace and spiritual self-care.

Another need is giving/generativity needs, which refers to the desire or necessity of giving to others and even oneself to achieve mental and emotional peace. This need becomes more important in old age because older people often go through life and may face regrets, resentments, or unresolved emotions that affect their mental and spiritual health. Self-forgiveness, which involves accepting oneself as a human being who has made mistakes and learned from these experiences, and forgiveness of others, which means letting go of negative emotions such as anger, resentment, or resentment toward people who may have harmed them, fall into this area. Giving solace is also one of the spiritual needs of older people, which, in the context of the need for forgiveness, means providing emotional support and comfort to a person who is involved in the process of forgiving themselves or others. This support helps older people to cope with difficult emotions such as anger, regret, guilt, or resentment and achieve mental and psychological peace.

5.3 The Impact of Spiritual Self-Care on Various Aspects of Older People's Lives

The effects of spirituality have been well-documented in numerous studies, which suggest that individuals with strong spiritual health demonstrate greater capabilities, resilience, self-control, and social support. For older people, spiritual self-care can cultivate a sense of integration and purpose, enriching their lives. Improved spiritual well-being also facilitates better adaptation to illness and life's challenges, fostering a more accepting approach to the later stages of life.

The benefits of spiritual self-care in older adults include reduced boredom, enhanced quality of life, increased longevity, alleviation of illness symptoms, and decreased feelings of loneliness and anxiety surrounding death. Below, we will categorize and outline the specific advantages of spiritual self-care.

5.4 Spiritual Self-Care Contributes to Physical Health

Many sources agree on the impact of spirituality on the ability to recover and on health- and disease-related conditions in older people. They suggest that progress in recovery is achieved more quickly with spirituality. Spirituality can enhance positive emotions and help neutralize negative emotions, acting as both a life-enhancing factor and a coping mechanism. Spiritual practices such as prayer, forgiveness, meditation, worship, and rituals, as well as spiritual guidance and self-care, have been found to be effective in reducing negative behaviors and improving physiological function. Spirituality also helps individuals cope better with adversity, whether external (such as harsh environmental conditions) or internal (such as genetic predisposition or vulnerability to mental disorders).

Studies have shown that attending spiritual ceremonies and engaging in spiritual self-care, both individually and in groups, can be somewhat protective for older people. Those who prioritize spiritual self-care report that using spirituality to strengthen their beliefs is very effective in their physical and mental recovery. Benefits of utilizing spirituality include gaining courage, learning how to cope with problems, embracing imperfection, believing in a higher power, understanding and accepting oneself better, transcending pain and suffering, and finding relaxation and coping mechanisms.

Research has shown that older people with HIV/AIDS consider spirituality a bridge between hopelessness, helplessness, and the meaning of life. Patients with HIV/AIDS tend to use spirituality to cope with their illness. Several studies have noted a significant relationship between spirituality and health-related outcomes. In the case of immunodeficiency diseases, it appears that the psychological health of older individuals, their coping mechanisms for stressors, social connections, and their beliefs and attitudes all play a significant role in the course of the disease. The results indicate that those who survive for an extended period tend to have significantly higher scores of spirituality compared to others.

Similarly, studies on older individuals with cancer have revealed that spiritual beliefs and practices contribute to promoting adaptation to cancer by addressing existential concerns such as the search for meaning in life and hope. They have also highlighted the importance of spiritual self-care in cancer treatment. Numerous studies on older cancer patients facing challenging conditions in terms of quality and meaning of life have shown that spirituality can be beneficial and effective. However, the fear of death may be easily triggered and can be somewhat controlled through spiritual self-care. The results of these studies have demonstrated that spirituality plays a crucial role when individuals are confronted with traumatic events.

Studies focusing on the significance of spiritual variables in cancer patients have concluded that these individuals find spiritual beliefs and spiritual self-care to be essential aspects of their lives that enhance their sense of worth. Some older individuals have reported that their spiritual self-care has increased significantly after being diagnosed with cancer compared to before the illness occurred. By incorporating spiritual self-care into their routines, they have generally experienced improvements in various aspects of their physical and mental health.

Studies have shown that individuals significantly associated with spirituality and health are less likely to experience health outcomes related to heart disease, such as myocardial infarction, and circulatory dysfunction, such as arterial hypertension or stroke. People who attend spiritual services frequently and engage in spiritual self-care practices like prayer, meditation, and scripture reading tend to have lower blood pressure. Additionally, various studies have found lower levels of C-reactive protein in individuals who practice spiritual self-care.

Furthermore, research has indicated that older adults who incorporate spiritual self-care into their routine may have a reduced incidence of atherosclerosis, leading to a decreased likelihood of developing cardiovascular disease in the future. Older adults who participate in spiritual self-care within groups and communities, engage in physical activity, attend social gatherings, and interact with others socially tend to have higher levels of physical activity and are less likely to be obese. As a result, they have lower risks of cardiovascular disease, high blood pressure, and high cholesterol.

Higher spirituality scores are associated with improved self-regulation and self-control, which leads to greater commitment to healthy behaviors such as regular exercise, balanced diets, and avoidance of harmful habits such as smoking and drug use. Studies have shown that spirituality protects against cardiovascular disease, largely by promoting health. There is growing interest in studying the role of spirituality on pain and functioning in people with chronic pain. Spirituality may reduce the negative effects of pain-related stressors, such as intensity and interference. Several studies have also shown that higher levels of spirituality are associated with better functioning, greater pain tolerance, and lower pain intensity. Spirituality influences how people interpret pain, which in turn influences their coping strategies. That is, having spirituality plays a role in shaping pain, how it is expressed, and how people evaluate their ability to cope with pain. This view is consistent with the interactional theory of stress and coping, which suggests that spirituality influences both primary appraisals (how pain is perceived) and secondary appraisals (evaluation of coping resources). Various studies also support this association, showing that people with higher spirituality experience less stress and tend to use more adaptive strategies. Spiritual self-care practices such as prayer, supplication, meditation, etc. have been associated with increased pain tolerance through positive cognitive reappraisal in older people. However, research on the relationship between spirituality, pain, functioning, and emotional responses is still emerging. Cultural factors also play an important role in how spirituality is associated with health outcomes, suggesting that findings from a study in one geographic region may not apply to another geographic region with a different culture.

There is a growing interest in studying the role of spirituality in pain and functioning among people with chronic pain. Spirituality may help reduce the negative effects of pain-related stressors, such as intensity and interference. Several studies have shown that higher levels of spirituality are linked to better functioning, increased pain tolerance, and lower pain intensity. Spirituality influences how individuals interpret pain, which in turn affects their coping strategies. In other words, spirituality plays a role in shaping how pain is experienced and expressed, as well as how individuals assess their ability to cope with pain. This perspective aligns with the interactional theory of stress and coping, which suggests that spirituality impacts both primary appraisals (perception of pain) and secondary appraisals (evaluation of coping resources). Numerous studies support this connection, indicating that individuals with higher levels of spirituality experience less stress and tend to utilize more adaptive strategies. Spiritual self-care practices, such as prayer, supplication, and meditation, have been associated with increased pain tolerance through positive cognitive reappraisal in older individuals. However, research on the relationship between spirituality, pain, functioning, and emotional responses is still developing. Cultural factors also play a crucial role in how spirituality influences health outcomes, implying that results from a study in one geographic region may not be applicable to another region with a different culture.

The role of spirituality in diabetes has been investigated as well. Spiritual growth and its dimensions in older people with diabetes can help them adapt to the stressful events of this disease. According to the theory of positive psychology, one effective treatment for increasing self-care in diabetic patients is the use of spirituality. Providing spiritual support for older people with diabetes, whose hope has been diminished by conventional treatment, can revive their hope for salvation. Controlling negative emotions that result from spirituality can be a suitable strategy for improving diabetes management in older people. The results of studies have shown that personal adjustment and self-care practices are related to spiritual beliefs, and spiritual beliefs are effective in choosing management strategies. Therefore, older people with diabetes can largely succeed in controlling diabetes by using spiritual self-care and applying this approach. Several studies have also indicated an increase in the immune system and in the number of white blood cells, such as neutrophils, lymphocytes, and monocytes, in older people with depression following spiritual therapy. Considering that spirituality is associated with better functioning of the autonomic nervous system, it has an impact on the physiology and health of the body by creating peace and hope and activating positive emotions. It also has a profound effect on the attitudes, beliefs, and behaviors of older people, as several studies have mentioned. The psycho-neuro-immuno-endocrine pathways and psychoneuroimmunology provide a framework for understanding the role of the mind over organic functions.

The brain performs these functions through autonomic efferent pathways that innervate active immune tissue and also through neuroendocrine hormones, such as corticotrophin-releasing hormone or substance P, which regulate cytokine balance, and these interactions are strongly modulated by psychological factors. Research has highlighted the importance of psychoneuroimmunological (PNI) factors in various diseases, demonstrating that emotional states and behaviors can significantly influence physiological functions and health outcomes. Chronic stress is associated with adverse biological processes that affect multiple organs and systems, which can ultimately reduce overall survival rates. Lifestyle choices and social stressors are important drivers of disease and affect lifespan. The stress response activates the sympathetic-adreno-medullary system and the hypothalamic-pituitary-adrenal axis, and cortisol is a key hormone in this process. Stress can lead to autonomic nervous system dysfunction and impair physical health. However, stress reduction techniques, particularly those involving belief systems, may help to reduce these physiological effects. Spiritual practices can positively influence multiple systems and promote autonomic balance by reducing sympathetic activity and enhancing parasympathetic activity. Engaging in spiritual self-care activities can enhance a sense of meaning in older adults' lives, helping individuals cope with hardships while increasing life satisfaction, optimism, and self-esteem. These practices are associated with virtues such as forgiveness, compassion, gratitude, wisdom, and altruism, all of which can help reduce the effects of stress and subsequent related illnesses and play a key role in older adults' lives.

Regular attendance by older adults (whether they are ill or not) at a religious or spiritual event can contribute to health stability through a variety of pathways, including modeling behavior, establishing social roles and interactions, or supporting a sense of self-esteem and purpose. Activities that encourage helping each other, such as volunteering, are common among older adults and have been shown to reduce mortality. The results of the study also show that spiritual beliefs and spiritual self-care of older people are significantly associated with a reduction in postoperative complications and mortality. Also, the use of spiritual self-care strategies has had a positive effect on increasing coping mechanisms to cope with the stress of surgery and illness and a sense of well-being at the end of the illness. Research indicates that spiritual self-care is effective for older people in managing various health conditions, including kidney and lung diseases, blood disorders, neurological issues, systemic lupus erythematosus, irritable bowel syndrome, musculoskeletal disorders, mental illness, bereavement, end-of-life challenges, general stress, and trauma from natural disasters or conflict. While definitive causality is not proven, there is strong evidence suggesting a causal relationship. Clinical and epidemiological studies reveal that seniors with strong spirituality enjoy better health and reduced healthcare needs. Furthermore, educating and incorporating spirituality enhances distress tolerance, resilience, spiritual experiences, positive coping skills, and overall quality of life among older people, contributing to improved mood. Thus, seniors and their families must prioritize and implement spiritual self-care both individually and in groups.

5.5 Spiritual Self-Care Is Essential for Mental Health

Mental health is crucial for overall well-being, encompassing emotional, psychological, and social aspects. It involves how individuals behave, perceive themselves, manage stress, and interpret life events. Older adults are especially susceptible to mental health issues, with one in five experiencing some form of mental illness later in life. Common disorders in this age group include depression, anxiety, and substance abuse, which can lead to disability and suicide, as well as high economic costs. The WHO has recognized mental health in older adults as a priority, yet it remains an area that is not fully addressed in medical science.

In the late nineteenth century, negative attitudes toward religion emerged in psychiatry and psychology, leading to the separation of religion from mental health care. This resulted in many patients' spiritual needs being overlooked. However, in recent decades, scientific research has started to explore the connection between spirituality/religion and mental health. Studies have shown a positive link between higher levels of spirituality/religion and lower rates of depression, suicide, and substance abuse. Individuals with strong spiritual beliefs often report better quality of life, increased optimism, and quicker recovery. Engaging in religious and spiritual activities has been shown to have a positive impact on mental health.

Therefore, acknowledging and addressing older adults' religious and spiritual beliefs can enhance their mental well-being. This section focuses on the importance of spiritual self-care in older adults and its impact on their mental health. Mental health decline is often associated with persistent negative emotions and thoughts in older people, which affects their quality of life. One strategy is to pay attention to spiritual self-care. Additionally, the detrimental effects of stress can be moderated by creating a spiritual support network and promoting healthy behaviors. This facilitates coping with stress by helping individuals understand the temporary nature of psychological distress and providing them with a sense of control. It also encourages older people to adopt health-promoting behaviors, which increases existential well-being.

Regarding depression, studies have shown that older people who practice spiritual self-care are less likely to experience depression and loneliness. Belief in a higher power as a source of comfort is associated with lower levels of depression. These findings suggest that embracing life with a belief in a divine presence, whether it be nature, energy, or God, may help reduce symptoms of depression in older adults.

Finding meaning in suffering is another way spirituality can help alleviate depression. Finding purpose in life is crucial for maintaining mental health and creating coherence in the lives of older individuals. This concept is a key component of many psychological theories. For example, in logotherapy, a form of psychotherapy developed by Frankl, finding meaning in life is seen as a fundamental motivator for humans. This perspective emphasizes taking control and responsibility for one's decisions rather than being passive.

Furthermore, the inability to find meaning in life can lead to various mental health issues, including depression. Erikson's theory of psychosocial development also supports the idea that older individuals who struggle to make sense of their life achievements may become frustrated, hopeless, and depressed.

Seniors can utilize spiritual self-care to find meaning in their lives through activities such as reading spiritual texts, meditating, praying, and engaging in community and spiritual events that provide a sense of purpose and fulfillment.

Spirituality plays a significant role in mental health, with ongoing research in the field. Studies on suicide among older individuals have shown that those with stronger spiritual beliefs are less likely to attempt suicide, as they have a greater sense of self-esteem, moral responsibility, and reduced feelings of loneliness. This suggests that spiritual self-care can be a protective factor against suicide among older adults.

Additionally, the findings on drug use mirror the original results on suicide. The studies have indicated that older individuals who participate in spiritual groups and incorporate a spiritual self-care dimension are less likely to engage in drug use. Spiritual components in self-help groups can also aid in recovery by building new social networks.

Furthermore, the research has demonstrated that spiritual self-care significantly reduces anxiety symptoms in older individuals. Anxiety in older adults may stem from physical and psychological changes, feelings of loneliness and isolation, confronting mortality, and a decrease in social roles. Anxiety, characterized by fear and apprehension, can lead to mental health issues if left unchecked. However, studies have shown that spirituality, which promotes healthy habits and discourages excessive consumption of harmful substances, can help manage anxiety and improve mental health in older individuals.

Moreover, understanding the connection between death anxiety and spirituality is crucial. Failing to grasp the meaning of life can create a psychologically stressful environment that exacerbates death anxiety. This concept was explored by Becker in the theory of death denial, which suggests that finding purpose in life serves as a defense mechanism against thoughts of mortality and, consequently, death anxiety.

Stress is a significant factor that affects the physical and mental health of older people. According to social experts, older individuals are one of the most vulnerable groups to various types of stress, second only to young people. Physical weaknesses and chronic diseases can be particularly stressful, leading to a lack of personal control and a decrease in life satisfaction. Older individuals who live alone often find themselves dwelling on thoughts of distant children, missing their deceased spouse, financial problems, and more. This isolation can easily lead to increased stress and depression. However, the absence of stress is a key indicator of good mental health. Spiritual resources among older individuals are considered crucial for adaptation during the aging process.

For instance, taking care of physical health with healthy nutrition, regular exercise, and sufficient sleep is important. Additionally, strengthening mental health through communication with family and friends, engaging in group spiritual activities, attending spiritual ceremonies, and more can be beneficial.

Studies have also shown that spiritual education can reduce psychological stress and increase distress tolerance and resilience in older individuals. Utilizing spiritual self-care can improve quality of life, happiness, and life expectancy while reducing psychological trauma and helping individuals adapt to circumstances, loneliness, depression, anxiety, and feelings of loneliness. It is evident that only a small number of older adults possess adequate psychological resilience and can adapt to age-related changes, with most feeling helpless when faced with challenging situations. Group and individual spirituality therapy has been found to be effective in enhancing the psychological resilience of older adults.

Psychological well-being is a complex construct that depends on emotional state, personality traits, and life experiences. Research indicates that spirituality can have a positive impact on the psychological well-being of older adults by influencing perceived control, positive emotions, social support, and coping mechanisms.

5.6 Enhancing Social Connections Through Spiritual Self-Care in Older People

Natural changes in older individuals lead to a decrease in their social roles and health status. These changes often result in job loss and feelings of disability, which can negatively impact their social interactions. Social interaction is a fundamental aspect of society that continues throughout one's life. Maintaining social connections can have a positive effect on the quality of life for older individuals, as it helps combat feelings of loneliness and isolation. Increased participation in society can also alleviate many of their concerns. Conversely, reduced social interaction can lead to feelings of isolation and depression, significantly impacting the overall quality of life for older individuals.

Various factors contribute to the quality of life for older individuals, including their relationship with their environment, physical health, psychosocial well-being, and level of independence. Social interaction, being a basic human need, not only enhances the quality of life for older individuals but also fosters a sense of belonging and connection with others. Engaging in social activities with a spiritual component can further improve their quality of life and overall health. These activities not only strengthen human relationships but also enhance spiritual self-care for older individuals.

Older individuals who maintain positive social interactions can uphold their social status through their social skills and experience a greater sense of belonging within social groups. One form of social interaction for older individuals involves spirituality, as it fosters human connections and can lead to increased happiness and satisfaction. Recognizing the significance of social interaction, researchers suggest that offering training courses to improve social skills in older individuals and focusing on spiritual activities can positively impact their quality of life. These initiatives can help expand human relationships, strengthen communication with a higher power, and ultimately enhance the overall well-being of older individuals.

Spiritual practices impact the health of older people through both tangible and intangible social support. Tangible support includes resources like financial assistance, transportation, and participation in spiritual group activities. Intangible support involves trust and a sense of belonging that comes from group membership. Spiritual community institutions and activities such as spiritual reading gatherings, sharing experiences, prayer, and meditation serve as self-care strategies that promote interaction, combat social isolation, and offer assistance during challenging times for older individuals. This collective participation strengthens family and social bonds, enhancing older people's sense of belonging and self-esteem. Providing social support to others in the community can act as a stress buffer for older individuals, and creating social interactions by helping others may reduce stress more effectively than receiving help. Active aging is a process that aims to improve the quality of life for older people by maximizing opportunities for health, social interactions, and security. Engaging in physical and social activities helps older individuals maintain their physical and cognitive abilities, fostering a sense of control over their lives and society, and influencing decision-making processes on important issues affecting older adults.

The results of the studies show that the effect of spiritual self-care on the social interactions of older people is well-known. For example, the meaningfulness of social relationships achieved through spiritual self-care is very important. Older people who benefit from spiritual self-care make their social relationships deeper and more meaningful. Their connections with others are often accompanied by feelings of empathy, forgiveness, and mutual respect, creating more stable relationships. Strengthening mental health in social interactions is another issue that many studies have pointed out. Spirituality can help older people be more patient and receptive when facing problems and challenges in social relationships. This reduces tension and increases the quality of interactions. The creation of spiritual social networks has also been of interest for a long time. Joining spiritual or religious groups, such as prayer groups or meditation sessions, provides opportunities for seniors to expand their social circles. In addition to providing spiritual support, these groups offer a platform for friendly interactions and new social connections. Increased social resilience is another benefit of spiritual self-care. Spiritual self-care helps seniors gain a deeper understanding of their own and others' social situations. This resilience allows them to meet new people with a broader perspective and enjoy social interactions. For seniors, spiritual self-care can be a way to find meaning and purpose in life, as well as improve social interactions.

5.7 Daily Practices for Nurturing Spiritual Self-Care in Older People

There are many ways to promote spiritual self-care in seniors, whether individually or in groups. For example, encouraging group spiritual activities such as attending religious services, meditation or yoga sessions, and forming spiritual book study groups can be beneficial. Using technology for spiritual social connections has also gained attention these days with the advancement of technology. Seniors can use social networks, video calls, or webinars to participate in online spiritual programs. Emphasis on volunteer activities with a spiritual approach is also of interest. For example, participating in charitable activities and helping others can strengthen a sense of meaning and purpose in seniors and create more opportunities for social interactions. Scheduling regular interactions with family and friends for spiritual self-care is very effective. Seniors can invite family members to discuss spiritual topics. Creating a schedule for regular meetings with friends and discussing calming topics can help seniors speak more about the issues that are causing them stress and anxiety and can reduce their isolation and loneliness. Reading books that emphasize spirituality and human values can foster a sense of peace and spiritual connection. Participating in charitable activities is also encouraged. Helping others not only strengthens a sense of meaning but also leads to greater social connection. Finding time to reflect and connect with nature is also beneficial. Nature is a rich source of spirituality. Seniors can experience deeper peace by taking a walk in nature, listening to the birds, or enjoying a sunrise. A quiet, loving environment for worship, meditation, or spiritual learning can significantly enhance seniors' well-being and promote spiritual self-care. Many seniors experience feelings of isolation, anxiety about mortality, or hopelessness as they age. Spiritual counseling can help alleviate these problems by providing a safe environment to share feelings and emphasize the positive elements of life, thereby reducing stress, anxiety, and depression.

Spiritual guidance is a beneficial process that helps seniors understand the importance of life, manage problems, and strengthen their spiritual connection. This guidance may include detailed discussions about personal beliefs, spiritual principles, and life purpose, which ultimately helps seniors increase their spiritual care. Spiritual guidance can help seniors discover new meaning at this stage by getting involved in charitable work, attending religious events, or supporting others, thereby strengthening their sense of purpose and significance in their lives. Spiritual connections enable individuals to cope more effectively with life's challenges and experience greater satisfaction in their lives, which increases their overall quality of life. Consider spiritual support programs, such as weekly gatherings to talk about spiritual matters. Prayer or group prayer. It is equally significant for seniors. These services aim to improve the spiritual and social connections of older adults and can be provided in a variety of settings, including private residences, nursing homes, or within the community. For example, spiritual retreats often include activities such as coordinated prayer, meditation, or reading of scripture. These initiatives not only encourage a sense of calm but also allow older adults to interact with others and experience a stronger sense of community. Research shows that many older adults may lack knowledge of effective self-care techniques. Practices such as meditation, deep breathing, and mindfulness can help reduce stress levels and increase focus. Holding hands-on classes to learn relaxation techniques can be a good solution. Creating support networks where older adults can share their spiritual experiences can be very effective. These programs may include social gatherings or group visits to religious sites. Some studies have shown that personal spiritual care also plays an important role in spiritual self-care. These services, usually provided in person, online, or by phone by spiritual counselors or psychologists with spiritual expertise, allow seniors to talk about their spiritual questions or concerns and receive specific guidance. The use of spiritual self-care is also associated with many positive outcomes that have been noted in numerous studies: increased self-confidence in interpersonal relationships, alleviating feelings of loneliness and isolation, creating a sense of participation in a broader community, strengthening family and friendship relationships, spiritual growth, and peace of mind in social interactions. Spiritual self-care also helps seniors maintain their independence in managing the spiritual aspects of their lives.

5.8 Arts-Based Spiritual Self-Care in Older People

The arts offer powerful alternative avenues for expression and healing and have long been associated with the sacred. As Picasso once said, "Art washes the dust of everyday life from the soul." Integrating art with spiritual care has the potential to incorporate the spiritual dimensions of care for diverse populations. This scoping review provides an overview of art-based spiritual care approaches in healthcare. Art and spirituality have been close allies throughout history in many faith and healing traditions and continue to be so today. A growing body of literature is emerging on the effectiveness and meaningfulness of arts-based initiatives not only for older adults but also for people of all ages seeking healing and spiritual self-care. These initiatives are creative therapies with a strong nonverbal component, such as art therapy, music therapy, dance therapy, and drama therapy. Each of these creative arts therapies has distinct training, theoretical foundations, processes, and professional identities that have evolved over time. For example, art therapy focuses on the visual arts and was originally based on art and psychological theories, but its theoretical underpinnings now include psychodynamic, humanistic, developmental, and family therapy perspectives. In addition, the field of expressive arts therapies encompasses a multidisciplinary approach, such as "visual arts, movement, drama, music, writing, and other creative processes to foster deep personal growth and community development." These are distinct from performing arts that are performed for an audience. Additionally, social or community art practices can have emancipatory goals and involve creative collaboration between artists, social institutions, and people and communities to strengthen social connections, embody and mobilize social action, or revive cultural traditions, all in the interest of promoting spiritual self-care in older adults. Research indicates that the arts enhance expression and transformation, aiding individuals in coping with illness, promoting well-being, supporting recovery, and ensuring older adults age successfully. The WHO affirms that the arts foster health, prevent mental and physical conditions, offer effective treatments for both acute and chronic issues, and affect social health determinants. There is a growing interest in integrating spiritual care and the arts as psychosocial-spiritual interventions in healthcare. The arts serve as a multisensory medium for expression and communication, significantly influencing spiritual well-being through various forms, including images, music, poetry, and storytelling. Art can be a tool for seniors to connect with their spiritual side, helping them cope better with life's challenges such as loneliness, illness, or the loss of loved ones, and find hope and inner peace. Seniors may not use words alone to express their spiritual feelings or thoughts; the arts, such as painting, music, or poetry, can be a language through which they communicate their inner messages to the world. Many seniors feel closer to God or the universe by creating images related to nature or spiritual concepts. Listening to or playing soothing music can enhance spiritual experiences and provide a space for meditation and reflection. Artistic activities, such as calligraphy, pottery, or drawing, focus seniors' minds on the present moment, reducing worries about the past or future and increasing connection with the present, a key aspect of spiritual self-care. Art allows seniors to continue feeling creative and make a meaningful impact, adding more meaning to their daily lives and strengthening their sense of self-worth. Art activities can also serve as a physical form of meditation or prayer. For example, calligraphy of religious verses promotes mental focus and spiritual peace.

Creating artwork with spiritual concepts, such as paintings inspired by religious or mystical ideas, is another form of spiritual self-care. Spiritual self-care goes beyond just connecting with oneself. Art can also connect seniors to communities that hold similar values. Engaging in art groups, exhibitions, or creative workshops can enhance a sense of unity and social support.

Box 5.1 Recommendations for Family Caregivers and Older Adults on Spiritual Self-Care

1. *Understand the Spiritual Needs of Seniors:*
   Seniors and their caregivers should be aware of the senior's beliefs, values, and spiritual needs.
   Listen empathetically to the senior's spiritual concerns and support them without judgment.
2. *Create a Positive Spiritual Environment:*
   Provide a quiet and inspiring space for prayer, meditation, or reading spiritual texts.
   Facilitate access to places of worship or online/physical religious programs.
3. *Support Social and Spiritual Activities:*
   Encourage participation in spiritual groups, yoga classes, or charitable programs.
   Use art, music, or poetry to enhance their sense of spirituality.
4. *Strengthen Emotional Connections:*
   Help maintain relationships with family and friends to strengthen their sense of belonging.
   Assist them in joining groups that share similar spiritual or social goals.
5. *Encourage Daily Spiritual Practices:*
   Encourage them to engage in daily activities such as meditation, gratitude journaling, or reading scripture.

Recommendations for Older Adults

1. *Dedicate time daily for reflection, prayer, or meditation.*

2. *Evaluate and reinforce your personal values and life philosophy.*
3. *Engage in artistic activities like painting, music, or poetry to encourage peace and spirituality.*
4. *List three things you appreciate every day.*
5. *Demonstrate kindness and gratitude to the people around you.*
6. *Become a member of social or spiritual organizations and participate in significant interactions.*
7. *Devote meaningful moments to family and friends.*
8. *Take a stroll in the outdoors or practice yoga to blend physical and mental well-being.*
9. *To enhance your energy and concentration, consume a nutritious diet and ensure adequate rest.*
10. *Explore spiritual literature or engage in spiritual learning initiatives to enhance your spiritual understanding.*
11. *Engage in charitable efforts or assist those who are less fortunate to foster a feeling of purpose and satisfaction.*

5.9 Summary of the Chapter

This chapter explores the concept of spiritual self-care in older people, their spiritual needs, the impact of spiritual self-care on various aspects of their lives (physical, mental, and social), the influence of art on spiritual self-care in older individuals, and daily practices for nurturing spiritual self-care in this population.

Older people often encounter challenges like anxiety, loneliness, memory loss, and retirement, which can result in issues such as depression, reduced quality of life, and increased anxiety. Spirituality can serve as a source of support, providing meaning, purpose, social support, stress reduction, and enhanced hope for older individuals.

Numerous studies have been conducted on spiritual self-care for older people, demonstrating that activities like engaging in social and spiritual ceremonies, meditation, prayer, contemplation, and helping others can enhance their quality of life. These activities not only alleviate symptoms of depression, anxiety, loneliness, and isolation but also foster feelings of hope and optimism, with positive effects on physical health.

In conclusion, readers are encouraged to utilize the information in this chapter to develop programs that enhance spirituality and spiritual self-care in older adults, taking practical steps to bring about positive changes in this area. Spiritual self-care in older adults not only enhances their well-being but also contributes to the creation of a society where older individuals experience fewer physical and mental health challenges.

5.10 Summary of Research Studies

An article titled “Importance of Spirituality in the Lives of Older People” was written in 2020 by Arti Kumari and Sheela Sangwan. This review article specifically focuses on the importance of spirituality for older individuals. In old age, spirituality becomes increasingly important due to various challenges such as physical illnesses, disabilities, loss of loved ones, loneliness, depression, and mortality. The study found that spirituality plays a vital role in managing chronic diseases and improving the overall quality of life for older adults. Regular participation in spiritual activities was linked to better health outcomes and quality of life. Additionally, engaging in spiritual practices like yoga and meditation was associated with improved sleep quality and a reduction in chronic disorders among older individuals.

A study titled “Benefits of Spirituality for Older People: A Literature Review” was conducted in 2021 by Lilyana, Maria Theresia Arie, et al. This study aimed to explore how spirituality impacts the ability of older adults to cope with and accept the changes that come with aging. The review highlighted the importance of incorporating spiritual care into support systems for older individuals, as it can significantly enhance their quality of life. Spirituality was found to help older adults cope better during times of illness or loss and contribute to overall life satisfaction. The authors concluded that spirituality has a positive influence on the physical and mental health of older adults.

A study titled "The Meaning and Role of Spirituality for Older Adults: A Qualitative Study" was conducted in 2020 by Yuksel Can Oz et al.

This study aimed to understand how individuals perceive the meaning and impact of religion and spirituality as they age. Through semi-structured interviews with 19 adults aged 65–88, the study identified four main themes: the meaning of spirituality, spiritual practices, the impact of spirituality, and the meaning of aging for the individual. Participants viewed aging as a process that increased social interaction, compassion, and helping behaviors. The study suggested that spirituality plays a crucial role in guiding the lives of older adults, helping them find meaning and cope with challenges. Spiritual support was also found to promote positive emotions and help older individuals manage stress. The authors recommended organizing training programs to raise awareness among health professionals about the spiritual needs of older adults.

A study titled "Social Interaction Using Spirituality Therapy to Improve the Quality of Life of Older People in the Community" was conducted in 2022 by Wachidah Yuniartika et al. This study aimed to assess the effectiveness of social interaction as a therapy to enhance the quality of life of older individuals. Reduced social interaction among older adults can lead to feelings of isolation, which may result in depression and impact their quality of life. The study, conducted in Gedongan Village, Baki District, Sukabumi Regency, Central Java Province, involved 40 respondents in a quasi-experimental design with pretest-posttest measurements and a control group. Social interaction therapy involved group sermons by an Islamic teacher, leading to improved quality of life for older individuals. The results indicated that social interaction using spiritual therapy can enhance the quality of life for older adults. The authors recommended incorporating spiritual approaches to improve social interaction as part of a comprehensive care program.

5.11 Critical Thinking (Scenario-Based)

5.11.1 Case Scenario 1

Emily, a 70-year-old woman who lives in a small house, starts her day with a simple spiritual practice. She sits in silence, takes a few minutes to breathe deeply, and writes thoughtful sentences in her journal about life, love, and gratitude. After breakfast, she reads books about higher powers, transcendence, and spirituality to expand her thoughts. She then meditates or focuses on gratitude in the present moment, trying to do each activity with mindfulness. Throughout the day, she engages in simple tasks like cooking or gardening with full attention.

In the evenings, she joins a small social group where people discuss their life experiences, meanings, and ways to maintain peace and hope. Before bed, she reflects on the meaningful moments of the day and writes about things that brought her peace.

Challenges in this scenario:

1. Lack of awareness of spiritual self-care techniques among seniors.
2. Loneliness and lack of support groups lead to feelings of isolation.
3. Loss of motivation or hope due to negative past experiences or physical conditions.
4. Physical or mental limitations hindering seniors from performing activities or focusing.
5. Difficulty in creating a quiet space for spiritual practices for seniors living in crowded or urban environments.

Critical Questions

1. Can spiritual self-care alone fulfill the emotional needs of older adults?

2. How can older adults living alone be motivated to engage in spiritual practices?
3. Can spiritual practices substitute social and emotional needs for older adults?
4. How can older adults with physical or mental limitations benefit from spirituality?
5. What role do family and community play in supporting older adults in spiritual self-care, and what measures are needed to strengthen these supports?

5.11.2 Case Scenario 2

David, a 68-year-old retired man, lives with his wife in a small apartment. Since retiring, he has established a routine to balance his body, mind, and spirit. He starts his mornings with gentle exercises and breathing exercises to bring calmness. He sets spiritual and psychological goals in a notebook for the day, including kindness, appreciation of small moments, and staying calm in challenging situations.

David reads books on philosophy and history to gain a deeper understanding of life. In the evenings, he and his wife take walks in the park, discussing their feelings and concerns. They also attend group sessions at a local community center where they engage in conversations about life's meaning, stress management, and gratitude.

Challenges in this scenario:

1. Limited access to social resources.
2. Family conflicts or lack of communication hindering emotional support.
3. Cognitive changes affecting engagement in activities like reading or mindfulness.
4. Resistance to change due to old habits or limiting beliefs.
5. Financial constraints preventing participation in activities like classes or social gatherings.

Critical Questions

1. How can we help seniors who do not have access to support groups for financial or geographical reasons?
2. Can social interactions be an adequate substitute for other spiritual dimensions?
3. What methods can be used to attract seniors who are not interested in new practices?
4. Can spiritual and psychological activities affect the improvement of family relationships in seniors? How?
5. How can we provide appropriate educational resources for spiritual and psychological self-care to seniors?

Bibliography

Anyfantakis D, Symvoulakis EK, Panagiotakos DB, Tsetis D, Castanas E, Shea S, et al. Impact of religiosity/spirituality on biological and preclinical markers related to cardiovascular disease. Results from the SPILI III study. Hormones. 2013;12:386–96.

Bae SM. Factors associated with depressive symptoms among older people Koreans: the role of health status, work ability, financial problems, living alone, and family relationships. Psychogeriatrics. 2020;20(3):304–9.

Becker E. (2024). Denial of death. Kepustakaan Populer Gramedia. (Original work first published 1973 by Free Press Paperbacks, USA; first published 2011 in Great Britain by Souvenir Press; this edition first published 2020 by Souvenir Press, an imprint of Profile Books Ltd, London).ISBN: 978-1-78816-426-9 (print), 978-0-28564-007-8

Best M, Butow P, Olver I. Do patients want doctors to talk about spirituality? A systematic literature review. Patient Educ Couns. 2015;98(11):1320–8.

Braam AW, Koenig HG. Religion, spirituality and depression in prospective studies: a systematic review. J Affect Disord. 2019;257:428–38.

Büssing A, Spalek R, Pikuła NG, Frick E, & Surzykiewicz J. (2021). Spiritual needs of older people. In Spiritual needs in research and practice: The spiritual needs questionnaire as a global resource for health and social care (pp. 369–395). Springer Nature Switzerland AG https://doi.org/10.1007/978-3-030-70139-0

Coelho-Júnior HJ, Calvani R, Panza F, Allegri RF, Picca A, Marzetti E, et al. Religiosity/spirituality and mental health in older adults: a systematic review and meta-analysis of observational studies. Front Med. 2022;9:877213.

Erikson EH. (1998). The life cycle completed (extended version) (Vol. 1). W. W. Norton & Company. Retrieved from https://philpapers.org/rec/ERITLC

Fegg MJ, Kramer M, Bausewein C, Borasio GD. Meaning in life in the Federal Republic of Germany: results of a representative survey with the Schedule for Meaning in Life Evaluation (SMiLE). Health Qual Life Outcomes. 2007;5:1–8.

Ferreira-Valente A, Damião C, Pais-Ribeiro J, Jensen MP. The role of spirituality in pain, function, and coping in individuals with chronic pain. Pain Med. 2020;21(3):448–57.

Foong HF, Hamid TA, Ibrahim R, Haron SA. The association between religious orientation and life satisfaction in older adults living with morbidity and multimorbidity: a gender perspective in Malaysia. Psychogeriatrics. 2020;20(6):891–9.

Fradelos EC, Tzavella F, Koukia E, Papathanasiou IV, Alikari V, Stathoulis J, et al. Integrating chronic kidney disease patient's spirituality in their care: health benefits and research perspectives. Mater Sociomed. 2015;27(5):354.

Frankl VE. (1985). Man's search for meaning: An introduction to logotherapy (4th ed., Part One translated by Use Lasch; Preface by Gordon W. Allport). Beacon Press. (Original work published 1946)

Gallardo-Peralta LP. The relationship between religiosity/spirituality, social support, and quality of life among older people Chilean people. Int Soc Work. 2017;60(6):1498–511.

Giancarlo Lucchetti MS, Peres MFP, Damiano RF, editors. Spirituality, religiousness and health. From research to clinical practice. Cham: Springer; 2019. isbn:978-3-030-21220-9; 265 Seiten; Preis: D 106, 99€(Hardcover); ISBN: 978-3-030-21221-6 E-Book 58, 84€. De Gruyter; 2022

Guerrero-Castañeda RF, Menezes TMO, Prado ML, Galindo-Soto JA. Spirituality and religiosity for the transcendence of the older people being. Rev Bras Enferm. 2019;72:259–65.

Hajihasani M, Naderi N. Death anxiety in the older people: the role of spiritual health and perceived social support. Aging Psychology. 2021;6(4):319–09.

Hayward D, & Krause N. (2014). Religion, mental health and well-being: Social aspects. In Religion, personality, and social behavior (pp. 255–280). Psychology Press. (1st ed., 2013). eBook ISBN: 9780203125359.

Heidari M, Ghodusi Borujeni M, Kabirian Abyaneh S, Rezaei P. The effect of spiritual care on perceived stress and mental health among the elderlies living in nursing home. J Relig Health. 2019;58:1328–39.

Jung JH. Attachment to god and death anxiety in later life: does race matter? Res Aging. 2018;40(10):956–77.

Khaleghipour S, Masjedi M, Ahmadi Z. Effectiveness of Islamic spiritual therapy on the lifestyle and the percentage of the white blood cells in the aged depressed people. J Res Psychol Health. 2016;10(3):16–29.

Kucinskas J, Wright BR, Ray DM, Ortberg J. States of spiritual awareness by time, activity, and social interaction. J Sci Study Relig. 2017;56(2):418–37.

Kumari A, Sangwan S. Importance of spirituality in the life of older people. Indian J Health Wellbeing. 2020;11(4–6):173–5.

McCombe G, Fogarty F, Swan D, Hannigan A, Fealy GM, Kyne L, et al. Identified mental disorders in older adults in primary care: a cross-sectional database study. Eur J Gen Pract. 2018;24(1):84–91.

Mitchell UA, Gutierrez-Kapheim M, Nguyen AW, Al-Amin N. Hopelessness among middle-aged and older Blacks: the negative impact of discrimination and protecting power of social and religious resources. Innov Aging. 2020;4(5):igaa044.

Mohammadi M, Alavi M, Bahrami M, Zandieh Z. Assessment of the relationship between spiritual and social health and the self-care ability of older people referred to community health centers. Iran J Nurs Midwifery Res. 2017;22(6):471.

Rieger KL, Reimer-Kirkham S, Burton B, Howell B, Liuta N, Sharma S, et al. Arts-based spiritual care in healthcare: a participatory, scoping review. Arts Psychother. 2023;84:102027.

Rosmarin DH, Koenig HG. Handbook of spirituality, religion, and mental health. London: Academic; 2020.

Sinha P, Hussain T, Boora NK, Rao GN, Varghese M, Gururaj G, et al. Prevalence of common mental disorders in older adults: results from the National Mental Health Survey of India. Asian J Psychiatr. 2021;55:102463.

Straßner C, Frick E, Stotz-Ingenlath G, Buhlinger-Göpfarth N, Szecsenyi J, Krisam J, et al. Holistic care program for older patients to integrate spiritual needs, social activity, and self-care into disease management in primary care (HoPES3): study protocol for a cluster-randomized trial. Trials. 2019;20:1–11.

Sytsma TT, Schmelkin LA, Jenkins SM, Lovejoy LA, Lapid MI, Piderman KM. "Keep the faith": spirituality as a contributor to resiliency in five older people people. J Relig Spiritual Aging. 2018;30(4):314–24.

Turner M. Can the effects of religion and spirituality on both physical and mental health be scientifically measured? An overview of the key sources, with particular reference to the teachings of Said Nursi. J Relig Health. 2015;54:2045–51.

Watkins YJ, Quinn LT, Ruggiero L, Quinn MT, Choi Y-K. Spiritual and religious beliefs and practices and social support's relationship to diabetes self-care activities in African Americans. Diabetes Educ. 2013;39(2):231–9.

Yuniartika W, Kartinah K, Sudaryanto A. Social interaction using spirituality therapy to improve the quality of life of the older people in the community. Evid Based Care. 2023;13(2):65–74.

The Role of Technology in the Self-Care of Older People

6

Fatemeh Bahramnezhad and Ali Khanipour-Kencha

In the end, the learner should be able to:

- Understand the impact of technology on self-care practices and overall well-being among older adults
- Identify key and emerging technology tools and applications that facilitate self-care in older people
- Select appropriate and usable technologies given the case scenarios, considering the conditions and limitations of older adults, and provide suitable technology-based solutions to help them and their families promote self-care behaviors and ensure safety
- Encourage caregivers, family members, and older adults themselves to adopt appropriate technology as a tool to improve self-care and independence
- Analyze the potential benefits and barriers to adopting technologies for self-care in the older people population
- Express ethical concerns, such as the loss of independence and privacy, related to the use of technology in elder care
- Explore real-world applications of successfully integrating technology into older adults' self-care routines

Older people need to engage in continuous and sustainable self-care practices. Chronic illnesses become more common as people age, with each disease requiring set conditions and care to manage. Patients are hence obliged to actively participate in personalized self-care. Furthermore, aging is often associated with deteriorating physical or cognitive conditions, encouraging the need for innovative approaches to support older people's self-care. It is necessary to provide independent living at home for vulnerable older people, as care for them is becoming a major social challenge and imposes high costs on the health care system. "Based on the World Health Organization (WHO) definition, long-term care (LTC) services are defined as services to ensure that people with or at risk of considerable loss of physical and mental capacity can maintain a functional ability consistent with their fundamental rights, freedoms, and human dignity" These services, provided by unpaid caregivers (mostly family and volunteers) and paid care workers, cover home, community, and facility (long-term residence) care. Care facilities include nursing homes or other group living facilities. Providing efficient and cost-effective home care services requires major changes in the current methods of monitoring and providing care to recipients. LTC services help people perform their daily activities and encourage social participation and management of chronic diseases. In other words, LTC provides various services designed to meet the chronic health and personal care needs of those

F. Bahramnezhad (✉) · A. Khanipour-Kencha
Tehran University of Medical Sciences, Tehran, Iran
e-mail: bahramnezhad@tums.ac.ir

F. Bahramnezhad (ed.), *Self-Care in the Elderly*, https://doi.org/10.1007/978-981-96-9021-3_6

who can no longer perform daily activities independently.

Healthcare providers providing LTC are facing some challenges in meeting the increased needs of older adults and their families owing to the significant increase in the older people population and the increasing burden of chronic diseases. LTC providers are often involved in duplicate tasks, many of which involve physical work, leading to a high risk of job stress, physical or emotional fatigue, burnout, and high mobility. All of these lead to poor quality of care. Thus, innovative solutions are required to meet the healthcare needs of LTC home residents and reduce the workload of healthcare providers.

Maintaining continuity of care for older people comes with several challenges. One of these challenges raised by today's modern life is the physical separation of some older people from their families. Additionally, family members might not be able to provide long-term or even routine supervision or assistance with the self-care activities of their older people. This is a very critical stage where advancing technologies can assist seniors and their families in initiating and improving self-care processes, alleviating barriers experienced by older individuals, and ultimately improving their self-care to make it a more enjoyable experience.

In other words, countries should meet the healthcare needs of the current and future older people population through innovative solutions and new technologies to achieve the Decade of Healthy Aging goals. We live in a time when technology is in its prime and continuing to grow at a rapid pace. The past few years, especially in the aftermath of the COVID-19 pandemic, have highlighted the growing significance of contemporary technologies—particularly Internet-based methods—in various therapeutic and caregiving contexts. Therefore, in our modern age, with the increasing penetration and promising scope of technology as a supportive and complementary strategy, healthcare practitioners are experiencing an ever-increasing number of patients who seek health information and communication through the Internet. In many developed countries, the application of technological support in medical consultations and health promotion can now be considered a common practice. Recent studies on home services for older people's care have been classified into different categories, including telehealth, artificial intelligence (AI), rehabilitation robots, mobile applications, and health monitoring.

On the other hand, family members often serve as the primary source of support for older people experiencing chronic illnesses and disabilities. According to estimates, 18.2% of the adult population in the United States, or about 43.5 million Americans, provided care to an adult relative in 2015. Of these, approximately 34.2 million were anticipated to be caring for people 50 years of age or older. Nonetheless, it is anticipated that by 2060, there will be a greater need for informal elder care providers than there are available. Family caregivers, unlike professional caregivers, usually assume this role without any official training or preparation, which leads to some difficulties related to caring responsibilities. Furthermore, the prolonged caregiving process typically imposes significant physical, psychological, emotional, social, and economic burdens on family caregivers, leading to considerable caregiving strain. Technologies have become an invaluable means of aiding caregivers in their duties as well as improving self-care practices among older people and members of the family. Examples of technologies that can help caregivers overcome some of these obstacles include robotic assistants for daily tasks, predictive analytics for identifying health risks, and AI-driven chatbots for companionship.

These advancements have improved caregiving services and eliminated temporal and spatial limitations inherent in traditional care models. In other words, technology has the potential to revolutionize older people's empowerment process and significantly impact their ongoing self-care practices. The integration of cutting-edge technologies into empowerment programs can encompass various aspects, including telehealth, social media, and streamlined communication devices, all of which facilitate the self-care process and its monitoring. This development has provided elders and their caregivers with numerous opportunities and diverse options to enhance self-care skills, although it may also present certain advantages and disadvantages. In this section, we will explore related concepts and their applications in older people's self-care, despite occasional difficulties in delineating clear boundaries between different technologies. We will also consider the opportunities and challenges they present, supported by recent studies conducted in this field.

6.1 Telehealth

The direct delivery of clinical care, including diagnosis, treatment, or consultation, using telecommunications and distant technology is known as *telehealth*. This concept dates back to the early 1900s and is an example of how new technology is being used to assist and deliver healthcare services. It includes a broad variety of remote services, such as patient care, education, and monitoring.

Many patients seek healthcare information online before or after their physician's appointments in light of access to the Internet. It is estimated that 69% of patients use the Internet first when searching for health information, and 35% of US adults use Internet resources to diagnose their medical conditions. Integrating telehealth with conventional outpatient and inpatient treatments has the potential to lower healthcare expenses while improving the quality of care, given the present unstable trends in rising medical prices and the growing demand for high-quality healthcare. Enhancing health outcomes, increasing patient participation, and improving access to treatment are the main goals of telehealth, especially for communities that might encounter obstacles to traditional healthcare methods. Telehealth is a comprehensive concept that encompasses a broad spectrum of activities, including telemedicine, telecare, telemonitoring, tele-empowerment, telerehabilitation, virtual consultations (text, audio, or video), Internet health communications, remote support networks, electronic health (e-health), and mobile health applications (m-health).

Despite being discussed in medicine for many decades, the integration of this concept into healthcare has progressed relatively slowly. Nonetheless, the COVID-19 pandemic has created opportunities for incorporating telehealth into healthcare systems by highlighting the optimal benefits of remote care and bringing innovative healthcare techniques to the public's notice. Telehealth involves providing procedures, examinations, and instructions through remote access and improving communication between patients and healthcare providers via smartphones or other devices. In this regard, the decision regarding whether in-person visits to a medical facility are necessary can be made on a case-by-case basis.

In recent years, seniors have been able to communicate with medical specialists from the comfort of their own homes using telehealth, which has completely changed their access to healthcare. This concept includes any method or piece of technology that provides healthcare remotely. Figure 6.1 depicts various telehealth applications in older people's self-care.

In this regard, the *Home Health* project is an advanced project in digital health and telecare. It aims to examine ways to enhance digital health infrastructure to improve patient care and evaluate new digital health interventions. Many tools apply AI methods to utilize collected symptom and clinical status measurement data to determine the patient's need for an earlier appoint-

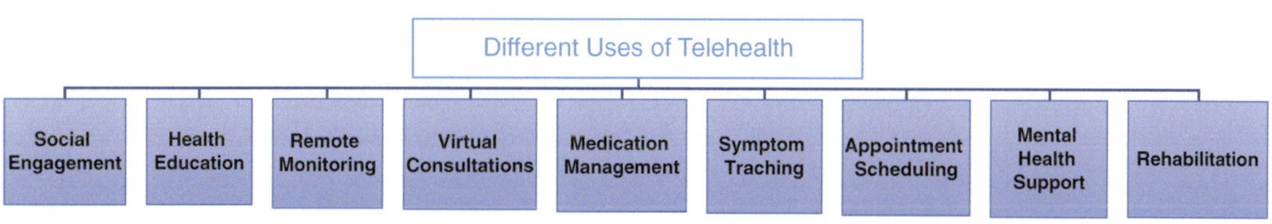

Fig. 6.1 Some applications of telehealth for older people's self-care

ment. Such an AI-based model dynamically schedules each patient's appointment with a GP or a related clinic for further assessment or treatment. This approach, along with the experience of healthcare professionals, enables timely clinical decision-making.

Wearable technology for chronic disease monitoring, mobile apps for medical instructions, and remote consultations with healthcare professionals are a few other examples of telehealth applications intended to improve elder self-care. Reduced transportation difficulties, increased convenience, and prompt medical consultations are some of the possible benefits of using telehealth services for seniors. In numerous studies involving older patients with various conditions, telehealth has been shown to promote self-care behaviors positively.

When seeking to enhance self-care among older adults through telehealth, it is recommended to guide them through five stages: (1) needs assessment; (2) goal setting; (3) structured learning of self-care behaviors; (4) development of an individualized self-care plan; and (5) evaluation of practice. Furthermore, providing telehealth services comprehensively and holistically to older people has become increasingly imperative in recent years. Many older people have multiple chronic conditions that affect every aspect of their lives. There are many telehealth solutions that enable caregivers to customize services based on the patient's unique situation. Additionally, when implementing telehealth, it is extremely important to assess and strengthen the digital literacy of older adults as needed. Otherwise, the program's efficacy can be jeopardized, which could result in unsuccessful outcomes.

Box 6.1 Digital Health Literacy: A Critical Component in the Effective Use of Health-Related Technology

Digital literacy refers to the competence required for the retrieval, assessment, and production of information through various digital technologies such as the Internet. It refers to one's capability and knowledge required to access and operate Internet-connected devices, successfully apply commonly available software, and the ability to read, understand, and responsibly interact with digital content.

Digital health literacy (DHL) combines elements of both digital literacy and health literacy. Competence in digital health refers to the capability of locating, comprehending, evaluating, and applying health information obtained from digital sources. This term is also referred to as e-health literacy and comprises a number of skills needed to access and locate relevant, applicable health information for health-related issues. There are many determinants that can influence digital health literacy, including age, geographical location, and socioeconomic status. This capability encompasses several broad categories, including acquisition of health information, resource evaluation, interpretation of health information, engagement in health matters, and understanding of confidentiality and safety measures in communication.

Prior to utilizing any telehealth services, it is important to assess the level of digital health literacy of the individual. There are several tools available to measure digital literacy among older adults, with the eHealth Literacy Scale (e-HEALS) and the Mobile Device Proficiency Questionnaire (MDPQ) being the most commonly used.

Therefore, when considering the application of empowerment of older people in terms of technology, it should be noted that their level of digital literacy needs to be assessed and improved over time, if necessary. Looking at the experience of the COVID-19 pandemic, people with low levels of digital literacy found it challenging to adopt and make use of digital health technologies, which translated into being socially excluded from seeking relevant health services.

6.2 TeleWellness

"Tele wellness," a growing concept in healthcare, involves using technology to enhance wellness and health practices to provide people access to health information, support, and services remotely from their homes. The roots of this concept can be traced back to the rise of telemedicine in the late twentieth century, which focused on enhancing overall well-being—including not only physical but also mental, emotional, and social dimensions of health—through remote health initiatives. As a comprehensive framework, tele wellness encompasses various dimensions of health and offers solutions tailored to individual needs. These days, it encompasses a broad range of services, including smartphone applications for managing chronic diseases, mental health counseling, online exercise courses, and dietary advice.

Because of their close relationship, the terms *"telehealth"* and *"tele wellness"* are occasionally used interchangeably. While both employ technology to enhance health outcomes, they can be distinguished from one another. Tele wellness generally emphasizes the improvement of health and general well-being through preventative measures and lifestyle modifications via remote means, whereas telehealth principally involves the remote delivery of clinical and medical treatment. Despite meeting distinct demands throughout the range of health management, both are important components of contemporary healthcare.

Telehealth typically encompasses interactions between patients and medical professionals. A few examples of telehealth applications include online therapy sessions with psychologists, remote blood pressure or glucose monitoring, and virtual consultations with physicians. Tele wellness, on the other hand, places more of a focus on lifestyle management and holistic health, giving priority to general well-being and preventative health measures. Virtual yoga or fitness courses, online dietary counseling, and virtual stress management sessions are some examples of tele wellness programs designed to encourage self-care practices among senior citizens.

6.3 Artificial Intelligence

The global information and communication technologies (ICTs) landscape has been reshaped by *artificial intelligence (AI)* over the past few years. AI refers to systems that analyze their surroundings and take actions with a degree of autonomy to achieve specific goals. The system may be based on software and operate in virtual environments (for example, conversational agents and facial recognition systems), or it may be based on hardware and operate in physical environments (for example, robots). In recent years, AI-enhanced interventions have been developed to support the health and capacity of older adults receiving in-home care, with the goal of expanding the scope of care, increasing its effectiveness, and reducing the workload of caregivers.

These technologies have the potential to improve workforce sustainability (e.g., act as additional support for caregivers), address service inequities (e.g., by providing services in remote areas where ITC availability is low and demand is high), and increase the efficiency of information systems and data analysis of people who need LTC. In some countries, home care for older people and/or nonself-sufficient patients is considered a priority for national health services. This type of care is mostly provided for two reasons. It meets the need to face the growing demand for health services related to the population aging by providing medical, rehabilitation, and nursing services to patients at home. Hence, it significantly improves the quality of life in their family. It also reduces the burden on hospitals, reduces emergency room admissions, and reduces inappropriate hospitalizations, leading to reduced costs for the national health system. AI can generate personalized recommendations adapted to each patient's unique conditions and needs by analyzing comprehensive medical history, socioeconomic and demographic data, symptoms, preferences, and outcomes. It can adapt to each patient's specific needs and enable a more purposeful and personalized approach to education. Thus, it increases patient engagement and is associated with more informed decisions and improved overall treatment outcomes. AI empowers patients to take an active role in their care, promotes a sense of independence, and improves adherence to treatment by adapting educational resources to the person. Additionally, caregivers develop a variety of skills through AI, which enhances their problem-solving abilities and aids in the management of disruptive behaviors.

The application of AI in home care can realize the combination of the Internet and wearable smart monitoring and increase the performance of home care services. Using intelligently collected user data can help government departments or retirement service institutions improve their efficiency, pave the way for interaction and communication between older people and their children, and improve the adherence and satisfaction of older people users. In the AI era, home care will be intelligent and of high quality. AI-equipped robots are a solution to the crisis in LTC homes, where workforce shortages are associated with a rapid increase in care demands. These robots have been used to support person-centered care for older people and to pay attention to the emotional, social, and physical needs of older people.

AI has a high potential in the area of home nursing for dementia. It provides a set of functions to help patients with dementia and their caregivers improve their daily productivity, quality of life, and daily care and reduce the burden on caregivers. These methods pave the way for cognitive stimulation and training, medication and task management, recreational activities, vital sign measurement, and remote consultation with healthcare professionals. Many countries are currently using telerobots for home intervention for dementia patients. They have shown promising results in intervention trials. *Social assistive robots (SARs)* can enhance or support the needs of dementia patients through noncontact interaction. They provide users with step-by-step instructions, task encouragement, event reminders, safety monitoring, and emergency help-seeking and make them socially active. Results of studies indicate that the robot reduces anxiety and depression and improves the well-being of dementia patients. For example, *PARO*, a social assistance robot, can interact with dementia patients and provide them with emotional support. Physical assistance robots can perform tasks such as dressing and supporting the transition from sitting to standing.

Evidence suggests that using AI-equipped robots in LTC homes can optimize resources, increase resident comfort, create patient-centered care, meet residents' needs, and improve healthcare provider workflow. Although AI-equipped robots may potentially reduce the burden on healthcare staff and increase efficiency in LTC homes, they are associated with some risks. The adoption and use of robotics are associated with ethical issues and technological risks such as safety, privacy and data security, responsibility, and impacts on the current workforce.

Furthermore, AI-enabled virtual assistants, such as AI-based reminders and tracking devices, can help patients with tasks such as reminding them to take their medications, adhering to their medical regimen, scheduling physician appointments, and monitoring vital signs and disease management strategies. Virtual assistants can also collect health data and report it to healthcare providers, leading to reduced workload and improved patient outcomes. AI algorithms can analyze a patient's treatment plan, medication regimen, and personal preferences to provide personalized notifications. These reminders can be customized based on the patient's preferred communication method, such as text messages or voice notifications. Additionally, feedback and reinforcement mechanisms integrated into AI-based platforms can provide ongoing support, leading to increased motivation.

Ambient intelligence (AmI) is considered a capable technology for a new generation of systems that provide services flexibly, transparently, and predictively. It requires minimum human-computer interaction skills. Many people desire to remain in their living environment, especially as they get older. In other words, they prefer to recover at home rather than in a hospital setting since it improves their quality of life and gives them confidence. AmI is concerned with the design of systems that can be embedded in the daily environments of older people, aiming to improve their quality of life. One aspect of this technology is *"empathetic technology,"* which refers to systems capable of detecting the emotional state of older people and responding appropriately by providing necessary care, which is often particularly beneficial for enhancing the lives of vulnerable individuals, such as older people. Older individuals, especially those living in care facilities, usually experience negative mood states. These states can include anxiety about being in the final stage of life or sadness due to missing family, friends, or pets. Consequently, equipping their living spaces—particularly in care facilities—with smart technology, which can detect and address these negative states, guiding them toward more positive emotions, can significantly enhance their well-being. As a simple example, one application of this technology is the use of smart lighting solutions to increase the comfort and mood within older people's living spaces. The rapid advancement in LED technology, along with the miniaturization and integration of sensors and electronics, has created numerous options for automatically generating light of any color and intensity at any time and place. Research has consistently shown that light and color can impact people's moods on a biological as well as a psychological level. For instance, different types of light and color can evoke varying levels of arousal (blue is more calming, while red is more energizing).

Ambient assisted living (AAL) can be considered a subfield of the broader field of AmI. It focuses on applying ambient intelligence techniques to improve the quality of life and independence of older people to increase the period they can live in their home environment, assist them with daily activities, promote the use of smart products, and *information technology (IT)* tools to provide remote care services. The European Union aims to strengthen the emergence of AAL services and systems for good aging at home, in the community, and in the workplace through the AAL Joint Program. These key objectives for AAL are defined as:

1. Increasing the time people live in their preferred environment by increasing their independence, confidence, and mobility
2. Supporting the maintenance of the health and functional ability of older people
3. Promoting a better and healthier lifestyle for people at risk
4. Increasing security, preventing social isolation, and maintaining support
5. Developing a multifunctional network around the person
6. Supporting caregivers, families, and care organizations
7. Increasing the efficiency and productivity of resources consumed in older people's communities

Any AAL system is based on pervasive devices, commonly applied in home automation systems. It helps to integrate devices and create a safe environment for people based on AmI technologies. The primary goal is to help people in their daily activities by creating a suitable, interconnected, adaptive, dynamic, and intelligent environment. These assistive technologies, which can complement human care rather than replace it, can improve the quality of life for both older people and their caregivers. A study conducted by Milella et al. (2023) confirms that AI-based technologies significantly enhance applications in AAL and improve remote monitoring by informal caregivers through the integration of home sensors.

AAL can also be considered a part of the smart home (SH) market, even if it is still a very small part of it. The older people's independence of ICT can be achieved in various ways by building *enhanced living environments (ELEs)* that are sensitive, adaptive, and responsive to human needs and habits. ELE is a term coined to refer to a place where AAL meets and uses ICT with algorithms, architectures, platforms, and systems appropriate to everyday life and the management of the personal environment. These enhanced environments require the development of processes that create a sense of comfort and security during interaction by making appropriate adjustments based on the people's needs and conditions.

As another usage of AI-enabled approaches, the data generated by the Internet of Things (IoT) sensor is utilized to make and design an advanced activity recognition (AR) model. Nowadays, traditional data analysis methods cannot cope with the increasing data growth in terms of variety and volume. Various types of big data, such as numerical, categorical, audio, visual, and textual data, are collected from different sources, which can be structured, unstructured, or semi-structured. Analyzing this type of data is mostly difficult using traditional data analysis tools, especially when the data grows over time, which can result in problems in maintaining the database. In this regard, AR is an application for recognizing ADLs through a learning process using machine learning (ML) and deep learning (DL) techniques. AR can significantly help in performing extensive data analysis and health-related indicators.

AI technology, now widely accessible at low costs, also has the potential to improve family caregivers' capacity for learning and providing care. These technologies can provide tailored training specific to the needs of each older people individual through advanced deep learning techniques. They can also help with mental health issues such as depression, stress, anxiety, sadness, and dysfunctional thinking among caregivers. This support ultimately contributes to improvements in life satisfaction, perceived self-efficacy, problem-solving behaviors, behavioral activation, and overall quality of life.

Generally, regardless of their location, patients and their caregivers can easily access educational materials anytime and anywhere. These materials enable them to learn at their own pace and convenience. Furthermore, AI can facilitate multilingual capabilities and ensure that educational content is adapted to different patient populations. AI-based platforms can provide translations, cultural adaptations, and explanations appropriate to different audiences. Accordingly, they facilitate effective communication.

However, healthcare providers should ensure that AI applications provide useful technology in supporting patient care. Thus, medical students should gain sufficient knowledge and skills about AI applications in medicine. They may even have to use applications that were not available during their studies.

6.4 E-Learning Platforms

Education for patients, especially older people, involves guiding them on the ways to prevent and manage medical conditions and diseases. This education is provided during healthcare interactions with the patient, structured courses, printed materials, videos, online public health communications, and other mechanisms. Patient education is an essential component of improving general health and promoting self-care in older people, as it offer multiple benefits. It empowers patients by enhancing their knowledge and skills to make decisions about their health and well-being. It improves health outcomes and increases patient satisfaction. Informed patients also develop improved health behaviors, such as increased adherence to medication regimens and healthier lifestyle choices. Proper education also has the potential to reduce the need for unnecessary medical interventions and, finally, reduce healthcare costs. Patients with chronic diseases can improve their capability to manage them by receiving proper education about their condition and how to promote self-care behaviors. It leads to better health outcomes and a reduced rate of using healthcare. Additionally, public health educational materials play a crucial role in improving population health. It helps to increase awareness about important health issues, such as the risks of communicable diseases, the importance of a healthy lifestyle, and even air pollution hazards.

Researchers argue that patients' awareness of their diseases is associated with self-care. Health education behaviors and guidelines can improve patients' awareness of the disease and improve their self-care capability. Studies have also revealed that health education positively affects patient cognition and enables them to act with self-efficacy after acquiring relevant knowledge from healthcare professionals. Health education and literacy are vital for patients to understand health guidelines, make personal health decisions, and care for family members. Health literacy refers to the level of knowledge and awareness that people can locate, understand, and apply health information to make appropriate health decisions.

Traditional approaches to patient education are unfortunately associated with some limitations in personalization and interaction. Today, the Internet and digital technologies provide invaluable educational resources for older adults and those who care for them. One of the most effective uses of information and communication technology in elder health is e-learning, referred to as Internet-based education or electronic learning. Webinars on health management, workshops on self-care practices, and digital literacy courses are some of the offerings available through e-learning platforms. These resources ensure that older adults have access to up-to-date scientific information and specialized training. Courses specifically designed for older adults address the individual needs of both older adults and their caregivers. Furthermore, by removing physical boundaries, this technology enables people to obtain professional guidance and instruction without the need for in-person visits.

In addition, recent developments in patient education involve adopting digital intelligence tools, including AI and machine learning (ML), which are rapidly changing the landscape. By providing personalized educational content, interactive interfaces, and real-time support appropriate to individual needs, these technologies are transforming education and engagement in the disease. Integrating AI into patient education provides promising solutions to address these challenges. Using AI, patient education can be enhanced, and personalized and interactive educational resources can be provided that meet individual needs and preferences. AI algorithms can personalize educational content by analyzing individual patient data and increase the effectiveness of educational materials. Interactive learning experiences with AI, such as chatbots and virtual assistants, engage patients in communication and immediate feedback.

AI also improves accessibility by providing mobile applications and multilingual capabilities. It also allows patients to learn at their own pace. AI applications in pain management education also include simplifying complicated pain mechanisms, providing evidence-based treatment recommendations, and supporting adherence through personalized reminders and reinforcement. As AI can play a vital role in predicting, treating, and monitoring a patient's disease management and progression, it can provide interactive information appropriate to the specific conditions and medical needs of patients. This can be integrated into digital health education platforms that offer a wide range of resources, including videos, authoritative articles, and interactive modules. These platforms can present evidence-based information in a more understandable way. It also enables patients to access educational content at their desired time.

In summary, AI in education is a combination of computer science, education, psychology, and learning sciences. Generative AI has also emerged as a promising tool for improving patient education and, thus, patient outcomes in various healthcare settings, including settings with limited resources. It uses algorithms to generate new data or content, such as images, audio, and video, similar to existing data. Generative AI in healthcare settings can be utilized to improve patient education and outcomes in various ways. For example, this technology can be utilized to create personalized educational materials for patients with chronic diseases such as diabetes. These models are developed based on a deep neural network that helps adjust responses to the user. The use of generative AI models may be useful for educating patients on various medical topics. In addition, physicians can utilize generative AI as a powerful tool for communicating with patients about their diseases or treatments.

In this regard, chat systems are automated attempts to mimic the human-to-human communication style to make an interaction with a computer system more intuitive for the user. These systems are easily accessible to the user via computer or mobile phone, unlike traditional oral and printed patient education media. A key feature of these systems is the flexibility of access to educational content since the user controls the topic. This is in contrast to paper educational materials (PEMs) or static websites where the information is prepackaged. Although such systems have been utilized for patient education limitedly, this educational medium has led to significant improvements in knowledge and self-management. Two types of chats are relevant to patient education. One is the information-seeking chat aimed at providing information to answer the user's question, and the other one is the inquiry chat, in which users seek to discover and verify evidence.

6.5 Virtual Space

The term *"virtual space"* refers to a digital or computer-simulated setting that allows senior citizens to interact with one another, socialize, access resources, collaborate with medical professionals, and share information. Because they enable users to access and interact with a wide range of informative resources, these virtual environments are crucial to the information-seeking process. Virtual activities are typically more participatory than educational activities in the physical world and have shown a high degree of efficacy.

With the help of this technology, older individuals and those who care for them may access a multitude of information that assists them in maintaining and improving self-care routines while fostering more relationships with peers and healthcare providers. The maintenance of self-care requires this element. Furthermore, a major concern for many seniors is *social isolation*; virtual platforms can help reduce feelings of *loneliness* by promoting and enhancing relationships with friends and family.

Virtual reality (VR), online communities for experience sharing, virtual support groups, and electronic communication platforms are a few examples of virtual space technologies that might help older adults with self-care.

"Virtual healthcare" encompasses a wide range of activities, including medical services delivery and remote patient-provider contact through virtual means, mobile applications, and video conferencing. Older individuals and their family caregivers can consult with healthcare professionals over the Internet using this method of healthcare delivery, eliminating the need to visit clinics or hospitals. It guarantees that older people receive ongoing education, counseling, supervision, and general self-care. Therefore, geographical distances or the time between visits do not affect healthcare quality.

Older folks can communicate directly with their doctors or nurses via audio or video during a virtual health appointment. Because it enables patients to obtain medical care without having to leave their homes, this is especially advantageous for people with mobility limitations or restricted access to transportation.

For seniors, direct communication and assistance from healthcare practitioners are also made easier by the usage of online meetings and video conferencing services. Additionally, these platforms allow peer information exchange and collaborative involvement among older people. The *"World Café Method"* is one of the cutting-edge interactive techniques that encourages user engagement and connection while promoting conversation in large groups. Geographically separated groups may debate certain subjects similarly to a café table, exchange ideas, and improve each other's ideas through a virtual World Café, which offers a platform for structured dialogue and collaborative thought. In order to foster a variety of viewpoints, World Café participants are treated as experts in their respective fields based on their lived experiences and empirical knowledge.

In this method, different levels of formality may be maintained in order to ensure that everyone has an opportunity to speak. Taking part in these conversations fosters relationships and a sense of belonging while encouraging and strengthening problem-solving and self-care skills. Through this process, older individuals' ties to their communities may be reinforced, and support networks beneficial to their mental and physical well-being can be established.

Even though studies have indicated that peer information exchange sessions have very positive outcomes, it is important to remember that older adults sharing knowledge and experiences virtually should be overseen by a trained healthcare professional. This supervision is necessary to ensure that debates stay based on scientific validity by preventing the spread of incorrect or pseudoscientific information that may be potentially inaccurate or harmful. Without this oversight, the outcome can be detrimental rather than advantageous.

One important use of digital technology is *virtual reality, or VR*. "*Virtual reality*" is a term that was first used in the late 1980s to describe the simultaneous display and experience of an interactive, computer-generated virtual environment. With the use of this technology, users may fully immerse themselves in computer-generated representations of certain settings, promoting both mental and physical engagement in learning and skill development.

VR, which is usually administered through immersive headgear, presents opportunities for interventions designed to enhance the social, psychological, and physical well-being of older people. As a result, VR technology has attracted a lot of interest lately because of its potential to manage pain, avoid accidents or falls, boost cognitive function and social interaction, improve motor skills and balance, and encourage physical exercise. VR can help older people with activities and some daily care responsibilities, whether it is implemented through specialist software or nonspecialized platforms (such as experimental and virtual reality games). This technology may be used to promote self-care and encourage active engagement in health practices, even if its primary use is in older individuals' rehabilitation. It has the potential to significantly improve older adults' capacity for self-care by encouraging learning and participation.

The use of virtual reality in the care and self-management of senior citizens has been the subject of several systematic evaluations. According to a systematic review by Corregidor-Sánchez et al. (2021), VR, as a rehabilitative strategy, can improve walking quality and endurance, hence enhancing functional mobility among older people. Nonspecialized VR technology sounds to be more effective in this situation despite its lower evidence quality, even though the quality of the evidence supporting specialized VR technology was determined to be greater. Another study by O'Connor et al. (2022) revealed that mindfulness interventions based on virtual reality could effectively serve as a self-care strategy for improving the self-management of chronic pain. Additionally, VR can be used to promote psychological self-care among older adults. The systematic review conducted by Pira et al. (2023) indicated that employing VR technology in therapeutic settings could yield beneficial effects on mental health, reducing stress and negative symptoms. According to the findings of Buele et al. (2023), VR technology may be valuable for enhancing cognitive functions and daily activities among older adults, including those with mild cognitive impairments and dementia.

Additionally, avatar-based technology may be used to provide instructions intended to institutionalize and promote self-care behaviors. An avatar is a dynamic online depiction or animation of a person that improves engagement in a virtual environment. With avatar-based educational technology, people may actively construct a distinctive online persona, which helps medical professionals conduct training more efficiently and encourages user engagement. Older adults with poor reading and health literacy skills may benefit most from this technology. By enhancing their knowledge, self-care practices, and general quality of life, older individuals might be better equipped to manage their chronic diseases through such technology.

6.6 Social Media Platforms

Social media platforms have profoundly changed the way people interact across generations. These digital tools facilitate connections and community-building among users, serving as vital resources for maintaining relationships with family, friends, and communities. Social media allows older adults to participate in a wide range of networking possibilities by improving peer connections. Seniors may learn self-care techniques and share their invaluable experiences through these platforms.

In this context, a systematic review conducted by Elnaggar et al. (2020) highlighted the promising future of using social media for self-care among diabetic patients, revealing significant interest and demand in recent studies regarding peer interaction related to self-management.

Social media platforms are essential for combating loneliness and isolation, two issues that are closely linked to aging. They make it possible for seniors to participate in conversations, exchange experiences, and maintain relationships with their loved ones. This connectivity lessens depressive symptoms and feelings of loneliness that might result from distance or mobility challenges. Furthermore, a lot of older people enjoy social activities; social media platforms enable them to participate in campaigns, express their opinions, support causes that are important to them, and maintain their social involvement. Furthermore, online groups focused on specific interests, such as gardening, travel, or health, allow older adults to connect with like-minded individuals. These communities can provide emotional support and a sense of belonging, which are essential for seniors' mental health and psychological self-care.

6.7 Large Language Models (LLMs)

Advanced artificial intelligence systems called *large language models (LLMs)* are designed to comprehend and produce human language, which makes communication and information retrieval easier. These models may perform a variety of tasks, including translation, summarization, question answering, and conversational interaction, by using extensive datasets to understand patterns, grammar, facts, and even the nuances of language. The concept of language modeling has been around for a few decades, with early attempts mainly focused on statistical techniques. However, the landscape significantly transformed with the introduction of deep learning techniques in the 2010s. One potential area of development is the integration of natural language processing (NLP), a field that uses computational linguistics and machine learning (ML) to process human language. It potentially improves conversational AI interfaces. NLP can enhance the capability of AI-based chatbots and virtual assistants to understand and respond to patient's questions and concerns more naturally. This advancement leads to more effective and engaging interactions between patients and AI systems, leading to enhanced learning experiences. Integrating NLP into AI-based patient education platforms provides new opportunities for improving conversational interfaces. AI solutions reflected in chatbots, which are complex language models, are promising tools for improving patient education and engagement. Chatbot is a large language model trained on large amounts of Internet-based text and enhanced with human feedback. It can answer questions and solve problems. It can play a vital role in complementing traditional patient–physician interactions and enhancing the overall patient education process. Interest in chatbots is growing due to their capability to provide direct access to information and provide accurate information in a personalized way anytime and anywhere.

These days, the emergence of models like OpenAI's GPT-2, followed by GPT-3 and GPT-4, as well as other examples like BERT and T5 (Text-to-Text Transfer Transformer), have shown unprecedented capabilities in producing content that is both coherent and contextually relevant. Developed by OpenAI in 2018, ChatGPT is a *pretrained generative transformer (GPT)* that has gained widespread popularity due to its capability to combine data from many sources and generate human-like responses. Recently, these GPT models have been used in experiments to impart medical reasoning and knowledge. Generative AI, such as that found in ChatGPT, can be effective in providing patient information, helping them understand diagnosis and treatment options, monitoring symptoms and adherence, providing feedback and encouragement, and answering their questions. ChatGPT can provide immediate, accurate, and understandable answers to patient questions thanks to its advanced language processing capabilities. This aspect of AI is particularly useful for the disambiguation of medical terms and for making post-operative guidelines more accessible to patients. Complementing the efforts of healthcare professionals by addressing common patient concerns and questions in telehealth, ChatGPT can serve as a first line of information.

LLMs have a wide range of possible uses in the healthcare profession, including research, education, consultancy, and patient care. By producing medical summaries, interpreting languages, and writing instructions, LLMs may facilitate patient communication. These models are also increasingly being used to improve clinical decision-making, decrease the workload of healthcare professionals, improve patient-provider communication, and increase diagnostic accuracy. These methods improve the overall healthcare process by fusing medical expertise with interpersonal communication. Through accurate real-time translations into many languages and the simplification of complicated medical terminology into plain language, they can enhance interactions between patients and healthcare practitioners. Additionally, this technology may provide patients, family caregivers, and healthcare professionals with accurate summaries of recent scientific studies.

In this regard, LLMs are viewed as practical approaches to elder care that provide promising opportunities to improve access, foster social contact, and improve self-care. These tools' primary advantages and widespread use lie in their user-friendly design, general availability, and human-like outputs. The appropriate incorporation of LLMs into older adults' daily lives has the potential to greatly enhance their quality of life. For instance, LLMs might help older people who may face mobility or cognitive challenges. LLM-powered chatbots can facilitate virtual consultations and offer prompt answers to health-related questions. Based on user inquiries about medical conditions or medication management, these models can provide appropriate recommendations, facilitating older adults' access to health information and enabling them to make knowledgeable decisions about their well-being. They can also help in monitoring daily activities, medication regimens, and eating habits through conversational interfaces, which promotes adherence to self-care practices. These models can also be integrated into applications that remind users about appointments or medications, thereby enhancing compliance with treatment regimens.

By facilitating social connection and diminishing feelings of isolation and loneliness, this technology can significantly contribute to the promotion of older individuals' mental self-care. According to earlier research, certain LLMs can be beneficial for mental health. For instance, compared to some healthcare team members, certain LLMs have shown better interpersonal skills and the ability to provide empathetic responses. In certain cases, artificial intelligence may perform better than some medical providers at recognizing emotional cues and reacting appropriately. Its accessibility and low cost are also advantages of this technology. These technologies can serve as a solution to mitigate discomfort and lessen the fear of being judged when talking about mental health difficulties, as treatment for psychological issues is frequently stigmatized in some societies.

Despite these positive aspects, LLMs should consider various aspects such as patients' familiarity with medical terminology, their level of anxiety when searching for healthcare information, and financial and other barriers, such as language. Thus, to achieve optimal results in each specific scenario, commands and guidance must be provided to these chatbots to ensure that the system's responses are consistent with each patient's needs. It is crucial to remember that AI may be unable to understand social quirks and cultural settings, which might result in the delivery of biased or erroneous information. Additionally, it necessitates Internet connectivity, which is unavailable in many rural places, like many other technologies, which exacerbates healthcare inequities.

Several educational factors must be taken into account to optimize the effectiveness of LLMs in elder care. Successful adoption of LLM-equipped gadgets depends on teaching older people how to utilize them. In addition, caregivers will need to receive training on how to use these technologies to effectively serve older individuals, tailoring their use according to individual abilities and needs. Models can be fine-tuned based on user feedback and their specific requirements to enhance usability and effectiveness. Further, it is necessary to be aware of the challenges and limitations associated with LLMs in order to minimize potential risks. The possibility of bias in the responses given to users is one issue with the use of this technology in elder self-care, which could pose risks in certain situations.

Although chatbots can provide valuable insights, they still cannot replace the understanding and expertise of medical professionals. Each patient, even with the same diagnosis, brings unique experiences, backgrounds, and levels of understanding. A chatbot may provide accurate data but fails to fully understand the emotional and user's cognitive state unless it is specified in advance. The health literacy of patients should be considered while presenting medical details to adjust their learning styles and levels. Adjusting the complexity and depth of information to the patient's understanding and comfort level is vital. It can also generate inaccurate or misleading information. Therefore, the precision and scientific validity of the information produced through language models should be confirmed by a healthcare expert prior to their use as caregiver support tools. In conclusion, while technology has the potential to greatly assist family caregivers in providing care for older people, caution must be taken to ensure that the data generated is accurate and scientific in order to guarantee the safety and efficiency of care practices for older people.

6.8 Health Monitoring Apps

Self-care and disease management among older people can be effectively achieved through diligent behavior monitoring. Technology has attracted a lot of interest lately in the field of health monitoring, especially for the senior population. It is acknowledged that the availability and development of smart platforms for ongoing health monitoring are critical technologies that support the transition to more proactive and cost-efficient healthcare. Numerous of these advances take a preventative stance, facilitating the early detection of adverse health conditions and thereby enhancing health care prevention and management.

One of the most critical functions of technologies such as smart homes and wearable devices is the continuous monitoring of health outcomes in older adults. Additionally, a wide array of mobile applications has been developed to assist users in tracking their health metrics and managing their overall well-being. Self-monitoring is considered a fundamental component of self-care.

Many studies have been carried out to design and examine innovative mobile applications for health monitoring that are especially suited to older persons, as mobile phones are among the most accessible technologies for them to learn and use. Examples of such applications include those for tracking calorie intake and blood sugar levels, step counters, daily activity logs, medication management and reminder systems, symptom tracking for chronic illnesses, and mood-tracking applications for mental health. Currently, there is a growing interest in applications that not only offer customization based on the specific conditions and comorbidities of older adults but also adopt a holistic and integrated perspective on their various health needs, encompassing physical, psychological, emotional, and social dimensions.

6.9 Wearable Technology

A potential development in healthcare technology is wearable technology, which refers to gadgets and devices worn on the body to track and record health parameters. These small electronic tools can be integrated into shoes, glasses, earrings, clothing, gloves, and watches, and they are continuously improving and evolving. In order to minimize interference with people's daily lives, some are even developing gadgets or chips that may be attached to the skin. In other words, a wearable care system using the Internet of Things (IoT) is an innovative and versatile application service system that can be worn on the body to monitor and manage personal health. So, IoT plays a key role in this technology. To link virtual products with real-world items, IoT integrates a number of significant methods, including wireless sensor networks, cloud computing, and measurement systems. These systems can monitor personal physical activity and record dietary habits and medication information. Using wearable devices, data can be collected and analyzed and provide feedback and more information about patient habits. Wearable technologies also provide real-time communication and locating functions for individuals and caregivers. The system supports multiple communication methods, such as voice, text, and video, for different needs and scenarios. The system can also determine personal locations through technologies such as GPS to better respond to and manage individual needs. The IoT-based wearable care system is an innovative, versatile, and secure application service system. It can help caregivers monitor and manage personal health well. It can also provide real-time communication and locating functions to manage and care for individuals well.

These advancements facilitate continuous monitoring of health-related outcomes, enhance self-care practices, and promote active lifestyles among older adults. As a result, they have attracted considerable interest in the fields of medicine and healthcare. Wearable technology is a prime example of remote monitoring capabilities, enabling the observation of physical activities and behaviors while recording physiological and biochemical parameters throughout older adults' lives. As a result, they make it possible to monitor the personal health of this vulnerable demographic for a continuous and long-term period.

The advantages of this technology include accessibility, cost-effectiveness, and user-friendliness. Wearable devices are commonly employed to monitor physical activity, weight, and energy expenditure; track vital signs and blood oxygen saturation while providing alerts for any anomalies; oversee cardiovascular health by measuring heart rate and blood pressure and recording their variations, alongside electrocardiogram (ECG) data; manage diabetes-related outcomes and monitor blood glucose levels; assess cognitive function and brain activity through electroencephalography (EEG); evaluate sleep quality and quantity; and detect falls, alerting caregivers when necessary. There are also several gadgets that can be used to track the whereabouts of older people and prevent their loss, especially those who are suffering from Alzheimer's disease or cognitive impairment. In the area of LTC services, electronic fences can be utilized to monitor and manage these patients. Caregivers can prevent older people from wandering outside a designated safe area by setting up an electronic fence while providing location monitoring and momentary alerts for timely intervention and management. This technology can help reduce the risk of harm to older people while providing peace of mind for family members and caregivers. Electronic fences can also be used to monitor the scope of activities and behavior of people in long-term care facilities or homes. It can help improve the safety and quality of care for people in long-term care settings.

Despite the fact that these smart gadgets are becoming increasingly popular, there are still many restrictions and difficulties when using them. For example, a large number of them fail to measure the intended outcomes accurately. There is still conflicting evidence about their validity and usefulness for evaluating particular health markers in older individuals. One primary reason for this is that these devices are predominantly designed and produced with younger individuals' physical and psychological characteristics.

6.10 Smart Home Technology

Older people may require frequent and immediate medical monitoring and interventions; failure to provide such care can lead to irreparable consequences. However, manually updating and processing daily activities can be difficult for older people. Thus, automated monitoring to track the activities of daily living (ADLs) of older people is the focus of the proposed methods. IoT-based sensors are embedded in smart devices that can automatically record events during human–machine interactions. Smart devices embedded in IoT can be integrated into a real-world environment by being deployed simultaneously, transforming the older people's home environment into a smart ecosystem.

For example, a home embedded with multiple sensors, known as a smart home, can enhance the capabilities of a simple home. A smart home (SH) can help and ensure robust monitoring regarding energy efficiency, healthcare, older people's safety, and behavior tracking. A smart home platform allows older adults to remain in the comfort of their own homes while maximizing their independence, thereby reducing the necessity for costly hospital visits and nursing home confinement. Smart home technology has transformed the interaction between individuals and their living environments, offering a range of tools designed to enhance safety, comfort, and independence for older adults. This technology includes various devices that can be remotely controlled or programmed, allowing seniors to operate independently and create a manageable, secure living space.

Consequently, smart home technology is seen to be among the most significant and promising developments for raising older people's quality of life as well as their safety and comfort. By facilitating better environmental management, this technology not only improves seniors' quality of life and self-care but also strengthens their sense of independence. Older adults can maintain a greater degree of self-sufficiency while maintaining their safety and well-being by incorporating these technologies into their everyday routines.

Such smart homes are equipped with environmental actuators and physiological sensors, both wearable and non-wearable, as well as advanced communication and information technologies. These include devices such as cameras and accelerometers. Through the IoT, these systems enable remote monitoring and management of home environments, encompassing factors such as temperature, humidity, smoke detection, and physiological indicators like heart rate. Furthermore, smart home systems possess the capability to communicate with healthcare centers and remote caregivers, allowing healthcare personnel to monitor the overall physiological status of seniors and implement necessary actions, including emergency interventions when required.

One of these systems is called Neo. It is a compact device that uses AI and assistive technology to identify household sounds that might indicate an emergency, such as a fall. Neo works like popular smart speakers, like Google Home. Its primary purpose is to listen for sounds that could signal potential problems, such as crying or the sound of breaking glass. The device records 10-second audio clips of various events for analysis and can engage in voice interactions to help occupants in an emergency. Upon detecting a worrying sound, Neo activates an older people care assistant who talks to the user to assess the situation through a set of questions. If a crisis is proven or no response is received, Neo contacts a caregiver or a relative's cell phone. The core algorithm that drives Neo's performance is a machine learning model trained on a large dataset of audio samples that represent various home sounds and events, including potential emergencies such as falls.

In terms of the benefits of SH technology, numerous aspects of life, such as safety, health, nutrition, physical activity, personal hygiene, social engagement, and leisure, are greatly enhanced by home automation systems. The applications of this technology include:

- Home monitoring systems designed to assess the physical condition of both the home environment and older people residents, including monitoring for incidents such as falls
- Voice-activated assistants that facilitate control over household devices, adjust temperature and lighting, provide medication reminders, and make voice calls—particularly

beneficial for seniors with mobility limitations
- Smart lighting systems that adapt according to the time of day, aimed at preventing falls.
- Smart thermostats that provide temperature control tailored to older adults, who may be more sensitive to temperature fluctuations
- Telehealth services that utilize health monitoring devices
- Security cameras and alert sensors that work collaboratively to ensure the health and safety of seniors, while also offering peace of mind to their families

Notwithstanding these many advantages, there are still issues with smart home technologies, including data volume, seamless connectivity, interoperability, and, most critically, privacy and data security.

6.11 Opportunities and Benefits of Technology in Older People's Self-Care

The technology's use in the self-care of older people is linked to numerous benefits:

- Technology has made it possible for older people to interact with their family, friends, and even their healthcare providers through video calls, social media, and messaging. This connection decreases the isolation that many seniors feel and, at the same time, provides them with valuable resources, up-to-date information, and instruction to help them take better care of themselves. More appropriate information and communications in the healthcare system reduce both temporal and spatial limitations, thus ensuring continuity in healthcare.
- A number of software applications allow older people to engage in personalized self-care processes. The new application provides opportunities for older people to actively participate in the self-care process and customize it according to their needs, such as living conditions, preferences, restrictions, and health problems.
- Devices can be designed and programmed such that older people can quickly contact emergency services or caregivers in urgent situations.
- There are also supportive applications and devices that can help to manage health. These include monitoring vital signs, level of activity, calories consumed, and sleeping patterns, thereby facilitating proactive health management.
- Many older adults take multiple medications throughout the day. Certain applications can remind them of the appropriate timing for medication intake, minimizing the risk of missed doses or medication errors. Smart pill dispensers are particularly helpful for seniors who manage multiple prescriptions, as they assist in organizing medications and provide reminders to take them on schedule.
- Voice assistants can aid them in performing household tasks, such as controlling ambient temperature and lighting. Furthermore, sensors can notify caregivers or family members in the event of unusual activities or emergencies within the home.
- Technology provides various games and applications tailored for older adults, facilitating their engagement in online communities and social groups of interest. Certain applications are specifically developed to stimulate cognitive function and maintain the mental activity of seniors with cognitive impairments.

6.12 Challenges and Limitations of Technology in Older People's Self-Care

Although technology may help older people take better care of themselves, become more independent, and have a better quality of life, it is pertinent to address the challenges and limitations that come with it:

- There are many technological barriers that prevent some older adults from utilizing many of these technologies. Factors such as financial constraints or lack of Internet access contribute to unequal access to technology among seniors.
- Some older people or their families may find the initial expenditure needed to access technology, as well as continuing expenses like updates and subscriptions, to be unaffordable.
- Some older adults exhibit reluctance toward new technologies. Older people typically accept and adapt to contemporary technology more slowly. Deficits in *digital literacy* are one of the most significant barriers to older adults' effective use of technology for self-care.
- Older people with physical restrictions, such as eyesight problems or mobility concerns, might not be able to use certain technologies.
- Technical issues or failures can cause annoyance and frustration, deterring people from using technology continuously.
- Certain technologies raise privacy issues by exposing private health information to possible breaches or misuse. Additionally, constant gadget monitoring might cause emotions of control or surveillance, which is detrimental to psychological health. These factors can result in a diminished level of trust and cooperation from some older adults toward new technologies.
- Overreliance on technology for daily tasks may undermine essential life skills and independence among seniors.
- While the use of technology can improve communication, it cannot replace the understanding and emotional support that arise from human interaction. Increased reliance on technology may lead to fewer in-person interactions, contributing to an increased sense of *physical loneliness*. It is important to note that one of the dangers older people may experience in this situation is *"skin hunger."* Box 6.2 provides further details on this concept.

Box 6.2 Beyond Touch: Exploring the Growing Concern of Skin Hunger Among Older People in Modern Society

Without a doubt, touch, as an essential feature of human existence, contributes to social, psychological, and emotional well-being. Physical contact between individuals is vital to strengthening social bonds and expressing emotions, significantly impacting physical and mental health. The orbitofrontal cortex and caudate nucleus can be activated by emotional touch, resulting in physiological and biochemical responses, including reduced blood pressure, heart rate, and cortisol levels. It also increases oxytocin and serotonin levels while decreasing substance P, which can alleviate pain. According to studies, touch can enhance immune function by boosting the activity of natural killer cells. Psychologically, an affectionate and caring touch has a relaxing effect that lessens stress, anxiety, depression, despair, fear, and concern. As a result of these findings, touch has been recognized as a prerequisite for good health and effective treatment in healthcare settings.

The physical loneliness experienced by older adults may result in a phenomenon known as *"skin hunger."* This term describes a deep-seated need for meaningful physical touch and human connection, characterized by feelings of loneliness and a longing for affection due to insufficient physical contact. Skin hunger is akin to the concept of *"touch deprivation"* and is linked to various emotional and psychological consequences, including despair, distress, anxiety, and depression. This issue, especially among older people, became more noticeable during the COVID-19 pandemic's social distancing measures.

In the contemporary era, modern technological developments have greatly facilitated remote communication; however, they have also exacerbated physical distances among individuals, even within families. While modern technology significantly improves older individuals' self-care, digital approaches cannot completely replace the emotional and psychological benefits derived from direct physical contact. Affectionate physical interactions—such as hugging, petting, holding hands, and kissing—cannot be adequately substituted by these technological advancements. Therefore, by making older individuals feel more physically alone, technology may contribute to the deterioration of the "skin hunger" condition. The consequences of this phenomenon might be more severe for older people who may face obstacles including physical limits and social isolation, jeopardizing their general health.

The quality of life for older people dealing with the difficulties of aging in a digital world can be considerably enhanced by acknowledging the significance of skin hunger and using tactics that promote physical connections. This section suggests several remedies that may alleviate these feelings among this population:

- To support older individuals' general well-being, a balance must be struck between opportunities for in-person interaction and technology solutions. In many cultures, family gatherings on different occasions are common and might lessen tactile deprivation. These meetings fulfill the needs of seniors for respect and acknowledgment.
- Arranging and coordinating frequent family get-togethers with the family members of older people might offer a break from the loneliness that the digital age frequently exacerbates. These gatherings can be facilitated by family members and caregivers, ensuring in-person contacts that mitigate tactile deprivation in older people.
- Sustaining social interactions and keeping in touch with friends and acquaintances is an essential part of aging well. Encouraging participation in social activities or support groups can create opportunities for physical interaction and connection, effectively countering the effects of isolation that may arise from reliance on digital communication. The importance of encouraging seniors to engage in face-to-face interaction cannot be overstated.
- The presence of a pet in the home can alleviate the discomfort associated with insufficient human interaction.
- Although the distancing effects of technology may cause skin hunger, creative solutions to overcome these constraints by incorporating touch into digital interactions are emerging. For instance, older people may find pleasure in robotic companions that mimic humans and devices that simulate warmth or gentle pressure. Certain gadgets with haptic feedback can replicate tactile feelings during virtual interactions, which may potentially alleviate skin hunger. However, despite the availability of these revolutionary technologies, a critical question still must be answered: Can any of these innovations genuinely replace human touch? Can they evoke feelings of humanity and empathy?

Despite the significance of skin hunger, it has not been extensively explored as a distinct phenomenon among older adults in academic research. Therefore, there is a pressing need for further studies to deepen our understanding of this concern using empirical data.

Recommendations for Family Caregivers and Older People

This section presents recommendations for the effective utilization of technology in the self-care of older people individuals:

- *Choosing Appropriate Technology:* As previously mentioned, a variety of technologies have been introduced to enhance the health and quality of life for older people, and these technologies are still being developed. It is essential to acknowledge that not every older person can use or benefit from every form of technology. For example, social media or self-monitoring apps may not be suitable for an older person who is suffering from Alzheimer's disease. Families should consider technologies that adequately meet the requirements of their older people family members, making sure that they are easy to use and not too complicated.
- *Preparing for Usage:* In order to help their senior loved ones, family caregivers need to take the initiative to educate themselves on how to use technology effectively. Before introducing and implementing any technology, it is crucial to improve older people's digital health literacy. A thorough awareness of both the benefits and drawbacks of a given technology is a prerequisite to its effective application. Furthermore, older people should be provided with proper training and sufficiently prepared to incorporate the necessary technology into their everyday lives.
- *Patience and Assistance During the Transition:* For older people, adapting and adjusting to new technology can sometimes be a tedious and drawn-out process. This transition requires patience, enabling older people to gradually adapt to and effectively integrate the technology into their daily lives. Family caregivers must be present and supportive throughout this period since neglecting older people in a technology-based environment would be like leaving a toddler alone in a deep pool!
- *Ongoing Support:* Family caregivers' presence and guidance are still required while using cutting-edge technologies for self-care and remote monitoring. Even while these technologies can reduce the necessity for constant supervision, older people still need their families' continuous support and attention. Physical, psychological, emotional, spiritual, social, and economic components should all be considered when providing this assistance.
- *Maintaining Balance:* Older people and their formal and informal caregivers must balance virtual interactions and in-person visits. However, even though technology makes it easier to communicate remotely and monitor an older person's condition, in-person care, physical contact, and a sincere connection must not be overlooked. Virtual connections cannot replace the value of in-person encounters.
- *Encouraging Independence:* Older people's autonomy and independence should not be hampered by new technology. This is a common misconception among families. Encouraging older adults to engage with technology gradually will help them maintain and improve their feelings of autonomy and self-efficacy.
- *Ensuring Regular Health Visits:* It is recommended that older adults continue to receive routine in-person medical checkups at healthcare facilities whenever possible. In a virtual setting, many tests and examinations are still impractical and might contain errors. Consequently, face-to-face discussions with medical experts should persist, tai-

lored to the unique requirements and situations of senior citizens.

- *Considering Regional and Cultural Differences:* This feature is especially crucial when using apps for self-care. To ensure usability and maximize efficacy, many programs are created regionally, taking into consideration the linguistic, cultural, socioeconomic, and climatic circumstances of particular areas or nations.
- *Addressing Ethical Considerations:* Even though the role of technology in senior health care is becoming increasingly prominent, there are a number of ethical considerations that need to be taken into account when incorporating various technologies into older people's daily lives. Protecting older people's privacy, social support, and autonomy are among the most important ethical principles. It must safeguard their independence, dignity, and respect, ensuring that users maintain control while preventing isolation from taking place. One major concern is that seniors may view family recommendations for technology use as a sign of neglect or rejection. They may also fear technology will diminish their control over their own lives. Accordingly, in order to successfully implement any technology, older adults must become familiar with the technology and develop trust in its use in advance. They ought to comprehend that technology is intended to provide supportive assistance rather than replace human affection, compassion, and care.

6.13 Summary of the Chapter

This chapter highlights the transformative impact that technology can have on self-care practices among the aging population. It discusses how technological tools such as telehealth, tele wellness, artificial intelligence, e-learning platforms, virtual spaces, social media, large language models, health monitoring apps, wearable technology, and smart home technology can enhance self-care and health promotion for older people. It describes the various ways in which self-care and the quality of life of older people can be improved through advanced technologies. It further examines the opportunities and challenges presented by technologies in the lives of older people today. Finally, recommendations aimed at empowering older people and their caregivers to navigate the technological landscape will be provided, along with a brief overview of existing research in this field.

6.14 Summary of Research Studies

One area of research that has gained significant attention and is rapidly evolving is the examination of how digital tools and innovations can enhance health management and independence in older adults. This field has become important due to the rising prevalence of chronic diseases in this demographic and the urgent need for new solutions that enable individuals to maintain their independence while effectively managing their health conditions. In recent years, numerous studies have investigated the impact of various types of technology on older adults' daily lives and health outcomes. Several randomized controlled trials (RCTs) have been conducted on the applications of various aspects of technology in self-care, and in some areas, due to the large number of studies conducted, high-quality systematic reviews have also been published. Examining the challenges and benefits of using technology is often achieved with anecdotal knowledge from qualitative studies of experts or even users.

Here, some examples of studies conducted in this field in recent years are presented. Despite the belief that telemedicine for older people is difficult or infeasible, a systematic review study by Batsis et al. (2019) showed that telemedicine is feasible and acceptable for providing care to older people and can improve health outcomes for them. In addition, Mac Eochagain et al. (2023) provided a comprehensive review of digital health applications, including remote assessment, monitoring, and intervention in geriatric oncology. They highlighted the potential of these technologies to enhance cancer care and improve patient outcomes. However, the review identified a lack of consensus regarding the correlation between remote digital assessments and health-related outcomes in older cancer patients. The authors underscored the necessity for collaborative studies to develop and evaluate technology specifically designed for this demographic. A systematic review by Forsman et al. (2018) of 21 studies demonstrated that technology-based interventions, including computer- and Internet-based education, positively impact the mental health of older adults, such as increased life satisfaction, improved social support, and reduced levels of depression. Some studies reviewed the uses of a specific type of technology in older adults. For example, Mattison et al. (2022) examined the impact of wearable devices (14 types of wearable devices) on healthcare outcomes in chronic disease management (18 chronic conditions) through a systematic review of 30 studies. They found that the findings showed mixed effects, with 50% of the studies showing positive effects on health outcomes such as pain management and exercise capacity, while the other half reported no significant improvements. In the systematic reviews conducted by Facchinetti et al. (2023) and Liu et al. (2019), which examined the effectiveness of smart homes in caring for older people with chronic conditions, it was found that smart homes have a positive impact on physical function and depression in this demographic. These findings highlight the significant potential of smart homes in supporting exacerbation control and enhancing patient safety by providing support in disease management. Another systematic review and meta-analysis by Al-Arkee et al. (2021) aimed to assess the impact of mobile health (m-Health) applications on medication adherence in cardiovascular patients by analyzing 16 RCTs. The review found that mobile apps significantly improved medication adherence, with 9 out of 12 studies reporting statistically significant improvements. The meta-analysis showed a mean difference of 0.90 (95% confidence interval [CI]: 0.03–1.78), albeit with high heterogeneity (I^2 = 93.32%). Additionally, 9 RCTs assessed clinical outcomes and reported improvements in systolic blood pressure, diastolic blood pressure, total cholesterol, and low-density lipoprotein cholesterol levels in the intervention group. Although the meta-analysis of these clinical outcomes from 6 RCTs favored app interventions, none were statistically significant. This suggests that while m-Health apps are effective, their effectiveness may vary based on app design and user engagement levels. Moreover, Wood et al. (2015) conducted a pilot study of the use of an iOS-based mobile app designed to improve diabetes self-management among rural older adults, which demonstrated increased diabetes knowledge and self-efficacy among participants. The reported ease of use suggests that interactive multimedia apps can be effective tools for older adults with health literacy. Studies by Esmaeilpour-BandBoni et al. (2021) and Ravari et al. (2021) have also shown that telephone-based telecare is an effective strategy in blood glucose management in older adults with diabetes. However, Toschi and Munshi (2020) discussed the benefits and challenges associated with using diabetes technology in older adults, emphasizing that while technology can reduce the burden of diabetes self-care and provide a sense of security, age-related cognitive and physical decline poses significant barriers to effective use. As previously mentioned, many studies have examined the applications of technology in improving self-care behaviors as well as its challenges among older people with various conditions, including cancer or cardiovascular, pulmonary, and musculoskeletal issues.

Moreover, recently, even studies on the applications of technology in palliative care have garnered increased attention. For example, Steindal et al. (2023) conducted a systematic review of 30 articles examining the use of telehealth in home-based palliative care. The findings indicated that telehealth facilitates stable support systems, enhances interpersonal relationships through visibility features, and optimizes the flow of information for appropriate care delivery. The study also noted barriers, including technological limitations, inflexible symptom reporting mechanisms, and privacy concerns. The review emphasizes the dual nature of telehealth, presenting substantial benefits while also posing significant implementation challenges. Therefore, as mentioned in this short discussion on studies, due to the breadth of this research, a detailed discussion on different studies in various patients is not feasible in this section.

In general, the findings of most of the studies suggest that technology can enhance the quality of life among older people by improving self-care behaviors, elevating their knowledge, enhancing health outcomes for seniors with chronic illnesses, and reducing costs associated with fewer hospital visits. Furthermore, research has demonstrated that technology can alleviate the burden on caregivers and reduce healthcare expenses through its supportive and assistive roles. However, there are challenges, including issues of digital literacy, accessibility, and potential privacy concerns that may impede widespread adoption. On the other hand, there is controversy regarding the effectiveness of these technologies in different older people populations.

Overall, although the intersection of technology and self-care among older adults represents a significant frontier in healthcare research, there exists a significant gap between hypothetical advantages and empirically demonstrated effects. Due to the rapid advancement of technology and the limited credible evidence regarding its impacts, the application of technology in home care has become a relatively new and popular area of research among researchers. Furthermore, it appears essential to design and conduct studies that assess both the positive and negative consequences of utilizing contemporary technology in older adults' self-care in future research.

6.15 Critical Thinking (Scenario-Based)

6.15.1 Scenario Case 1

Mr. Jack is a 76-year-old man with diabetes and Parkinson's disease. Although he is able to perform his daily activities independently, he uses a walker to move within the home. Furthermore, he has a hearing impairment and uses a hearing aid. Following the loss of his spouse, he resides with his only daughter, Rose, a nurse by profession. As a nurse, Rose's work requires her to be at the hospital on certain nights a week. While the health care team has educated Jack on some basic self-care behaviors concerning his conditions, he sometimes neglects some self-care activities due to fatigue. Most importantly, he sometimes does not take his medication when he should or takes it inappropriately. Furthermore, Jack is reluctant to accept technology and seems concerned with its complexity. Rose, who is also the family caregiver in this case, feels overwhelmed by her responsibilities.

Discussion Points

1. How can technology enhance and sustain Jack's self-care behaviors?
2. Which technologies could alleviate some of Rose's caregiving burden while ensuring that Jack receives appropriate care?
3. What strategies can be employed to encourage Jack to embrace technology?

Bibliography

Aanesen M, Lotherington AT, Olsen F. Smarter elder care? A cost-effectiveness analysis of implementing technology in elder care. Health Informatics J. 2011;17(3):161–72.

Al-Arkee S, Mason J, Lane DA, Fabritz L, Chua W, Haque MS, Jalal Z. Mobile apps to improve medication adherence in cardiovascular disease: systematic review and meta-analysis. J Med Internet Res. 2021;23(5):e24190.

Alhuwail D, Abd-Alrazaq A, Al-Jafar E, & Househ, M. (2022). Telehealth for the geriatric population: Uses, opportunities, and challenges. In Smart home technologies and services for geriatric rehabilitation (pp. 107–122). Elsevier. https://doi.org/10.1016/B978-0-323-85173-2.00008-4.

Bala B. Chatbots are not clinicians: addressing misconceptions about large language model use in psychiatric care. Acad Psychiatry. 2025;49(1):44–5.

Batsis JA, DiMilia PR, Seo LM, Fortuna KL, Kennedy MA, Blunt HB, Bagley PJ, Brooks J, Brooks E, Kim SY, Masutani RK. Effectiveness of ambulatory telemedicine care in older adults: a systematic review. J Am Geriatr Soc. 2019;67(8):1737–49.

Buele J, Varela-Aldás JL, Palacios-Navarro G. Virtual reality applications based on instrumental activities

of daily living (iADLs) for cognitive intervention in older adults: a systematic review. J Neuroeng Rehabil. 2023;20(1):168.
Cammisuli DM, Taurisano P, Schuller BW, Qian K. Digital health and virtual health care for adults and older adults: innovative technological solutions for diagnosis, management, and rehabilitation. Front Med. 2024;11:1417069.
Chandrasekaran R, Katthula V, Moustakas E. Too old for technology? Use of wearable healthcare devices by older adults and their willingness to share health data with providers. Health Informatics J. 2021;27(4):14604582211058073.
Clina J, Ferguson C, Rimmer J. Eight week telewellness program improves nutrition knowledge among people with physical disabilities. Arch Phys Med Rehabil. 2022;103(12):e126.
Connolly C, Hernon O, Carr P, Worlikar H, McCabe I, Doran J, et al. Artificial intelligence in interprofessional healthcare practice education–insights from the home health project, an exemplar for change. Comput Sch. 2023;40(4):412–29.
Corregidor-Sánchez AI, Segura-Fragoso A, Rodríguez-Hernández M, Jiménez-Rojas C, Polonio-López B, Criado-Álvarez JJ. Effectiveness of virtual reality technology on functional mobility of older adults: systematic review and meta-analysis. Age Ageing. 2021;50(2):370–9.
Dermody G, Whitehead L, Wilson G, Glass C. The role of virtual reality in improving health outcomes for community-dwelling older adults: systematic review. J Med Internet Res. 2020;22(6):e17331.
Elguera Paez L, Zapata Del Río C. Older people users and their main challenges usability with mobile applications: a systematic review. In: Design, user experience, and usability. design philosophy and theory: 8th international conference, DUXU 2019, held as part of the 21st HCI international conference, HCII 2019, Orlando, FL, USA, July 26–31, 2019, proceedings, part I 21. Springer International Publishing; 2019. p. 423–38.
Elnaggar A, Ta Park V, Lee SJ, Bender M, Siegmund LA, Park LG. Patients' use of social media for diabetes self-care: systematic review. J Med Internet Res. 2020;22(4):e14209.
Esmaeilpour-BandBoni M, Gholami-Shilsar F, Khanaki K. The effects of telephone-based telenursing on glycated hemoglobin among older adults with type 2 diabetes mellitus: a randomized controlled trial. J Nurse Pract. 2021;17(3):305–9.
Facchinetti G, Petrucci G, Albanesi B, De Marinis MG, Piredda M. Can smart home technologies help older adults manage their chronic condition? A systematic literature review. Int J Environ Res Public Health. 2023;20(2):1205.
Field T. Touch for socioemotional and physical well-being: a review. Dev Rev. 2010;30(4):367–83.
Floyd K. What lack of affection can do to you. Psychology Today. 2013. https://tinyurl.com/y8dfclz9.
Forsman AK, Nordmyr J, Matosevic T, Park AL, Wahlbeck K, McDaid D. Promoting mental wellbeing among older people: technology-based interventions. Health Promot Int. 2018;33(6):1042–54.
Frennert S, Östlund B. Narrative review: technologies in eldercare. Nord J Sci Technol Stud. 2018;6(1):21–34.
Gajarawala SN, Pelkowski JN. Telehealth benefits and barriers. J Nurse Pract. 2021;17(2):218–21.
Grandi LC, Bruni S. Will the artificial intelligence touch substitute for the human touch? NeuroSci. 2024a;5(3):254–64.
Grandi LC, Bruni S. COVID-19 and human touch, two sides of the same coin: an opinion article about touch deprivation and future directions. BioMed. 2024b;4(4):366–71.
Grgurić A, Mošmondor M, Huljenić D. The SmartHabits: an intelligent privacy-aware home care assistance system. Sensors. 2019;19(4):907.
Hajijama S, Juneja D, Nasa P. Large language model in critical care medicine: opportunities and challenges. Indian J Crit Care Med. 2024;28(6):523–5.
Haun JN, Alman AC, Jean-Baptiste E, Melillo C, McMahon-Grenz J, Paykel JM. Delivery of complementary and integrative health using virtual health resources: a scoping review. J Integr Complement Med. 2022;28(11):851–61.
Huh J, Le T, Reeder B, Thompson HJ, Demiris G. Perspectives on wellness self-monitoring tools for older adults. Int J Med Inform. 2013;82(11):1092–103.
Jensen CM, Overgaard S, Wiil UK, Clemensen J. Can tele-health support self-care and empowerment? A qualitative study of hip fracture patients' experiences with testing an "App". SAGE Open Nurs. 2019;5:2377960819825752.
Khanipour-Kencha A, Ghiyasvandian S, Mohammadi S, Khabazkhoob M, Mirshahi A, Wells R, Zakerimoghadam M. Effectiveness of a comprehensive tele-empowerment programme on self-care behaviours, uncertainty and readmission of patients with heart failure: protocol for a randomised controlled trial. BMJ Open. 2023;13(8):e074256.
Khemapech I, Jitrong V. Elder care—importance technologies and opportunities. In: Proc. Int. Conf.; 2021. p. 1–16.
Kim S, Chow BC, Park S, Liu H. The usage of digital health technology among older adults in Hong Kong and the role of technology readiness and eHealth literacy: path analysis. J Med Internet Res. 2023;25(1):e41915.
Kinnunen T, Parviainen J, Haho A. Technology-mediated touch. In: The skills and ethics of professional touch: from theory to practice. Singapore: Springer Nature Singapore; 2023. p. 107–42.
Kon B, Lam A, Chan J. Evolution of smart homes for the older people. In: Proceedings of the 26th international conference on world wide web companion; 2017. p. 1095–101.
Kriegel J, Grabner V, Tuttle-Weidinger L, & Ehrenmüller, I. (2019). Socially assistive robots (SAR) in in-patient care for the older people. In IndHealth 2019 – From eHealth to dHealth (Vol. 260, pp. 178–185). IOS Press. https://doi.org/10.3233/978-1-61499-971-3-178
Kuijsters A, Redi J, De Ruyter B, Heynderickx I. Lighting to make you feel better: improving the mood of

older people with affective ambiences. PLoS One. 2015;10(7):e0132732.

Kulurkar P, Kumar Dixit C, Bharathi VC, Monikavishnuvarthini A, Dhakne A, Preethi P. AI based older people fall prediction system using wearable sensors: a smart home-care technology with IOT. Meas Sens. 2023;25:100614.

Lee HY, Ju M, Kang M, Lee H, Choi J, Oh J. Preparedness, challenges, and opportunities for digital intervention for chronic disease management: a qualitative study in rural areas of South Korea. Health Syst Reform. 2024;10(2):2378503.

Liao Y, Thompson C, Peterson S, Mandrola J, Beg MS. The future of wearable technologies and remote monitoring in health care. In: American Society of Clinical Oncology educational book. American Society of Clinical Oncology. Annual Meeting, vol. 39. NIH Public Access; 2019. p. 115.

Lin B, Wu S. COVID-19 (coronavirus disease 2019): opportunities and challenges for digital health and the internet of medical things in China. Omi a J Integr Biol. 2020;24(5):231–2.

Liu L, Stroulia E, Nikolaidis I, Miguel-Cruz A, Rincon AR. Smart homes and home health monitoring technologies for older adults: a systematic review. Int J Med Inform. 2016;91:44–59.

Liu P, Li G, Jiang S, Liu Y, Leng M, Zhao J, Wang S, Meng X, Shang B, Chen L, Huang SH. The effect of smart homes on older adults with chronic conditions: a systematic review and meta-analysis. Geriatr Nurs. 2019;40(5):522–30.

Liu S, Wright AP, Mccoy AB, Huang SS, Genkins JZ, Peterson JF, Kumah-Crystal YA, Martinez W, Carew B, Mize D, Steitz B. Using large language model to guide patients to create efficient and comprehensive clinical care message. J Am Med Inform Assoc. 2024;31(8):1665–70.

Loveys K, Prina M, Axford C, Domènec ÒR, Weng W, Broadbent E, et al. Artificial intelligence for older people receiving long-term care: a systematic review of acceptability and effectiveness studies. Lancet Healthy Longev. 2022;3(4):e286–e97.

Lyndon H, Tyas D. Telehealth enhances self care and independence in people with long term conditions. Nurs Times. 2010;106(26):12–3.

Mac Eochagain C, Senac NM, Cavanagh M, Roy M, Ciccone AS, Contreras B, Testa GD, Velasco R, Marinho J, Serrano AG, Schiaffino MK. Digital health in geriatric oncology: a Young International Society of Geriatric Oncology review. J Geriatr Oncol. 2023;14:101649.

Maher C, Dankiw KA, Singh B, Bogomolova S, Curtis RG. In-home evaluation of the NeoCare artificial intelligence sound-based fall detection system. Future Internet. 2024;16(6):197.

Majumder S, Aghayi E, Noferesti M, Memarzadeh-Tehran H, Mondal T, Pang Z, Deen MJ. Smart homes for older people healthcare—recent advances and research challenges. Sensors. 2017;17(11):2496.

Maswadi K, Ghani NB, Hamid SB. Systematic literature review of smart home monitoring technologies based on IoT for the older people. IEEE Access. 2020;8:92244–61.

Mattison G, Canfell O, Forrester D, Dobbins C, Smith D, Töyräs J, Sullivan C. The influence of wearables on health care outcomes in chronic disease: systematic review. J Med Internet Res. 2022;24(7):e36690.

McGrath C, Kennedy MR, Gibson A, Musse S, Kosar Z, Dawson S. World Cafés as a participatory approach to understanding research agendas in primary care with underserved communities: reflections, challenges and lessons learned. Res Involv Engagem. 2023;9(1):101.

Milella F, Russo DD, Bandini S. How Artificial Intelligence can support informal caregivers in their caring duties to older people? A systematic review of the literature. Artif Intel Ageing Soc. 2023;3623:18–39.

Mueller SM. Social touch and touching patients. In: Human touch in healthcare: textbook for therapy, care and medicine. Berlin, Heidelberg: Springer Berlin Heidelberg; 2023. p. 171–218.

Nahm ES, Zhu S, Bellantoni M, Keldsen L, Russomanno V, Rietschel M, Majid T, Son H, Smith L. The effects of a theory-based patient portal e-learning program for older adults with chronic illnesses. Telemed J E Health. 2019;25(10):940–51.

Noone C, McKenna-Plumley PE. Lonely for touch? A narrative review on the role of touch in loneliness. Behav Chang. 2022;39(3):157–67. https://doi.org/10.1017/bec.2022.12.

O'Connor S, Mayne A, Hood B. Virtual reality-based mindfulness for chronic pain management: a scoping review. Pain Manag Nurs. 2022;23(3):359–69.

Olufokunbi KC. Technology devices for eldercare. In: ICT4AWE; 2018. p. 299–306.

Onthoni DD, Sahoo PK. Artificial-intelligence-assisted activities of daily living recognition for older people in smart home. Electronics. 2022;11(24):4129.

Park HY, Yeom IS, Kim YJ. Telehealth interventions to support self-care of stroke survivors: an integrative review. Heliyon. 2023;9(6):e16430.

Parmanto B, Aryoyudanta B, Soekinto TW, Setiawan IM, Wang Y, Hu H, Saptono A, Choi YK. A reliable and accessible caregiving language model (CaLM) to support tools for caregivers: development and evaluation study. JMIR Form Res. 2024;8:e54633.

Peeters JM, Wiegers TA, Friele RD. How technology in care at home affects patient self-care and self-management: a scoping review. Int J Environ Res Public Health. 2013;10(11):5541–64.

Pira GL, Aquilini B, Davoli A, Grandi S, Ruini C. The use of virtual reality interventions to promote positive mental health: systematic literature review. JMIR Ment Health. 2023;10(1):e44998.

Pirzada P, Wilde A, Doherty GH, Harris-Birtill D. Ethics and acceptance of smart homes for older adults. Inform Health Soc Care. 2022;47(1):10–37.

Qi J, Wu C, Yang L, Ni C, Liu Y. Artificial intelligence (AI) for home support interventions in dementia: a scoping review protocol. BMJ Open. 2022;12(9):e062604.

Ravari A, Sheikhoshaqi A, Mirzaei T, Raeisi M, Hassanshahi E, Kamiab Z. Effect of tele-nursing on blood glucose control among the older people with diabetes: a randomized controlled trial. Evid Based Care. 2021;11(2):54–63.

Rimmer JH, Wilroy J, Galea P, Jeter A, Lai BW. Retrospective evaluation of a pilot eHealth/mHealth telewellness program for people with disabilities: Mindfulness, Exercise, and Nutrition To Optimize Resilience (MENTOR). mHealth. 2022;8:15.

Rimmer JH, Young HJ, Bachiashvili V, Baidwan NK, Mehta T. Enhancements to a telewellness program for people with physical disabilities: mindfulness, exercise, and nutrition to optimize resilience (MENTOR 2.0). Prev Chronic Dis. 2024;21:E02.

Schlegel C, Geering A, Weber U. Learning in virtual space: an intergenerational pilot project. GMS J Med Educ. 2021;38(2):Doc37.

Schulz R, Beach SR, Czaja SJ, Martire LM, Monin JK. Family caregiving for older adults. Annu Rev Psychol. 2020;71(1):635–59.

Schwamm LH. Telehealth: seven strategies to successfully implement disruptive technology and transform health care. Health Aff (Millwood). 2014;33(2):200–6.

Shahbazi M, Bagherian H, Sattari M, Saghaeiannejad-Isfahani S. The opportunities and challenges of using mobile health in older people self-care. J Educ Health Promot. 2021;10:80.

Shibata T, Hung L, Petersen S, Darling K, Inoue K, Martyn K, Hori Y, Lane G, Park D, Mizoguchi R, Takano C. PARO as a biofeedback medical device for mental health in the COVID-19 era. Sustain For. 2021;13(20):11502.

Snoswell CL, Chelberg G, De Guzman KR, Haydon HH, Thomas EE, Caffery LJ, Smith AC. The clinical effectiveness of telehealth: a systematic review of meta-analyses from 2010 to 2019. J Telemed Telecare. 2023;29(9):669–84.

Steindal SA, Nes AA, Godskesen TE, Holmen H, Winger A, Österlind J, Dihle A, Klarare A. Advantages and challenges of using telehealth for home-based palliative care: systematic mixed studies review. J Med Internet Res. 2023;25:e43684.

Teixeira E, Fonseca H, Diniz-Sousa F, Veras L, Boppre G, Oliveira J, Pinto D, Alves AJ, Barbosa A, Mendes R, Marques-Aleixo I. Wearable devices for physical activity and healthcare monitoring in older people: a critical review. Geriatrics. 2021;6(2):38.

Thomas E, Skeie KB, Huang H. Inclusion of older people users via virtual spaces in the early stages of the innovation process. R&D Manag. 2024;54(2):214–26.

Toschi E, Munshi MN. Benefits and challenges of diabetes technology use in older adults. Endocrinol Metab Clin. 2020;49(1):57–67.

Tuena C, Pedroli E, Trimarchi PD, Gallucci A, Chiappini M, Goulene K, Gaggioli A, Riva G, Lattanzio F, Giunco F, Stramba-Badiale M. Usability issues of clinical and research applications of virtual reality in older people: a systematic review. Front Hum Neurosci. 2020;14:93.

Turjamaa R, Pehkonen A, Kangasniemi M. How smart homes are used to support older people: an integrative review. Int J Older People Nursing. 2019;14(4):e12260.

Van Agteren J, Ali K, Fassnacht DB, Iasiello M, Furber G, Howard A, et al. Testing the differential impact of an internet-based mental health intervention on outcomes of well-being and psychological distress during COVID-19: uncontrolled intervention study. JMIR Ment Heal. 2021;8(9):e28044.

Wang X, Luan W. Research progress on digital health literacy of older adults: a scoping review. Front Public Health. 2022;10:906089.

Wang W, Lin B, Mei Y, et al Self-care interventions in stroke survivor–caregiver dyads: a protocol for systematic review and meta-analysis BMJ Open 2021;11:e051860. https://doi.org/10.1136/bmjopen-2021-051860.

Wilmink G, Dupey K, Alkire S, Grote J, Zobel G, Fillit HM, Movva S. Artificial intelligence–powered digital health platform and wearable devices improve outcomes for older adults in assisted living communities: pilot intervention study. JMIR Aging. 2020;3(2):e19554.

Wong AK, Bayuo J, Wong FK, Yuen WS, Lee AY, Chang PK, Lai JT. Effects of a nurse-led telehealth self-care promotion program on the quality of life of community-dwelling older adults: systematic review and meta-analysis. J Med Internet Res. 2022;24(3):e31912.

Wong KLY, Hung L, Wong J, Park J, Alfares H, Zhao Y, et al. Adoption of artificial intelligence–enabled robots in long-term care homes by health care providers: scoping review. JMIR Aging. 2024;7(1):e55257.

Wonggom P, Kourbelis C, Newman P, Du H, Clark RA. Effectiveness of avatar-based technology in patient education for improving chronic disease knowledge and self-care behavior: a systematic review. JBI Database System Rev Implement Rep. 2019;17(6):1101–29.

Wood FG, Alley E, Baer S, Johnson R. Interactive multimedia tailored to improve diabetes self-management. Nurs Clin. 2015;50(3):565–76.

Wu M. (2019). Wearable technology applications in healthcare: A literature review. On-Line Journal of Nursing Informatics, 23(3). Retrieved from https://www.himss.org/resources/wearabletechnology-applications-healthcare-literature-review

Yu L, Chan WM, Zhao Y, Tsui KL. Personalized health monitoring system of older people wellness at the community level in Hong Kong. IEEE Access. 2018;6:35558–67.

Yu DS, Li PW, Yue SC, Wong J, Yan B, Tsang KK, Choi KC. The effects and cost-effectiveness of an empowerment-based self-care programme in patients with chronic heart failure: a study protocol. J Adv Nurs. 2019;75(12):3740–8.

Zheng Zhonghua, LIAO Lizi, DENG Yang, QIN Libo, and NIE Liqiang. Self-chats from large language models make small emotional support chatbot better. (2024). Proceedings of the 62nd Annual Meeting of the Association for Computational Linguistics, Bangkok, Thailand, 2024 August 11-16. 11325–11345.

Self-Care in Minor Ailments and Chronic Diseases

7

Ali Khanipour-Kencha

By the end of reading this chapter, learners should be able to:

- Understand the importance of self-care in managing minor ailments and chronic diseases among older adults
- Identify common minor ailments and chronic diseases affecting the older adult population
- Provide effective self-care strategies for managing minor ailments and chronic diseases in seniors
- Assess the needs of older adults and suggest tailored self-care techniques
- Foster a holistic approach to self-care that encompasses all dimensions of health
- Explore available resources and support systems that can enhance older adults' self-care practices in various aspects of their lives
- Understand the potential barriers and challenges to self-care and strategies to overcome them in older adults

The aging process causes the body to weaken, the individual's functioning to decline, and general health to deteriorate. Thus, it is not surprising that many minor ailments and chronic diseases are more prevalent among the older population compared to other age groups, highlighting the significance of self-care for older adults. The importance of self-care has never been more salient, especially as we live in an era where healthcare systems are often overburdened with unforeseen demands. Accordingly, this chapter explains how self-care can be applied to the management of minor ailments and chronic conditions in older individuals. Besides discussing the common health problems of seniors, practical recommendations will be provided regarding self-care improvements in this context.

7.1 Minor Ailments in Older Adults

Minor ailments are often uncomplicated medical issues such as simple colds, headaches, backaches, insect bites, heartburn, and nasal congestion, which resolve on their own and usually do not require specialized medical interventions. They can reasonably be self-diagnosed and managed with minimal self-care, using over-the-counter (OTC) medications or simple home remedies. In general, these conditions are self-limiting and short-term in nature; laboratory results are not required, and there is no significant medical history or potentially serious symptoms that indicate a more dangerous condition, so they carry a low risk and need only minimal or temporary follow-up. Nonetheless, some patients choose to see a doctor for minor ailments, while others do not. This difference in help-seeking behavior in dealing with minor ailments is usually rooted in three factors: (1) medical need (the type of disease and its severity), (2) enabling

A. Khanipour-Kencha (✉)
Tehran University of Medical Sciences, Tehran, Iran

F. Bahramnezhad (ed.), *Self-Care in the Elderly*, https://doi.org/10.1007/978-981-96-9021-3_7

factors (access to care, individual resources), and (3) predisposing factors (demographic, social structure, health beliefs, psychological characteristics). On the other hand, these minor health problems are dealt with differently in various countries. In most developed countries, community pharmacists have been successfully integrated into a variety of public health programs, including providing treatment and counseling for minor ailments. However, the lack of standard instructions for managing these conditions in developing countries is one of the factors hindering the provision of such services.

Due to the minor nature of these conditions, many individuals opt to self-medicate rather than consult a physician. Nonetheless, unnecessary visits to the emergency department (ED) or general practitioners for minor issues can result in a substantial burden on the patient's medical expenses and travel costs. Thus, they can become a major source of clinical and financial burden in primary, secondary, tertiary, and emergency care. In this regard, approximately 8% of emergency department visits are for minor ailments, which results in an estimated cost of £136 million per year. Certainly, patient attitudes regarding minor ailment management have changed significantly in recent years. However, some groups of patients, including older people, poorly educated individuals, and non-Western patients, have lagged behind this trend and continue to consult general practitioners for minor ailments.

During advanced age, these conditions may be more common and last longer due to age-related changes such as body weakening, but they usually do not require extensive medical intervention. While they may cause discomfort or irritation, they are typically not life-threatening. In spite of this, minor ailments should not be underestimated in older people, as their quality of life and daily routines can be disrupted while experiencing uncomfortable symptoms related to these conditions. One concern with minor ailments in older people is that self-care is often associated with self-treatment. This can be more serious and have greater consequences for the older generation, who may have diminished physical function and a potentially less effective system for detoxifying drugs from their bodies. In addition, seniors usually suffer from several underlying health problems and consume a wide variety of medications. Self-medication with OTC medicines or even herbal remedies, which is common in some cultures, can cause drug interactions or worsen the underlying disease in older people.

7.2 Self-Care for Common Minor Ailments in Older Adults

A thorough understanding of minor ailments and employing self-care techniques to manage them can help older individuals maintain their health and ensure that they seek specialized medical care when necessary. In the following, some of the most common minor ailments in older people and related self-care tips will be discussed:

7.2.1 Common Cold

The common cold is a benign and self-limited syndrome distinct from viral influenza, acute bronchitis, bacterial pharyngitis, sinusitis, and allergic rhinitis. It refers to a group of diseases caused by members of several virus groups. This condition indicates a mild infection of the upper respiratory tract associated with different degrees of nasal congestion and discharge, sneezing, runny nose, sore throat, cough, mild fever, and fatigue. Most individuals recover with rest and hydration and do not need special medical treatment. Some major training on self-care for this disease includes:

Self-Care Tips

- It is better to avoid exposure to very cold weather, closed environments with large numbers of people, and communication with infected individuals, and to take prophylactic measures to prevent contracting the disease.
- Enough rest and proper sleep are critical. Sleeping with the head at an angle of 45

degrees can prevent the accumulation of mucus in the sinus cavities.

- If not prohibited (such as in heart and kidney failure), drinking warm liquids is helpful. Water, clear broth, or warm lemon juice with honey (with restrictions for diabetic patients) can help relieve throat congestion. Warm liquids, including chicken soup or tea, may relieve congestion by increasing mucus flow. Alcohol, coffee, and carbonated drinks with caffeine are not appropriate and can exacerbate dehydration.
- Encourage older adults to wear warm clothes and to make the home environment warm and moderate. They should avoid exposure to cold air (by using a mask).
- Advise the patient to add cool moisture to the air. A cooling vaporizer or humidifier can relieve nasal congestion.
- Using supplements such as zinc and vitamin C can be beneficial. Using these supplements can reduce the duration of the disease. There is conflicting information in the studies concerning the role of vitamin D in the prevention of respiratory infections.
- Foods should be consumed while observing nutritional restrictions. Fatty foods are not advisable.
- Pharmacotherapy with medications such as decongestants, antihistamines, and painkillers must be used under the supervision of a physician and after ensuring that there is no interaction with the medications being consumed. Many brands produce age-appropriate medications, such as cold medications that are safe for individuals with hypertension, making them suitable for older people.
- Some studies have revealed that using probiotics can reduce the rate of acute respiratory infections or reduce the need for antibiotics in these individuals. However, the evidence in this area is not strong, and high-quality studies are required.
- Gargling with salt water can help loosen mucus and reduce sore throat and nasal congestion.
- To relieve an irritated nose or cracked lips, moisturizers or Vaseline can be used.
- In the case of fever (body temperature above 37.5 degrees Celsius), it is better to wear cool clothes. However, in the case of chills, it is better to wear warm clothes until the shivering stops. Then, light clothing can be worn again. Bathing during fever and chills is not recommended and can exacerbate the symptoms.
- Using acetaminophen tablets or suppositories can be useful in reducing fever, if not prohibited. Using aspirin or other Non-Steroidal Anti-Inflammatory Drugs (NSAIDs), such as ibuprofen, without the approval of a physician or pharmacist is not appropriate.
- Meditation can reduce the disease symptoms and duration (see Chap. 3).
- Concerning the impacts of physical activity in preventing and recovering from colds, there are conflicting reports. Due to the limitations for older people, high-intensity activities that exacerbate fatigue are not recommended.
- Recommend that the patient refer to healthcare providers in case of exacerbated symptoms or prolonged illness.

7.2.2 Allergic Reactions

Allergic conditions are mostly considered childhood disorders. However, their prevalence is growing in older people. The increase in the prevalence of allergic disorders in older people has been associated with efforts to ensure the best possible quality of life for this age group. This issue leads to increased attention to diseases that were previously ignored. The immune system changes with aging, and these changes can cause allergic reactions in this population. Immunosenescence can reduce resistance to infection, weaken the response to vaccination, and contribute to the development of age-related diseases. Thus, the most severe clinical impact of this phenomenon seems to be the loss of diversity in T-cell and B-cell receptors, occurring due to the accumulation of dysfunctional cells and reduced output of the thymus and bone marrow. In other words, immunosenescence seems to reflect dysregulation in the innate immune system. These changes in the immune system affect the way in which the body reacts to allergens and often make the diagnosis and treatment of allergies different in older adults compared to younger individuals. Additionally, weakness, concomitant medical problems, memory problems, and the use of multiple prescribed and non-prescribed medications can affect the occurrence of reactions in this age group. Allergies can cause other health problems, such as respiratory problems, or reduce the quality of life, making it essential to identify and treat allergies, especially among older people. During allergy season, older people may experience different clinical symptoms ranging from itching, congestion, watery eyes, runny nose, and sneezing to hives, swelling, or breathing problems. Seasonal allergies are regarded as a common minor ailment in older people, primarily associated with mild symptoms such as sneezing, runny nose, and tears. We will now refer to some training provided in the area of self-care for allergic conditions:

Self-Care Tips

- Since allergies can be a threat to older adults, it is crucial to refer to an allergist or healthcare provider in the case of symptoms such as hives, swelling, or breathing problems.
- It is essential to be aware of environmental stimuli such as dust, plant and flower pollen, animal fluff, and hair and to minimize exposure to them. Washing hands, taking a shower, changing clothes after going out, and using a mask can reduce exposure to pollen, especially in spring.
- Observing hygiene in the house is essential. Dusting and vacuuming can minimize dust and allergens in the house. Throw away things that collect dust.
- Mold is one of the common causes of seasonal allergies, so try to keep the humidity in your house below 50% if possible.
- It is advisable not to open the windows during allergy season and to use air conditioners instead.
- Eating healthy, vitamin C-rich, immune-boosting foods like leafy greens, apples, walnuts, and fatty fish can help control seasonal allergy symptoms.
- Antihistamines are considered among the most common medications for controlling allergy symptoms. However, some antihistamines may interfere with other medications or cause adverse side effects such as drowsiness, dizziness, and dry mouth in older people. Thus, it is necessary to consult a physician before prescribing any medicine.

7.2.3 Mild Headaches

The prevalence of headaches seems to decrease with aging, but the one-year prevalence of headaches in patients over 65 years of age has been reported to be about 51%. Additionally, older people experience headaches in their daily lives due to polypharmacy, several comorbidities, and possible intolerance to painkillers. Different types of headaches may occur among older adults. Based on the International Classification of Headache Disorders, third edition, headaches are generally divided into primary and secondary causes. The primary causes include migraine, tension-type headaches (TTHs), cluster headaches, trigeminal autonomic cephalalgias (TACs), and hypnic headaches, accounting for almost two-thirds of headaches in this population. “Primary headache” is a headache in the absence of another organic disorder that causes it. The prevalence of tension-type headache (TTH), as the most common primary headache, is 35.8% in older people worldwide. Migraine is the second most common primary headache disorder, with a prevalence of 5.7% in older adults, although its prevalence mostly decreases with aging. Unlike the primary headaches, up to 19.7% of new daily persistent headaches in older people are secondary to a serious cause that should be followed up seriously. The following tips can be helpful in self-care for older adults in case of primary mild headaches:

Self-Care Tips

- Older people and their caregivers should be aware of the red flags associated with secondary headaches and take them seriously. Warning signs include sudden onset of headaches, the presence of systemic symptoms such as weight loss, loss of appetite, fever, night sweats, extreme fatigue, changes in a previously persistent primary headache pattern, falls, walking disturbances, seizures, memory problems, urinary incontinence, neurological deficits identified during clinical examination, and positional changes in headaches. Another notable complaint is new persistent headaches or thunderclap headaches. These severe headaches start suddenly and peak within 60 seconds. They may fade after one hour but can also last for more than a week.
- Regular exercise within the tolerance limit can be useful as an alternative to relaxation therapy or medication for migraine headaches.
- Adhering to a healthy, high-fiber, and balanced diet and drinking adequate fluids (within the patient's tolerance and allowed limit) can be helpful since dehydration can cause headaches.
- Adequate rest and sleep can be helpful.
- Exposure to intense light, high noise, and environments with heavy air should be avoided.
- Consumption of caffeine and tobacco can exacerbate headaches.
- Relaxation methods and appropriate stress control approaches can reduce the occurrence of headaches in older people. Massage can also be helpful in this regard.
- Pharmacotherapy is very useful in relieving mild headaches. However, it should be used with the prescription and permission of the physician in older adults.
- There are some recommendations concerning warm and cold compresses to relieve headaches. A cold compress on the forehead helps to improve tension headaches and migraines. Warm compresses can help reduce muscle tension and relieve some headaches.
- Weight correction can be effective in reducing the occurrence of headaches, especially migraine headaches, since the odds of migraine in people who are morbidly obese increase more than twice compared to people who have a normal body mass index (BMI).

7.2.4 Dyspepsia (Indigestion)

The digestive system and stomach become vulnerable in old age. At this age, the mucosal defense system is weakened, the digestion of food is disturbed due to reduced saliva, stomach acid, and digestive enzymes, and the risk of *Helicobacter pylori* infection also increases. Foods are not chewed sufficiently due to the loss of teeth or inappropriate dentures, so digestive tract movements are reduced due to the decreased mobility of older people. All these factors contribute to the occurrence of dyspepsia in this population. Additionally, the use of certain drugs, especially non-steroidal anti-inflammatory drugs (NSAIDs), and most importantly aspirin, can exacerbate this condition.

Self-Care Tips

- Dyspepsia is associated with conditions such as discomfort after eating, early satiety, abdominal bloating, epigastric pain or discomfort, and loss of appetite. It affects the quality of life of older adults. The following tips are recommended for self-care for this condition:
- Some of the warning signs that make it essential to refer to a healthcare professional include symptoms such as the presence of blood in stool, vomiting, dysphagia, unplanned weight loss, anemia, pain in the chest, jaw, neck, or arm, severe and persistent abdominal pain, jaundice, and shortness of breath.
- If the dyspepsia symptoms persist, older people must be examined to rule out organic diseases or serious conditions such as peptic ulcers, cancer, celiac disease, or autoimmune

gastritis. Upper gastrointestinal endoscopy is a very useful and safe method in this regard.

- Foods that worsen dyspepsia should be avoided. Foods such as fried, fatty, and spicy foods; alcohol and caffeine; and carbonated drinks exacerbate dyspepsia.
- Educate older adults to chew their food slowly and thoroughly.
- Eating heavy food should be avoided. Five or six small meals daily instead of three large meals can be beneficial.
- Based on some studies, the consumption of probiotics can be beneficial.
- To reduce the feeling of fullness, drinking large amounts of liquids while eating should be avoided.
- Educate older adults to avoid eating 2 to 3 hours before bedtime and not to lie down immediately after eating. Encourage them to raise the head of the bed or keep the head and shoulders elevated with a pillow while sleeping.
- Keeping the weight in a healthy range is also important. Excessive weight puts pressure on the abdomen, pushing up the stomach and causing acid to leak up to the esophagus.
- Advise them to reduce everyday stress, anxiety, and mental pressure through relaxation and stress control methods.
- Regular exercise appropriate for older people's conditions will help them lose excess weight and have better digestion.
- Advise older people to quit smoking and assist them in this process.
- Wearing tight clothing is better to be prevented.
- Educate them to avoid taking certain painkillers such as aspirin, ibuprofen, naproxen sodium, or other NSAIDs without a physician's approval.
- Some herbal remedies, including simple peppermint or a combination of peppermint and cumin oil and the Japanese herbal formula Rikkunshito, can be beneficial if approved by the physician.

7.2.5 Gastroesophageal Reflux Disease (GERD)

This condition, known as *pyrosis* or simply *heartburn*, is the most common disorder of the upper digestive system among older adults. Symptoms of GERD mostly include heartburn with burning epigastric and retrosternal pain, acid regurgitation, belching, and nausea. Based on reports, older patients with GERD experience fewer symptoms. However, their disease is often more severe and is associated with esophageal complications (such as erosive esophagitis, esophageal stricture, Barrett's esophagus, and adenocarcinoma of the esophagus) and extraesophageal complications (such as chest pain, ear, nose, and throat manifestations such as globus sensation, laryngitis; dental problems; and lung problems such as chronic cough, asthma, and pulmonary aspiration). Therefore, older patients are referred to physicians with unusual symptoms such as chest pain and pulmonary and laryngeal symptoms rather than the classic symptoms of heartburn, which can delay diagnosis. Serious attention should be paid to GERD in older people since it reduces their quality of life and increases the possibility of serious gastrointestinal problems, such as esophageal cancer. The following tips are recommended for self-care of this problem:

Self-Care Tips

- Many antacids are commonly available over the counter. They are very beneficial in improving the symptoms of this condition. Some of them include magnesium hydroxide agents (which can cause diarrhea) and aluminum hydroxide (which can cause constipation). The consumption dose is about 30 ml half an hour after meals and at bedtime. However, these drugs should not be used for long times, and due to the possibility of electrolyte disorders or drug interactions in older

people, they should be used with caution and under the supervision of a physician.
- Consuming fatty, spicy, and sour foods, sauces, and carbonated and caffeinated drinks exacerbates the symptoms.
- Refer to the tips presented in the dyspepsia section to receive more information regarding lifestyle modifications.

7.2.6 Dry Skin (Xerosis)

The epidermis and dermis become thinner, the sweat glands and subcutaneous fat are lost, and the volume of connective tissue containing collagen and elastin decreases as the skin age increases. In addition, the skin's mechanical strength decreases, and generally, the skin's capability to maintain moisture, control temperature, and sense the surrounding environment decreases. Thus, xerosis is a common skin condition in older adults caused mostly by water loss from the stratum corneum. This affects 30 to 99.1% of people aged over 60 years. In addition to the body's physiological changes, older people suffer from various diseases, such as diabetes or thyroid and kidney problems. They often receive many medications, such as diuretics, which can exacerbate the development of xerosis. This condition, reported mostly in the lower legs, elbows, and arms, can cause cracks on the skin of older people and lead to itching, bleeding, infection, and asteatotic dermatitis. The following tips are recommended in the area of self-care in managing xerosis in older adults:

Self-Care Tips

- Older adults should refer to specialized centers in case of bruises, infections, and serious skin problems.
- Exposure to intense and direct sunlight, as well as dry and cold air, must be avoided.
- A balanced diet that includes sufficient intake of protein, vitamins, and beneficial fatty acids should be followed.
- Drinking enough water daily, if there are no restrictions, is also recommended.
- Older people should be encouraged to reduce the time spent taking a bath or shower. They can take a bath with warm water, but should avoid a bath with very hot water since it increases the loss of skin fat and may cause skin irritation.
- The use of spicy and fragrant soaps and alkaline detergents can exacerbate skin dryness. Appropriate and milder detergents are recommended.
- Excessive immersion in water can exacerbate skin dryness.
- Using bath oils is not recommended since they increase the risk of falls in older adults.
- They can use appropriate lotions and moisturizers, especially after bathing.
- If older adults intend to use vegetable oils for skin lubrication, they should be aware that not all oils are beneficial for the skin. A study revealed that although sunflower seed oil is beneficial for moisturizing the skin, olive oil may be harmful to skin hydration in adults and negatively affect skin integrity.
- Wearing loose clothing and avoiding woolen clothing can reduce skin irritation.
- Smoking must be stopped or limited.

7.2.7 Constipation

As a functional disorder of the digestive system, constipation is common in older people due to reasons such as dietary changes, pelvic floor dysfunction, reduced physical activity, and polypharmacy. It occurs frequently and sometimes chronically, affecting the patient's quality of life. It mostly appears as persistent hard or lumpy stools, reduced frequency of defecation (less than three times a week), the need to strain to defecate, a feeling of incomplete evacuation, or a feeling of anorectal obstruction or obstruction with 25% of bowel movements. Based on a systematic review by Salari et al. (2023), the overall prevalence of constipation in older adults was reported to be 18.9%. The highest prevalence of constipation is in older adults in Africa (32.3%), while the lowest is in Asia (13.6%). Its causes in older patients are often multifactorial. It may be due to primary factors (slow transit due to primary colonic smooth muscle dysfunction, dyssynergic defecation, and irritable bowel syndrome) or secondary factors (endocrine or metabolic disorders, neurological disorders such as Parkinson's disease and stroke, medications, and opioid use), or chronic idiopathic constipation. This condition may even be associated with certain characteristics of aging or comorbidities. For example, a cross-sectional study by Wang et al. (2021) on 11,743 older people showed that the constipation prevalence was significantly higher in older people with dementia, one of the diseases of aging. In older adults, constipation may be associated with fecal impaction, fecal incontinence, and even stercoral ulcers, bleeding, and anemia. Management measures include lifestyle modifications (such as increasing fluids, fiber, and exercise), discontinuation or reduction of unnecessary medications if permitted by the physician, and, as a next step, appropriate laxatives. Some self-care tips for older people suffering from constipation are presented here:

Self-Care Tips

- Physical activity increases gastrointestinal motility, and a sedentary lifestyle or complete rest contributes to the exacerbation of constipation in older adults. Thus, encourage the patient to stay active and, for example, regularly walk or do resistance training.
- Teach older people to use a healthy diet high in fiber (such as fresh fruits and vegetables, cooked or raw, cereals, and whole grain breads). A dietary fiber intake of 20–25 grams per day is beneficial. However, increased fiber intake may cause problems such as bloating and flatulence.
- Dehydration can exacerbate constipation. Advise older adults to drink enough fluids (usually six to eight cups of water per day) if there is no restriction. Drinking enough water, fruit juice, and other fluids can help patients have regular bowel movements.
- Some studies have indicated that probiotics can improve bowel function and reduce symptoms of constipation. Older people should use probiotics in their diet.
- It is recommended to establish a routine and regular pattern for bowel movements. The onset of bowel movements is a conditioned reflex to some extent. People with a normal bowel pattern mostly empty their bowels at about the same time each day. Colonic motor activity is highest after waking up and after eating. Thus, the first two hours after waking up and after breakfast can be the best time for bowel movements.
- Teach older people about bowel movements. Teach them to go to the toilet on time and have at least two bowel movements, usually 30 minutes after eating. Diaphragmatic breathing and body posture (for example, sitting, bending forward, and raising the legs 8 to 12 inches off the floor) may also affect the ease of bowel movements.
- Laxatives can be useful in patients who do not respond to lifestyle modifications. These drug combinations in older adults should be noted by considering the patient's history (heart and kidney disease), drug interferences, cost, and individual side effects, and in consultation with a healthcare professional.
- Laxatives have different functions and effectiveness, so they should be selected by the physician. Uncontrolled and indiscriminate use of these drugs can cause complications. Bulk laxatives, osmotic laxatives, and stimulant laxatives, respectively, can be used with physician approval in the short term for 3 months with reasonable safety in older patients. Although stimulant laxatives are effective, chronic use of them should be avoided as long-term safety in older adults is unknown. Bisacodyl suppositories can only be used once a week without physician advice.
- Milk of magnesia is a mild laxative and can be used in doses of two tablespoons (30 cc) once or twice daily for a short period if approved.

- Glycerin suppositories have limited efficacy and are used for the short term. Stool-softening edible oils, such as paraffin oil, are not recommended for older adults, especially if they have swallowing problems, due to the risk of aspiration.
- Studies have provided conflicting results regarding laxative products and teas containing senna. Although these products have good laxative effects, they mostly cause other intestinal problems if used regularly.
- Studies have indicated that polyethylene glycol seems to be safe and effective when used long-term for about 6 months in older patients.
- Some studies have revealed the positive effects of some other methods, such as acupressure (ear acupressure) or fermented oat drinks (for example, those containing *B. Llongum* and *B. Llactis* fermentation), but they are not enough, and more studies are needed.
- Cognitive retraining of the pelvic floor and abdominal wall muscles, recommended as biofeedback therapy, is a painless and noninvasive method to facilitate bowel evacuation. In this technique, electromyographic surface electrodes on the anal plug and the surface electrode of the abdominal wall are used to improve muscle control. It is recommended mostly in pelvic floor dysfunction, especially dyssynergic defecation.
- The patient should see a physician if changes are not effective or he experiences symptoms such as pain, blood in the stool, hemorrhoids or fissures, severe weight loss, or suspicion of fecal impaction and incontinence.

7.2.8 Diarrhea

Diarrhea in older people is one of the annoying conditions that may occur due to multiple comorbidities, immunodeficiency, weakness, and poor nutritional status. Diarrhea caused by some infectious agents, such as *C. difficile* colitis, is associated with significant complications such as malnutrition and mortality in this population. Thus, this condition should be considered in older adults. Careful follow-up of this condition is vital to ensure adequate hydration, electrolyte replacement, and infection control measures to contain the outbreak. Diagnosing the type of diarrhea and the cause of its occurrence is also crucial in treatment. Diarrhea treatment can range from dietary changes to medication (such as loperamide, diphenoxylate, and bismuth subsalicylate) to hospitalization and broad-spectrum antibiotics. The following self-care points should be considered for older people suffering from diarrhea:

Self-Care Tips

- Oral fluids and electrolyte replacement are essential in mild to moderate diarrhea. Oral rehydration solutions (ORSs) are common and may be beneficial in some cases.
- Color and frequency of urination are ways to judge hydration. Infrequent urination (less than every three to five hours) or dark yellow urine is a sign of dehydration.
- Encourage the patient to take appropriate rest periods to restore energy and recovery.
- Adequate nutrition is vital during an episode of acute diarrhea. If the patient has no appetite, you can give them more soup and fluids for a short time. Starches and cooked grains (such as potatoes, noodles, rice, wheat, and oats) or crackers, bananas, and soups are also helpful if not prohibited.
- The *BRAT diet* can help to firm up stools. This diet includes *bananas, rice, applesauce, and toast.*
- Advise the patient to eat small, frequent meals and gradually add semi-solid and low-fiber foods to the diet.
- Probiotics may help restore intestinal flora balance and reduce the diarrhea duration. However, there is some controversy in this regard. A meta-analysis by Jafarnejad et al. (2016) reported that probiotic supplementation was associated with a reduced risk of antibiotic-associated diarrhea in adults but not in older people (aged 65 years and older).
- Advise older adults to avoid dairy products, high-fat, spicy, high-fiber foods, and foods

and beverages containing artificial sweeteners during this period.

- A *low-FODMAP* diet is recommended for patients with Irritable Bowel Syndrome with Diarrhea (IBS-D). FODMAPs are poorly absorbed, osmotically activated in the small intestine, and increase gastrointestinal motility.
- This leads to diarrhea and fermentation in the large intestine, which causes gas, bloating, cramps, and abdominal pain. Milk, yogurt, and dairy-based ice cream; some wheat-based products; beans and lentils; some vegetables such as artichokes, asparagus, onions, and garlic; and some fruits such as cherries, pears, and peaches are high in FODMAPs. Table 7.1 provides explanations about foods containing FODMAPs.
- Teach older people to avoid using alcohol, cigarettes, and caffeine.
- Diarrhea can cause irritation, burning, and even sores in the anal and perineal areas. Visit a physician if pain, irritation, or sores occur in these areas.
- It is best to avoid wearing tight pants or underwear. Cotton underwear helps to ventilate the body and prevents irritation or sores.
- The patient can start over-the-counter antidiarrheal medications, such as loperamide and bismuth subsalicylate, under the supervision of a healthcare professional if infectious diarrhea is ruled out. Explain these medications and how to take them to the patient.
- The older person should be taught to observe basic hand hygiene and encouraged to wash their hands regularly during diarrhea, especially if it is infectious. Hands should be wetted with plain soap and water and rubbed together for 15 to 30 seconds.
- The patient should visit the physician if diarrhea persists or worsens (more than 2 days) or if symptoms such as fever (more than 38.5 °C), severe abdominal pain, or bloody stools are experienced.

Table 7.1 Details on FODMAP

Fermentable	They include foods that intestinal bacteria feed on and convert into gas in a chemical process called fermentation.
Oligosaccharides	They include soluble plant fibers found in onions, garlic, beans/lentils, and many wheat products, also known as prebiotics.
Disaccharides	They include lactose, the sugar found in dairy products. Lactose intolerance is one of the most common food intolerances worldwide.
Monosaccharides	The sugar in fruits or fructose is a fermentable sugar found in certain amounts in some fruits.
Polyols	These are sugar alcohols used commonly as artificial sweeteners or that occur naturally in some fruits.

7.2.9 Fatigue

"Fatigue," often confused with *"asthenia"* and *"weakness,"* is a subjective state characterized by a feeling of reduced energy and a perception of reduced physical or mental work capacity. It is a commonly reported symptom in older adults, especially those with chronic diseases, with a reported prevalence of 15–75%. Fatigue in older people can be caused by physical factors (e.g., chronic diseases, anemia, effects of medications), psychological factors (e.g., depression, anxiety), or lifestyle factors (e.g., poor sleep hygiene, inadequate nutrition). Identifying the underlying cause is vital for effective management. Fatigue may be a sign of a reduction in inherent reserves and capacity in old age, leading to negative health outcomes. Some of these outcomes include the inability to perform activities of daily living, physical decline, worsening of medical conditions, readmissions, and mortality. Some self-care strategies for fatigue include:

Self-Care Tips

- Inadequate sleep can cause fatigue. Implementing sleep hygiene behaviors can help older people in this regard.
- Teach older adults to distribute their energy throughout the day and avoid doing heavy tasks that require a lot of energy all at once.

They can do heavy tasks in several stages with rest periods between them.

- Advise them to avoid being sedentary and to engage in light but regular exercises to maintain energy throughout the day. Walking, yoga, and tai chi can be helpful.
- Teach older people that inadequate intake of essential nutrients (e.g., vitamins B12, D, and iron) can help improve the feelings of fatigue. Paying attention to older people's food intake and malnutrition is vital. A balanced diet rich in whole grains, vegetables and fruits, lean proteins, and healthy fats can help maintain energy levels. Certain nutrients such as iron, vitamin D, and B vitamins are also essential in energy metabolism.
- Drinking adequate fluids throughout the day (if not restricted) is helpful since dehydration can cause fatigue in older adults.
- Chronic pain in older adults due to neuropathy, arthritis, etc., can cause sleep disturbances or fatigue. Recommend pain management strategies to older people.
- Increasing social relations and avoiding loneliness can help reduce feelings of fatigue to a limited extent.
- In the case of continuous fatigue, visit a physician to find the underlying cause.
- Recent studies have indicated that taking nicotinamide mononucleotide (NMN) in the afternoon may effectively improve lower limb function, reduce sleepiness in older people, and potentially prevent a decline in physical performance and improve fatigue. Additionally, branched-chain amino acids (BCAAs), along with exercise, may reduce fatigue by affecting tryptophan metabolism and enhancing physical and mental performance. However, more high-quality studies are needed in this area.

7.2.10 Insomnia and Sleep Disorders

Adequate and high-quality sleep is vital for the overall health and well-being of older people. Sleep for 7 to 8 hours is considered appropriate for this population. However, many older people, even with adequate sleep, report dissatisfaction with the quantity and quality of sleep due to difficulty falling asleep, staying asleep, or waking up early. Although sleep disorders are not normal, their prevalence increases with aging.

Despite the high prevalence of insomnia in the older population, reported to be about 50% in many studies, there is a wide variation in reports from different parts of the world (from 6% in Taiwan to 62.1% in Egypt). A systematic review and meta-analysis by Endomba et al. (2023) reported the pooled prevalence of insomnia disorder in older adults according to the Diagnostic and Statistical Manual of Mental Disorders (DSM) at 19.6%. Insomnia in this population was associated with female gender, depression, anxiety, cardiovascular and respiratory conditions, and pain. Older people may have difficulty falling asleep (sleep onset insomnia) in 35–60% of cases, staying asleep (sleep maintenance insomnia) in 50–70% of cases, or both. These problems in older adults can be a symptom of a medical problem (such as pain, enuresis, dyspnea, obstructive sleep apnea [OSA], restless legs syndrome [RLS], circadian rhythm disorders, or psychiatric problems) or a side effect of various factors. Some chronic diseases in older people also exacerbate this problem. For example, about 80% of patients with Parkinson's disease experience sleep problems, with sleep maintenance insomnia being the most common among them.

Prolonged insomnia can have serious consequences, such as increased memory problems and impaired health outcomes in older people. Sleeping less than 4–5 hours or more than 10 hours per night may be associated with increased mortality. Thus, cognitive behavioral therapy for insomnia (CBT-I), pharmacological treatments (from melatonin to benzodiazepines and zolpidem), or even methods such as acupuncture can improve sleep problems, but they should be prescribed by a specialist for the patient. Some studies suggest that bright light therapy may be beneficial for daytime sleepiness and insomnia in older people, especially those with Parkinson's disease or circadian rhythm disorders. Some self-care points to improve sleep health are presented below:

Self-Care Tips

A regular sleep schedule and adherence to it are essential for people with insomnia. Advise the patient to go to bed only when they feel sleepy. If they are unable to fall asleep within 20 minutes, suggest that they leave the bedroom, engage in some activity, and return when they are sleepy.

- Older people should get up every morning and avoid napping regardless of how much sleep the patient gets during the night.
- The bedroom environment should be designed in a way appropriate for sleep. It should be dark and quiet, have a comfortable temperature (between 15.6 and 20 °C (60 and 68 °F)), and have effective ventilation.
- Encourage older people to be physically active during the day and, if possible, exercise regularly. Adequate aerobic exercise improves the ability to fall asleep. However, exercise before bedtime is not recommended.
- Teach older people to avoid heavy and fatty meals within two hours of bedtime.
- Fluid intake should be limited before bedtime, as frequent urination during sleep can disrupt sleep.
- Smoking and alcohol consumption before bedtime should be stopped. Alcohol may induce sleep but will cause inappropriate sleep.
- Advise the patient to avoid caffeine (green tea, cola, coffee, and chocolate) 6 to 8 hours before bedtime.
- Teaching relaxation techniques such as deep breathing exercises, progressive muscle relaxation, biofeedback, and guided images helps reduce stress and tension during the daytime.
- Using electronic devices and looking at screens 30 to 60 minutes before bedtime can prevent sleeping.
- Listening to your favorite relaxing music and humming it can relax the brain and vagus nerve and improve sleep.
- The patient should be taught to avoid uncontrolled taking of sleeping pills or suddenly stopping prescribed medications.
- A specialist should be consulted to begin appropriate treatment if sleep problems are not resolved.

7.2.11 Mood Swings

Mood swings in older people may manifest as increased irritability, sadness, unexplained crying, insomnia, restlessness, anxiety, and rapid transitions from happy to sad or content to aggressive. The prevalence of these mood swings increases with aging and in older population, especially those who are hospitalized. Mood swings in this age group can be associated with several factors, including life changes, loss of loved ones, depression, chronic conditions, and cognitive decline. Negative perceptions of health and frailty can also cause this condition.

Many older people, especially when hospitalized, lose interest in enjoyable activities (estimated at 15% in one cross-sectional study). Older people in healthcare facilities often experience negative mood states, such as anxiety or sadness.

These moods are often caused by feelings of approaching the end of their lives or missing their family, friends, or even pets. Since positive moods are associated with increased health and well-being, older adults should cope with these negative moods. Some self-care approaches may help manage these mood swings:

Self-Care Tips

- Social participation and maintaining social relations are beneficial for the emotional well-being of older adults and can help stabilize their mood.
- Helping older people manage their chronic diseases and create a sense of control over their diseases positively affects their mood regulation.
- Insufficient sleep and rest can exacerbate mood swings. Additionally, not receiving healthy and nutritious meals timely can make any person's mood worse and create hangry

(hungry + angry) states. It is necessary to pay attention to these basic needs of older adults.

- Engaging in mentally stimulating activities such as puzzles, reading, or learning new skills can enhance cognitive function and improve mood.
- Teaching mindfulness techniques and practicing meditation or relaxation techniques is vital in this population. Mindfulness can help regulate mood and reduce symptoms of anxiety and depression (see Chap. 3).
- Encourage the patient and his family to make positive changes in their living environment. The decoration and color combinations used and the rate of using flowers and ornamental plants often affect people's moods.
- Some new technologies, such as various aspects of ambient intelligence and "empathic technology," can be useful by recognizing the emotional state of the person and providing the necessary care solutions. One of these solutions is the use of intelligent lighting. A study by Kuijsters et al. (2015) showed that exposing older adults to lighting ambiance with bright and positive emotional meaning improved their mood. Sad older people can benefit from an arousing and activating ambiance, and anxious older people from a cozy ambiance.
- Encouraging the patient to have regular physical and mental screenings is crucial. Conditions such as thyroid disorders or vitamin deficiencies can significantly affect mood and require medical intervention.
- Families should be taught ways to strengthen social support for older people and identify risk factors.
- Help from a mental health professional is needed in the case of continuous mood changes and self-destructive thoughts such as self-harm or suicide.

7.3 Chronic Diseases in Older Adults

Chronic diseases such as diabetes, hypertension, and heart failure (HF) are noncommunicable and mostly incurable conditions that are often not immediately life-threatening and accompany the patient for a long time. As a multidimensional experience, they expose the patient to debilitating conditions and limitations. Evidence suggests that the number of chronic conditions a person has is positively associated with the number of emergency department (ED) visits. About 80% of all hospital admissions are attributed to chronic conditions. These diseases also affect normal daily life activities and consequently the quality of life. They naturally increase the level of demand for medical services and the economic burden imposed on the patients, healthcare systems, and societies, as they require a long period of treatment and care. In this regard, the World Health Organization (WHO) defines chronic diseases and multiple diseases as major challenges facing health systems worldwide. Longer life expectancy makes the body more susceptible to disease. Thus, the prevalence of chronic diseases in older adults is high. Chronic diseases in older adults are mostly associated with disabilities such as mental health problems, mobility problems, poor cognitive function, falls and accidents, wounds and injuries, malnutrition, and communication problems. They can lead to dependence in performing daily life activities and associated problems. Population aging has been a worrying phenomenon in recent decades. It is predicted that the population of older people aged over 65 years will reach about 1.5 billion by 2050. It is also estimated that over 90% of older people aged over 65 years will have at least one chronic disease, and 50% will have two chronic diseases. Healthcare costs for older patients with multiple chronic conditions are 5.5 times higher than for other older patients. This is an alarming sign for healthcare systems. Given what was stated above and the fact that chronic disease care is a challenging issue for older adults, promoting self-care for older people with chronic diseases is a promising solution and is the focus of many current interventions.

7.4 Holistic Perspective in Self-Care Programs for Older People

Chronic diseases will change many aspects of the life and health of older adults. Thus, self-care is a multidimensional behavior and will be beneficial if there is a holistic perspective among the patients and caregivers of those with chronic diseases.

A holistic perspective on self-care acknowledges the multidimensional nature of health and wellness and integrates the different physical, mental, emotional, social, and spiritual dimensions. This approach is especially crucial for older people, who often face complex health challenges and a reduced overall quality of life. Holistic healthcare focuses on the whole person and dates back to Florence Nightingale, the founder of modern nursing, as she taught nurses to focus on the principles of wholeness, unity, health, and the link between people and their environment.

Based on the definition of the World Health Organization (WHO), health is not merely the absence of disease, but it is a state of complete physical, mental, and social well-being. Thus, a holistic perspective on self-care for older adults is essential to achieving complete well-being. Unfortunately, many studies and methods of empowering self-care focus only on the physical and, in some cases, psychological dimensions of patients. Overall well-being, self-efficacy, and independence of a patient depend on their capability to self-care in all aspects of life. Attention to older people's needs in the various dimensions should be considered in the development of a comprehensive care plan. Considering the needs and increasing awareness regarding how to promote well-being in each dimension is the most essential step in the active participation of older adults in self-care. Guiding and assisting older people in strengthening each of these areas may require the involvement of specialists and professionals. Box 7.1 provides a guide outlining the dimensions that should be considered in holistic self-care and the items that should be addressed in each dimension.

Box 7.1 A General Guide Outlining the Dimensions for the Development of a Holistic Self-Care Program

Physical

- *Identifying the disease and its symptoms:* What is the disease? How does it develop, and what happens? What are the stages and symptoms? What are the available treatments? What tools or methods can help track health?
- *Monitoring and managing symptoms:* How to monitor the symptoms of the disease? How is each of them managed? What are the warning and dangerous signs? What are the necessary measures when dangerous symptoms appear?
- *Diet modification:* What is the appropriate diet? What are the fluid and food restrictions? What are the dos and don'ts of the diet according to the diseases? What foods interfere with prescribed medications?
- Improving physical activity: What is the appropriate level of activity and appropriate exercise? How much and when is it allowed? What is the necessary monitoring before, during, and after exercise? What are the methods of maintaining energy? What are the methods of improving rest and sleep health? What are the considerations related to sexual activities?
- *Medication adherence:* What are the available treatments? What are the prescribed medications, and what are their

uses? What is the appropriate way and time to use medications, and what are the strategies to avoid mistakes or forgetting to take them? What are the expected and dangerous complications? When is the next visit with the physician and routine checkups? When and how to access healthcare professionals?

- *Modifying unhealthy habits:* What are unhealthy behaviors? How can they be stopped (such as smoking)?
- *Improving the safety of the living environment*: What are home safety modifications, such as fall prevention measures and appropriate home temperature, and how are they evaluated? What are the technologies needed to improve the safety of older people's home environment?
  - *Professional Support Resources*
    Specialist physician, nurse, nutritionist, physiotherapist, occupational therapist, rehabilitation specialist

Psychological

- *Identifying mental health concerns:* What are common mental health issues (e.g., anxiety, depression)? What are the signs and symptoms of each? What are the signs that indicate a need for support? What are the danger signs that require serious measures?
- *Monitoring and managing mental well-being:* How can you regularly assess your mental state? What are appropriate relaxation techniques, and how are they performed? What are stress management methods such as mindfulness and cognitive behavioral strategies?
- *Engaging in cognitive activities:* What activities provide mental engagement (e.g., puzzles, reading)?

  - *Professional support resources*
- Psychologist or therapist, psychiatrist, geriatric mental health counselor

Emotional

- *Identifying emotions*: How to identify, label, and express your emotions? What triggers emotional reactions in your life?
- *Managing emotional health:* What strategies help regulate emotions (e.g., taking daily notes, talking to friends)? How to practice self-compassion and resilience? What support networks (e.g., support groups) are there, and how to access them?
- *Developing and maintaining healthy relationships:* How to maintain and strengthen relationships with family and friends? How do you develop trustful, supportive relationships?
  - *Professional support resources*
    Licensed therapist/counselor, social worker, support groups, life coach

Spiritual

- *Promoting spirituality and practicing related actions:* What practices can enhance spiritual well-being (e.g., meditation, prayer)? How does participating in religious events or personal reflection (depending on the patient's preference) help the patient?
- *Finding purpose and meaning:* What are the values and purpose of life? What activities are consistent with the patient's spiritual and religious beliefs?
- *Relation with nature:* How does spending time outdoors or in nature help the old person relax?
  - *Professional support resources*
    Spiritual leader/clergy, religious counselor, wellness coach

Personal

- *Creating appropriate daily routines:* How to develop a consistent daily schedule that includes self-care activities? What is an appropriate routine for personal health and hygiene?

- *Paying attention to hobbies and interests:* What are the interests that bring happiness and satisfaction to older people? What are new hobbies available considering the limitations of aging?
- *Enhancing self-reflection and awareness:* What are personal goals and aspirations? What areas of life need more attention? What are advance directives, and how should they be set?
- *Setting goals:* What are achievable goals that feel satisfying? How can SMART (Specific, Measurable, Achievable, Relevant, Time-bound) goals be created? What steps can be taken to achieve personal growth?
- *Time management:* How to prioritize tasks and responsibilities? What tools can help improve productivity?
  - *Professional support resources*
    Life coach, educated mentor, geriatric care manager

Professional

- *Skills development:* What skills and hobbies can lead to personal growth? What training opportunities are available to enhance specific aging skills?
- *Participation in voluntary activities:* How to find opportunities for meaningful involvement in work or community service?
- *Work-life balance:* How to set boundaries between work and personal life? What self-care practices can be integrated into the workday?
  - *Professional support resources*
    Career counselor, occupational therapist, professional mentor, volunteer coordinator

7.5 Self-Care for Common Chronic Diseases in Older Adults

Chronic diseases are managed rather than cured. Thus, patients are often responsible for implementing many aspects of their treatment plan. Promoting self-care through various methods is one response to the high prevalence of chronic disease among older people. The requirements for self-care when living with the challenges of aging and chronic conditions are sometimes more complex, as self-care is an integral aspect of the lives of older people with chronic diseases.

According to the conceptual model presented by LeBlanc and Jacelon (2018) regarding the concept of self-care in older adults suffering from chronic disease, self-care is a multidimensional concept that has multilevel effects (individual, social, and systemic levels) and is mediated by the aging contexts and processes. Self-care originates and is learned throughout an individual's life and is provided based on the care needs when living with chronic health conditions. Adequate self-care is essential to reduce ED visits, hospitalizations, and early death. However, the rate of successful self-care varies widely among patients with chronic disease, and interventions to increase self-care have yielded conflicting results. One reason that self-care varies among patients with chronic disease is that individuals have different perceptions of their disease, its management, and their role in the treatment plan. Nurses' attention to the concept of self-care and methods for promoting it provides an opportunity for these patients to increase their authority and engage more in decisions about their treatment and care. Engagement in self-care and adherence to these behaviors requires high knowledge, motivation, and skills in older adults. The following section discusses common chronic diseases in older people and also highlights self-care tips for each disease:

7.5.1 Cancer

Cancer is typically defined as a disease in which the body's cells grow uncontrollably and spread to other parts of the body. The more advanced the cancer is, the more severe the symptoms and disabilities. Several treatment options have been introduced and are being implemented. However, cancer has become one of the major health challenges of society. Almost 52,900 cases of cancer are diagnosed every day worldwide, and 27,000 people die from this disease. It is estimated that about 28 million new cases of cancer will be diagnosed and 16.2 million people will die from this disease by 2040. Cancer can be considered a kind of age-related disease, as the incidence of most types of cancer increases with aging. Its incidence in people over 65 is 11 times higher than that in younger people. It is predicted that about 6.9 million new cancers will be diagnosed in adults aged 80 years or older worldwide by 2050. Cancer is also associated with gender. The lifetime probability of cancer is 44.85% for males and 38.08% for females, indicating that males are more likely to develop cancer despite their shorter life expectancy. The mortality rate for cancer patients is higher, especially in older adults and those with comorbidities. A general estimate reports that about 60% of cancers occur in people aged 65 years or older. About 70% of cancer deaths occur at this stage. The cancer types that commonly affect older adults include breast, lung, and colon cancer in older women, and prostate, lung, and colon cancer in older men. They are mostly classified as carcinomas, forming in the cells that make up the skin and lining of internal organs. In this regard, breast cancer is the most commonly diagnosed cancer in women, affecting about 1 in 8 females, while prostate cancer is more common in males.

Generally, cancer can affect all aspects of the quality of life. Studies have indicated that quality of life in cancer patients is significantly reduced in terms of physical, mental, and overall health. Physical symptoms of cancer vary depending on its type and the treatments. However, they can include sleep disturbances, pain, nausea and vomiting, diarrhea, neuropathy, skin rashes, cachexia, muscle and joint pains, swollen lymph nodes, sexual dysfunction, and cognitive impairment. Fatigue is also a major symptom, which can manifest as chronic fatigue syndrome (CFS), also known as myalgic encephalomyelitis. Older people with cancer often have comorbidities, such as dementia, that complicate their health outcomes and self-care. They also often face challenges in finding a coherent healthcare plan. Additionally, these patients experience anxiety and stress related to their health conditions, which can lead to disease progression. Disease progression also leads to pain and other symptoms of cancer that can affect daily activities, health, and overall well-being. Thus, self-care and education are particularly crucial for these patients to manage pain and symptoms. Table 7.2 presents a summary of self-care recommendations for cancer patients.

7.5.2 Diabetes Mellitus

Diabetes mellitus (DM) is a metabolic disorder caused by reduced insulin production by the pancreas, impaired insulin action, or both, leading to elevated blood sugar levels (normal blood sugar: 70–100 mg/dL). There are different types of diabetes. Type 1 diabetes is caused by impaired insulin production, while type 2 diabetes occurs when the body does not use insulin effectively or when the insulin produced by the pancreas is insufficient. There are many non-modifiable and modifiable risk factors for type 2 diabetes. Non-modifiable risk factors include age, genetics, and social determinants of health (including education level, socioeconomic status, and exposure to noise and arsenic). Modifiable risk factors include obesity, diet, smoking, sleep duration, sleep quality, and physical inactivity. Based on the guidelines provided by the American Diabetes Association, this disease can be diagnosed in several ways:

- Suffering from primary symptoms of diabetes along with a physician's diagnosis
- Fasting sugar of 126 and above
- Random sugar of 200 and above
- Postprandial sugar of 200 and above
- Hemoglobin A1C of 6.5% and above, indicating the mean blood sugar level over the past two to three months

Diabetes is nowadays one of the most important public health concerns worldwide, with a high prevalence. It is estimated that 642 million people will struggle with this disease by 2040. With aging, insulin production decreases, fat

Table 7.2 Self-care tips for older adults with cancer

Familiarization with the disease and clinical manifestations monitoring	Educate the patient about their disease and physiology, as well as the available diagnostic methods and treatments, in a simple and comprehensible manner. Explain the clinical manifestations associated with the disease to the patient. In cases of cancer, the manifestations may vary depending on the affected area of the body and the stage of the disease. However, some common signs and symptoms may include: Chronic fatigue Persistent and recurrent gastrointestinal issues Changes in bowel or bladder habits Rashes, skin lesions, or alterations in the affected tissue Significant weight loss and cachexia Chronic pain, including muscle and joint pain Swelling of lymph nodes Cognitive impairments Inform the patient about warning signs and emergency actions. For instance, persistent changes in bowel or bladder habits that lead to complications such as retention, a wound that does not heal, unusual bleeding or discharge from any part of the body, thickening or lumps in the breast or elsewhere, indigestion or difficulty swallowing, noticeable changes in warts or moles, and persistent cough or hoarseness. In these situations, it is essential to consult healthcare professionals. Patients may experience alterations in blood cells due to the nature of certain cancers, particularly those related to the hematologic system, or as a result of chemotherapy. A reduction in white blood cells (leukopenia) heightens the risk of infection; therefore, patients should be educated on infection control measures. Similarly, a decrease in platelet levels (thrombocytopenia) increases the risk of bleeding, and patients should be trained in methods to prevent bleeding as well as to recognize potential symptoms. Pain management in these patients is one of the most critical components of enhancing self-care. Screening for pain, addressing moderate to severe pain with strong opioid medications, managing bone metastasis pain through radiotherapy and bisphosphonates, and supporting patients in learning self-care techniques for pain management are strongly recommended by studies. Encourage the patient to maintain a symptom diary to document treatment side effects and any changes in their health status. This can facilitate timely communication with healthcare providers. Educate the patient on the importance of undergoing routine checkups and tests as recommended by their healthcare providers. Emphasize the necessity of attending all scheduled appointments with their physician and primary care providers for monitoring disease progression and effectively managing side effects.

Diet modification	Encourage the patient to adhere to a balanced diet that includes foods from the four main food groups: fruits and vegetables, carbohydrates, dairy, and proteins. Older people should ensure adequate hydration by drinking sufficient fluids (within the limits advised by their healthcare provider), especially if they experience side effects such as nausea or diarrhea. In cases of decreased appetite, it is advisable to consume smaller meals more frequently throughout the day. The adoption of neutropenic diets (particularly those that eliminate raw fruits and vegetables) is not recommended for cancer patients as a means of preventing infections during treatment. Harmful diets, such as the Western diet or fast foods and excessive consumption of certain food categories (foods high in saturated fats and full-fat dairy), can worsen treatment outcomes in cancers. Consuming outside food due to concerns regarding the hygiene of food preparation or thorough cooking may elevate the risk of infection in these patients. Animal proteins, such as fish, poultry, red meat, and low-fat dairy products, should not be eliminated from the diets of cancer patients (unless directed by their healthcare provider). One of the most common complications in these patients is muscle loss, which can lead to decreased functional capacity, increased risk of chemotherapy toxicity, and higher rates of hospitalization and disease-related complications. Dietary interventions for cancer patients should ideally begin at the early stages of diagnosis to positively influence treatment processes and outcomes. Total parenteral nutrition (TPN) is not routinely recommended for cancer patients but may be temporarily utilized for specific groups of patients, such as those experiencing reversible bowel obstruction. Currently, there are no FDA-approved pharmacological interventions specifically aimed at improving cancer-related cachexia. However, a short course of treatment with progesterone analogs or corticosteroids may be suggested for these patients, contingent upon a careful evaluation of the potential benefits and risks. It is advisable for the older patients to consult with a nutritionist to develop a personalized dietary plan that addresses specific nutritional needs and manages side effects. Encourage the older patients to quit smoking and avoid alcohol consumption.
Physical activity improvement	Cancer patients should engage in aerobic and resistance exercises during their treatment to help mitigate the side effects of cancer therapy. These exercises can lead to reduced fatigue, improved cardiovascular and respiratory health, enhanced physical performance, and increased strength. In certain populations, such activities may also improve quality of life and reduce anxiety and depression. Encourage the patient to participate in gentle activities such as walking, stretching, or yoga, within their tolerance levels. If possible, it is advisable to incorporate light resistance training two to three times a week to help maintain muscle mass and strength. Exercises that improve balance and flexibility and reduce the risk of falls (such as yoga or tai chi) can be beneficial. Preoperative exercise programs for patients with lung cancer may contribute to shorter hospital stays and a reduction in postoperative complications. Encourage the patient to prioritize daily activities. They should distribute various tasks throughout the day to prevent activity intolerance, take breaks between activities, and practice breathing exercises. They should avoid performing all energy-demanding activities in one day or consecutively and refrain from bending or standing for prolonged periods during activities. Educate the older patients to pay attention to how their body responds to physical activity and to adjust the intensity and duration accordingly. They should avoid overexertion and rest if they notice any significant changes in vital signs. It is essential to consult with a healthcare provider before starting any new exercise program to ensure its safety and appropriateness. Teach the patient about the importance of adequate rest, sleep hygiene practices, and strategies for maintaining energy levels.

(continued)

Table 7.2 (continued)

Medication management	Educate the patient about chemotherapy and supportive treatments during the chemotherapy regimen, including the overall function of the medications, the purpose of their administration, potential side effects, and the timing and method of their use. Provide information regarding radiation therapy, including how it is performed, its duration, potential side effects, and posttreatment care. In older people with cancer, managing medication use is particularly important due to the complexity of their regimens. Adverse drug effects can be significantly more dangerous in this population. Recent studies indicate that ongoing communication with a pharmacist, coordinated by the healthcare system and the patient's treatment team, can be effective in managing their medications and preventing unwanted side effects across all healthcare settings, including hospitals, emergency care, and palliative care. For older patients, it is essential to periodically review all medications with healthcare providers to ensure that they are necessary, effective, and do not cause adverse interactions. Any side effects or concerns regarding medications should be promptly communicated to healthcare providers for adjustment or substitution. Advise older patients to avoid self-medicating with any new drugs or abruptly discontinuing prescribed medications and altering dosages without consulting their physician. Recommend that patients utilize pill organizers, reminders, or medication management programs to track their medications and dosages and ensure timely administration.
Other considerations	Teach the patient stress management techniques, such as yoga, meditation, and deep breathing exercises (see Chap. 3). Encourage participation in activities they enjoy. To address the emotional challenges arising from a cancer diagnosis, familiarize older patients with useful resources for counseling, therapy, and emotional support. Encourage them to join support groups for older individuals facing this illness, allowing them to share their experiences and learn from others who are confronting similar challenges. The early integration of palliative care services is beneficial for effectively managing symptoms and enhancing the quality of life alongside medical treatments. Introduce the patient to local palliative care providers in their area. It is advisable for older people to become acquainted with advance care planning and take appropriate steps in this regard. This process facilitates discussions about future medical care priorities with family members and healthcare providers, ensuring that their wishes are respected. Prepare older patients to utilize new and appropriate technologies that can enhance their self-care behaviors (refer to Chap. 6 for further details).

mass relative to muscle tissue increases, and insulin resistance increases. Additionally, increased cortisol production reduces muscle mass and increases liver cell resistance to insulin. Factors such as inactivity, obesity, increased stress associated with aging, reduced renal function, and the use of diuretics, beta-adrenergic agonists, and corticosteroids lead to impaired glucose metabolism and diabetes in older adults. Thus, diabetes is one of the most common diseases of old age. Based on estimates in the United States, about 40% of adults with diabetes are 65 years of age or older. In this age group, about 21.4% are diagnosed with diabetes, while an estimated 16% remain undiagnosed. This indicates a vital gap in awareness and management of the disease among older people. Among people 65 years of age and older, about one in three suffers from this chronic disease, mostly type 2 diabetes (90 to 95% of cases).

In old age, factors such as taking various medications, cognitive impairment, depression, urinary incontinence, falls, persistent pain, and weakness can lead to reduced self-care in this population. Additionally, the presence of age-related comorbidities and reduced physical activity may complicate the management of this disease. Thus, the complications of diabetes in older adults can be more severe and lead to an increased risk of cardiovascular disease, kidney problems, neuropathy, visual impairment, and diabetic foot ulcers. A comprehensive approach to managing the complications of diabetes in old age is vital. Older people with diabetes are recommended to consider nutritional counseling, regular blood sugar checks, consultation with a physician to simplify the medication regimen, regular position changes for sedentary older people, attention to physical and social activity, and continuous examination of the feet to prevent ulcers. In this regard, Table 7.3 presents some of the most important self-care tips for older people suffering from diabetes.

7.5.3 Hypertension

Hypertension is a condition in which blood pressure (BP) in the arteries is persistently high. In other words, normal blood pressure is usually less than 120/80 millimeters of mercury (mmHg), and hypertension is diagnosed when systolic blood pressure is 140 mmHg or higher or diastolic pressure is 90 mmHg or higher. The American College of Cardiology and the American Heart Association divide blood pressure status in people into four general categories, as presented in Table 7.4.

Hypertension can be asymptomatic for years, which is why this disease is called the *"silent killer"* and is usually asymptomatic until blood pressure has increased to a dangerous level. In addition, hypertension over a long period can affect organs such as the brain, heart, kidneys, and eyes. If hypertension is not diagnosed and treated, it can lead to heart disease (heart failure, myocardial infarction (MI)), stroke, kidney failure, and vision loss.

Statistics on the prevalence of this disease vary. However, it is estimated that hypertension affects more than one billion people worldwide. Its prevalence increases significantly with aging. The Centers for Disease Control and Prevention (CDC) reports a prevalence of 63.1% in older people, making it one of the most common chronic diseases in this age group. This is due to age-related physiological changes and the concomitant occurrence of other diseases in older adults. With aging, structural and functional changes occur in blood vessels, including the accumulation of atherosclerotic plaques, impaired vascular dilation, and reduced vascular elasticity. These factors prevent blood vessels from regulating blood pressure, and thus, the likelihood of developing hypertension increases. Age-related reduction in kidney function, reduced effectiveness of the renin-angiotensin-aldosterone system, and increased activity of the sympathetic

Table 7.3 Self-care tips for older adults with diabetes

Familiarization with the disease and clinical manifestations monitoring	Educate the patient about their disease and physiology, as well as the type of diabetes and the available diagnostic methods and treatments, in a simple and comprehensible manner. Resources from the American Diabetes Association or local diabetes education programs can be appropriate. Explain the clinical manifestations associated with the disease to the patient. Such as: Elevated blood glucose levels beyond the normal range (as previously described) Unusual increase in urination (polyuria) Dry mouth and excessive thirst (polydipsia) Increased hunger (polyphagia) Feelings of fatigue Blurred vision Frequent infections and wounds that heal slowly Tingling, pain, or numbness in the hands and feet Inform the patient about warning signs and the need for emergency action. For instance, recurrent hypoglycemia and hyperglycemia, excessive urination with a lack of control, severe weight loss, persistent hunger and thirst, blurred vision and visual disturbances, numbness or tingling in the hands or feet, development of foot ulcers, and nonhealing or slow-healing wounds are among these symptoms. In such cases, it is essential to seek care from healthcare professionals. Educate the patient on how to use a glucometer for daily blood glucose monitoring at home. Encourage them to check their blood glucose levels according to their healthcare provider's recommendations, especially if they are taking insulin. This should be done when fasting, before meals, at bedtime, before exercise, and whenever there is suspicion of elevated or low blood glucose levels. However, the frequency of blood glucose monitoring may vary among patients and should be discussed with their physician. It is advisable to maintain blood glucose levels within the normal range and avoid fluctuations. Instruct the patient to recognize the signs of high and low blood sugar (hyperglycemia and hypoglycemia): *Hyperglycemia*: Symptoms include those mentioned above, such as polyuria, polydipsia, and polyphagia. In more severe cases, nausea and vomiting, shortness of breath, fruity-smelling breath (in cases of diabetic ketoacidosis), and hyperglycemic hyperosmolar state (HHS) with blood glucose levels exceeding 600 mg/dL may occur. *Hypoglycemia:* Symptoms include sweating, trembling, palpitations, nervousness, hunger, difficulty concentrating, headache, dizziness or lightheadedness, weakness or fatigue, blurred vision, irritability, and in more severe cases, seizures and loss of consciousness may occur. Advise the patient to inform their doctor if they experience recurrent episodes of low blood sugar. In cases of diabetic ketoacidosis or hyperglycemic hyperosmolar state, prompt medical attention is required. Encourage the patient to undergo routine checkups and tests (monitoring A1C levels, kidney function, and cardiovascular health) as recommended by their healthcare providers. Emphasize the importance of attending all scheduled appointments with their physician and primary care providers to monitor treatment effectiveness and manage potential side effects.

(continued)

Table 7.3 (continued)

Diet modification	Encourage the patient to follow a balanced diet that includes foods from the four main food groups (fruits and vegetables, carbohydrates, dairy products, and proteins). Carbohydrate intake should be minimized. Instead, they should focus on whole grains, lean proteins, healthy fats, fruits, and vegetables. The Plate Method—filling half of the plate with non-starchy vegetables, one-quarter with lean protein, and one-quarter with whole grains—can serve as a practical guide for these individuals. Including fruits in the diet is crucial as they provide essential vitamins and minerals. Diabetic patients should learn how to count carbohydrates to manage their blood glucose levels effectively. Instruct the patient to reduce their intake of sugary foods, desserts, and snacks (such as chips, chocolate, and cookies) that can cause rapid increases in blood sugar levels. If possible, opt for natural sweeteners or fruits (within limits set by their physician). It is advisable to minimize the consumption of high-fat, processed, and fast foods. Low-fat dairy products should be preferred. Oils used should be unsaturated and liquid, such as olive oil or sunflower oil. Encourage the older patients to stay hydrated by drinking adequate fluids (within limits advised by their healthcare provider). Sugary beverages (sodas and commercial fruit juices) or excessive caffeine should be limited in these patients. Recommend that the patient always carry fast-acting sugars that can quickly raise blood sugar levels in case of hypoglycemia. Encourage the older patients to quit smoking and avoid alcohol consumption.
Physical activity improvement	Any activity that can elevate heart rate and metabolism contributes to weight loss, blood pressure reduction, and blood sugar control. Encourage the patient to engage in gentle activities such as walking, stretching, or yoga within their tolerance levels. Aim for approximately 150 minutes per week or 30 minutes on most days. Walking outdoors is beneficial. On warmer days, a daily walk of 20 minutes indoors, with consideration for rest periods, can be an effective alternative. If possible, it is advisable to incorporate light resistance training two to three times a week to help maintain muscle mass and strength. Exercises that improve balance and flexibility and reduce the risk of falls (such as yoga or tai chi) can be beneficial. Exercising while hungry may lead to a drop in blood sugar levels, which can be dangerous. Therefore, a snack should be consumed prior to exercising. Educate the patient on methods to lose and maintain weight within a healthy range. Educate the older patients to pay attention to how their body responds to physical activity and to adjust the intensity and duration accordingly. They should avoid overexertion and rest if they notice any significant changes in vital signs. It is essential to consult with a healthcare provider before starting any new exercise program to ensure its safety and appropriateness. Teach the patient about the importance of adequate rest, sleep hygiene practices, and strategies for maintaining energy levels.

(continued)

Table 7.3 (continued)

Medication management	Familiarize the patient with oral and injectable diabetes medications, including their general functions, intended purposes, potential side effects, and the timing and methods of administration. Explain to the patient that weight loss, nutrition, and exercise are crucial alongside medication therapy. If insulin is prescribed, the patient or their caregiver must learn the injection technique. Insulin should be administered subcutaneously, with suitable sites including the abdomen, arms, and thighs. Additionally, the injection site should be rotated regularly. Different insulin types have varying peak effects; some must be injected before or during meals, while others are to be administered after meals. Correct and timely insulin use is essential for diabetic patients. For older patients, it is essential to periodically review all medications with healthcare providers to ensure that they are necessary, effective, and do not cause adverse interactions. Any side effects or concerns regarding medications should be promptly communicated to healthcare providers for adjustment or substitution. Advise older patients to avoid self-medicating with any new drugs or abruptly discontinuing prescribed medications and altering dosages without consulting their physician. Recommend that patients utilize pill organizers, reminders, or medication management programs to track their medications and dosages and ensure timely administration.
Other considerations	Teach the patient stress management techniques such as yoga, meditation, and deep breathing exercises (see Chap. 3). Encourage participation in activities they enjoy. Chronic stress can lead to elevated blood sugar levels. Encourage them to join support groups for older individuals facing this illness, allowing them to share their experiences and learn from others who are confronting similar challenges. Prepare older patients to utilize new and appropriate technologies that can enhance their self-care behaviors (refer to Chap. 6 for further details). *Foot care:* Given that wound healing is impaired in individuals with diabetes, consistent foot care is of utmost importance: Individuals with diabetes should wear comfortable shoes with a wide toe box to prevent pressure on the feet and reduce the risk of injury. Before wearing shoes, check the inside to ensure it is smooth and free of foreign objects such as pebbles. Feet should be inspected daily for wounds, injuries, and blisters. Those who cannot accurately assess the soles of their feet should use a mirror or seek assistance from another person. Feet should be protected from extreme temperatures. Therefore, when checking water temperature, especially in the bath, avoid placing feet directly in water. Feet should be washed daily with mild soap and water and then dried carefully with a soft towel. Pay special attention to drying between the toes. Proper nail trimming is important to ensure that edges do not harm the toes. Preventing dry skin on the feet by using moisturizing creams is beneficial; however, these creams should not be applied between the toes.

nervous system also affect blood pressure in seniors. The effects of years of unhealthy lifestyles and environmental and socioeconomic risk factors should also not be overlooked.

Hypertension in older adults is associated with a rapid decline in health status and frailty. This condition is defined as increased vulnerability to stressors leading to a reduced ability to cope with potentially acute negative events and a reduced ability to maintain homeostasis, which can increase the risk of adverse health outcomes. Management of hypertension in older adults requires a multidimensional approach that includes lifestyle modification, medication adherence, and regular healthcare visits. However, its management in older individuals is particularly complex due to the presence of multiple comorbidities, cognitive decline, and the potential for polypharmacy, which can complicate treatment regimens and adherence. Studies indicate that many older people do not adhere well to self-care behaviors associated with this disease. Consequently, self-care education and lifestyle changes for seniors seem essential. Table 7.5 presents self-care tips related to hypertension in older adults.

Table 7.4 Blood pressure classification

Blood pressure classification	Systolic blood pressure		Diastolic blood pressure
Normal	<120	And	<80
Prehypertension	120–139	Or	80–89
Stage 1 of hypertension	140–159	Or	90–99
Stage 2 of hypertension	≥160	Or	≥100

Table 7.5 Self-care tips for older adults with hypertension

Familiarization with the disease and clinical manifestations monitoring	Educate the patient about their disease and physiology, as well as the available diagnostic methods and treatments, in a simple and comprehensible manner. Reliable sources in this area include healthcare providers, the American Heart Association, the National Heart, Lung, and Blood Institute, and educational materials from reputable organizations. Explain the clinical manifestations associated with the disease to the patient. Hypertension is often asymptomatic; however, patients may experience the following symptoms: Headaches Dizziness Chest pain Nausea and vomiting Palpitations or irregular heart rhythms Shortness of breath Blurred vision Nosebleeds (epistaxis) Inform the patient about warning signs and the need for emergency action. In general, when hypertension is accompanied by symptoms, it is essential to consult healthcare professionals, as it may increase the risk of cardiovascular complications, kidney disorders, or stroke. Teach the patient and their family caregivers how to measure blood pressure at home. Measuring blood pressure twice daily (morning and evening) can help older individuals gain a better understanding of their disease management. Instruct the patient to undergo regular checkups and routine tests, particularly cardiovascular and kidney examinations, as recommended by their healthcare providers. Emphasize the importance of attending all scheduled appointments with their physician and primary care providers to monitor treatment effectiveness and manage potential side effects.

(continued)

Table 7.5 (continued)

Diet modification	Encourage the patient to follow a balanced diet that includes foods from the four main food groups (fruits and vegetables, carbohydrates, dairy products, and proteins). Introduce the DASH diet (Dietary Approaches to Stop Hypertension) to older patients with hypertension and encourage them to adhere to it. The DASH diet emphasizes fruits, vegetables, whole grains, lean proteins, and low-fat dairy while reducing saturated fats and cholesterol (see Fig. 7.1). The goals of this diet include: Consuming four to five servings of fruits and vegetables daily Consuming six to eight servings of whole grains Eating two servings or less of lean meat, fish, or poultry Educate the older patients to limit sodium intake to less than 2,300 mg per day (or 1,500 mg for further blood pressure reduction). It is advisable to eliminate salt from the dining table and use alternative seasonings such as pepper, thyme, and fresh lemon juice to enhance the flavor of foods. Reading food labels and prioritizing low-sodium options while shopping can be helpful. Inform the patient about hidden sources of sodium, such as canned foods, processed meals, ready-made soups, sauces, soy sauce, peanut butter, even bread, and many cheeses. Foods rich in potassium (such as bananas, oranges, spinach, and potatoes) can help lower blood pressure (potassium intake should be around 4.7 grams for patients without hyperkalemia risks). High potassium intake may be contraindicated for certain patients (e.g., those with kidney issues or those taking specific medications). Encourage the older individuals to drink adequate fluids to stay hydrated (within the limits set by their physician). Dehydration can affect blood pressure levels. Teach the patient to limit consumption of sugary beverages, processed drinks, and those containing caffeine. Consumption of fast food can lead to increased blood pressure and may be associated with cardiovascular complications; therefore, it should be eliminated or minimized. Encourage the patient to quit smoking and avoid alcohol consumption.
Physical activity improvement	Any activity that can elevate heart rate and metabolism contributes to weight loss, blood pressure reduction, and blood sugar control. Engaging in at least 150 minutes of moderate-intensity aerobic exercise each week (such as brisk walking or swimming) can help reduce blood pressure and enhance cardiovascular health. Recent guidelines published by the American Heart Association recommend that all seniors aged 65 and older engage in moderate-intensity aerobic activity for at least 30 minutes on five days a week, or vigorous aerobic activity for at least 20 minutes on three days a week, if there are no contraindications. If possible, it is advisable to incorporate light resistance training two to three times a week to help maintain muscle mass and strength. Exercises that improve balance and flexibility and reduce the risk of falls (such as yoga or tai chi) can be beneficial. Educate the patient to pay attention to how their body responds to physical activity and to adjust the intensity and duration accordingly. They should avoid overexertion and rest if they notice any significant changes in vital signs. Advise the patient to seek ways to incorporate more movement into their daily routine, such as taking the stairs instead of the elevator or participating in gardening when possible. Educate the patient on methods to lose and maintain weight within a healthy range. It is essential to consult with a healthcare provider before starting any new exercise program to ensure its safety and appropriateness. Teach the patient about the importance of adequate rest, sleep hygiene practices, and strategies for maintaining energy levels.

(continued)

Table 7.5 (continued)

Medication management	Educate the patient about antihypertensive medications, including their mechanisms of action, the purpose of their prescription, potential side effects, and the appropriate timing and method of administration. Monitoring vital signs, particularly blood pressure and pulse, prior to medication administration is crucial. Explain to the patient that weight loss, nutrition, and exercise are crucial alongside medication therapy. For older patients, it is essential to periodically review all medications with healthcare providers to ensure that they are necessary, effective, and do not cause adverse interactions. Any side effects or concerns regarding medications should be promptly communicated to healthcare providers for adjustment or substitution. Advise older patients to avoid self-medicating with any new drugs or abruptly discontinuing prescribed medications and altering dosages without consulting their physician. Explain to the patient that some medications, such as cough syrups, laxatives, sedatives, and alkalizing agents, contain significant amounts of sodium and should not be taken without medical advice. Recommend that patients utilize pill organizers, reminders, or medication management programs to track their medications and dosages and ensure timely administration.
Other considerations	Teach the patient stress management techniques such as yoga, meditation, and deep breathing exercises (see Chap. 3). Encourage participation in activities they enjoy. Chronic stress can lead to elevated blood pressure. Encourage them to join support groups for older individuals facing this illness, allowing them to share their experiences and learn from others who are confronting similar challenges. Prepare older patients to utilize new and appropriate technologies that can enhance their self-care behaviors (see Chap. 6).

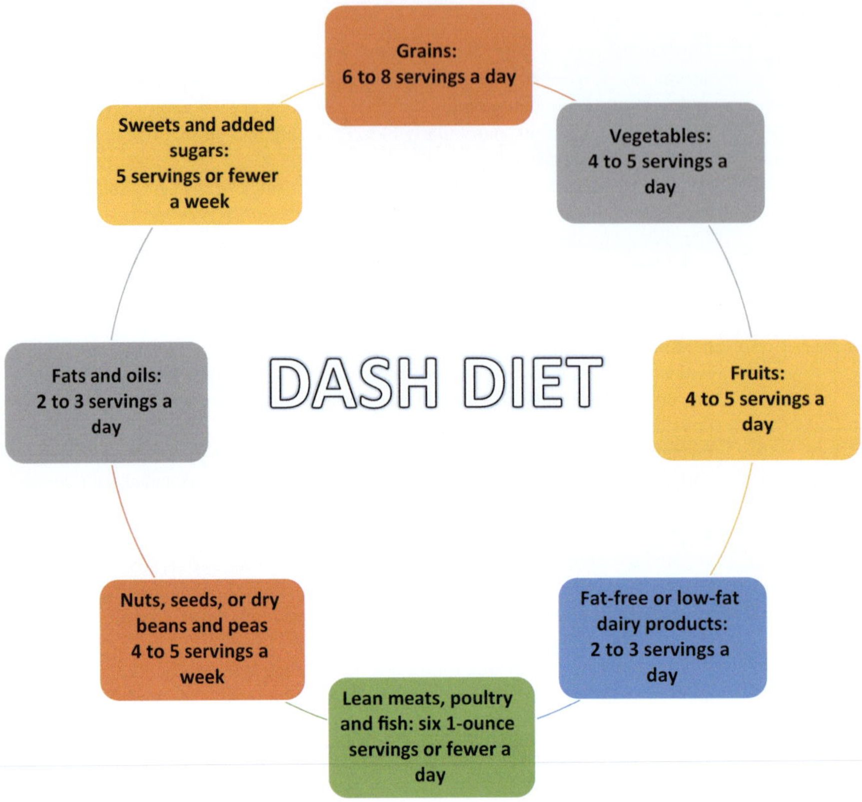

Fig. 7.1 The DASH diet

7.5.4 Coronary Artery Disease

Coronary artery disease (CAD), also known as coronary heart disease (CHD) or ischemic heart disease (IHD), is the most common cardiovascular disease. It leads to reduced blood flow to the heart muscle due to the accumulation of atheromatous plaque in the arteries of the heart. With increasing age, factors such as age-related physiological changes, including arterial stiffening and reduced cardiac efficiency, altered blood pressure control, dyslipidemia, increased oxidative stress and inflammation levels, impaired renal function, and impaired glucose metabolism put older adults at increased risk of developing this disease. It manifests through symptoms ranging from angina to heart attacks. Thus, CAD is a leading cause of mortality and morbidity in this population. It can lead to serious complications such as heart attack, abnormal heart rhythms, or heart failure in patients.

More than 70% of adults will develop CAD by the age of 70, making the prevalence of this disease high in older adults. Based on an update from the American Heart Association (AHA) published in 2019, 31% of males and 25.4% of females over the age of 80 have CAD. Additionally, some autopsy studies indicate a prevalence of about 60% of obstructive CAD in patients over the age of 80. Treatments for this disease in patients include lifestyle modification, appropriate drug therapy, and revascularization. Although percutaneous coronary intervention (PCI) is the preferred treatment for older patients with STEMI, physicians must weigh the benefits against the risks of revascularization for those with NSTEMI and stable CAD, considering the specific conditions and functional status of the patient. Moreover, frailty, sarcopenia, multiple comorbidities, cognitive impairment, delirium, and polypharmacy are syndromes of older people that affect their prognosis with CAD and complicate their management. Additionally, older patients are still less included in clinical trials examining treatment and care approaches for CVD. Many studies have excluded older patients and included merely those who are at lower risk. The lack of strong evidence and the related conditions associated with aging make the management of older patients with CAD more complex. Self-care of CAD in older adults requires a multidimensional approach that includes lifestyle modification, stress management, maintaining a heart-healthy diet, adherence to medication, engaging in regular physical activity, and regular healthcare visits that empower older individuals to take control of their cardiovascular health and improve their overall quality of life. Table 7.6 presents the most important self-care behaviors in older adults with CAD.

Table 7.6 Self-care tips for older adults with coronary artery disease

Familiarization with the disease and clinical manifestations monitoring	Educate the patient about their disease and physiology, as well as the available diagnostic methods and treatments, in a simple and comprehensible manner. Reliable sources in this area include healthcare providers, the American Heart Association, the National Heart, Lung, and Blood Institute, and educational materials from reputable organizations. Explain the clinical manifestations associated with the disease to the patient. Such as: Chest pain, pressure, or discomfort (angina) Fatigue Palpitations or a rapid heartbeat Shortness of breath Swelling in the hands or feet Lightheadedness or dizziness Inform the patient about warning signs and the need for emergency action. Symptoms such as severe chest pain that may radiate to the back, jaw, teeth, or left arm and shoulder, lasting 15–30 minutes and not improving with sublingual nitroglycerin, along with severe shortness of breath, cold sweating, nausea, and dizziness, can all be indicative of a heart attack or myocardial infarction (MI). In such cases, it is essential to seek emergency medical attention or visit the nearest healthcare facility. Teach the patient and their family caregivers how to measure blood pressure and pulse at home. Educate them about the normal ranges for these measurements. Instruct the patient to undergo regular checkups and routine tests, particularly cardiovascular examinations, as recommended by their healthcare providers. Emphasize the importance of attending all scheduled appointments with their physician and primary care providers to monitor treatment effectiveness and manage potential side effects.
Diet modification	Encourage the patient to follow a balanced diet that includes foods from the four main food groups (fruits and vegetables, carbohydrates, dairy products, and proteins). A diet rich in fruits, vegetables, whole grains, lean proteins (such as fish and poultry), and healthy fats (such as those found in nuts and olive oil) is beneficial. The Mediterranean diet is often recommended for heart health. Obesity, high blood pressure, and elevated cholesterol levels are three significant risk factors for this condition. To manage obesity, the patient should follow weight loss strategies suggested by healthcare providers or a registered dietitian. For blood pressure management, refer to the information provided in Table 7.5. Controlling sodium intake, being mindful of hidden sources of sodium, and adhering to the DASH diet (as illustrated in Fig. 7.1) are crucial for managing blood pressure in these patients. Instruct the patient to reduce their consumption of red meat, high-fat dairy products, foods high in cholesterol such as egg yolks, and processed foods containing saturated or trans fats. Instead, low-fat dairy options, unsaturated fats like olive oil and sesame oil, and lean cuts of meat are appropriate choices. Encourage the patient to use smaller plates or portion measurements to avoid overeating. Small but nutritious and frequent meals can be beneficial. Educate the patient to avoid heavy and gas-producing foods. Encourage older individuals to drink adequate fluids to stay hydrated (within the limits set by their physician). Teach the patient to limit consumption of sugary beverages, processed drinks, and those containing caffeine. Consumption of fast food can lead to increased blood pressure and may be associated with cardiovascular complications; therefore, it should be eliminated or minimized. Encourage the patient to quit smoking and avoid alcohol consumption.

(continued)

Table 7.6 (continued)

Physical activity improvement	Any activity that can elevate heart rate and metabolism contributes to weight loss, blood pressure reduction, and blood sugar control. Engaging in at least 150 minutes of moderate-intensity aerobic exercise each week (such as brisk walking or swimming) can help enhance cardiovascular health. Recent guidelines published by the American Heart Association recommend that all seniors aged 65 and older engage in moderate-intensity aerobic activity for at least 30 minutes on five days a week, or vigorous aerobic activity for at least 20 minutes on three days a week, if there are no contraindications. If possible, it is advisable to incorporate light resistance training two to three times a week to help maintain muscle mass and strength. Exercises that improve balance and flexibility and reduce the risk of falls (such as yoga or tai chi) can be beneficial. Advise the patient to avoid exercising in extremely hot, cold, or humid environments. Educate the old patient to pay attention to how their body responds to physical activity and to adjust the intensity and duration accordingly. They should avoid overexertion and rest if they notice any significant changes in vital signs. Educate the patient on methods to lose and maintain weight within a healthy range. It is essential to consult with a healthcare provider before starting any new exercise program to ensure its safety and appropriateness. Teach the patient about the importance of adequate rest, sleep hygiene practices, and strategies for maintaining energy levels.
Medication management	Familiarize the patient with prescribed medications such as antianginal agents, antihypertensives, antiplatelet drugs, and anticoagulants. Explain the overall function of these medications, their intended purpose, potential side effects, and proper timing and methods for administration. Monitoring vital signs, particularly blood pressure and pulse, prior to medication administration is crucial. If antithrombotic medications (such as antiplatelet and anticoagulant drugs) are prescribed, educate the patient about the risk of bleeding, its symptoms, and important drug and food interactions. Explain to the patient that weight loss, proper nutrition, and lifestyle modifications are critically important alongside pharmacotherapy. For older patients, it is essential to periodically review all medications with healthcare providers to ensure that they are necessary, effective, and do not cause adverse interactions. Any side effects or concerns regarding medications should be promptly communicated to healthcare providers for adjustment or substitution. Advise older patients to avoid self-medicating with any new drugs or abruptly discontinuing prescribed medications and altering dosages without consulting their physician. Explain to the patient that some medications, such as cough syrups, laxatives, sedatives, and alkalizing agents, contain significant amounts of sodium and should not be taken without medical advice. Recommend that patients utilize pill organizers, reminders, or medication management programs to track their medications and dosages and ensure timely administration.
Other considerations	Teach the patient stress management techniques such as yoga, meditation, and deep breathing exercises (see Chap. 3). Encourage participation in activities they enjoy. Encourage them to join support groups for older individuals facing this illness, allowing them to share their experiences and learn from others who are confronting similar challenges. Prepare older patients to utilize new and appropriate technologies that can enhance their self-care behaviors (refer to Chap. 6 for further details).

7.5.5 Heart Failure

Heart failure (HF) is a complex clinical syndrome in which the heart does not pump blood as it should, leading to a lack of oxygen and nutrients throughout the body, along with distressing symptoms for the affected individual. It is commonly characterized by shortness of breath, fatigue, exercise intolerance, dizziness, weakness, pulmonary and extremity edema, chest pain, and palpitations. It is the leading cause of hospitalization in people over 65 years of age. The functional capacity of the heart muscle decreases with aging. Hence, it is considered a fundamental syndrome of aging. Thus, heart failure is highly prevalent in older adults, which may be due to a complex interplay of diseases and age-related physiological changes. Among the 5.7 million adults with HF in the United States, it is estimated that 92% are 60 years of age or older, and more than 50% are 80 years of age or older. Older adults also show a high tendency for the development of HF with preserved ejection fraction (HFPEF), creating some challenges for diagnosis. The rate of HF also increases with aging for both genders. For example, the annual rate of new cases per 1000 person-years for white men aged 65 to 74 years is 9.2, 22.3 for those aged 75 to 84 years, and 43.0 for those aged 85 years and older. The corresponding rates among white women are 4.7, 14.8, and 30.7 per 1000 person-years, respectively.

Heart failure is mostly treated by a combination of medications and lifestyle modifications or, in severe cases, surgery, ventricular assist devices (VADs), and heart transplantation. However, the rate of rehospitalization is also significantly higher in these patients, imposing substantial cost on patients and the healthcare system. In this regard, engaging in self-care is one of the most critical efforts to reduce rehospitalization rates. Self-care in HF is a complex set of behaviors that includes adherence to treatment regimens, interpretation of heart failure symptoms, decision-making about appropriate treatment measures during exacerbations, and the ability to perform primary care and work with caregivers. Generally, the available evidence suggests that the status of self-care in the general population of patients with heart failure is inadequate. This issue is even worse in seniors who face natural age-related disabilities and comorbidities (such as fatigue syndrome, physical limitations, and cognitive impairment). Considering the importance of using self-care in controlling symptoms and preventing HF progression, Table 7.7 presents some important self-care tips for this disease.

Table 7.7 Self-care tips for older adults with heart failure

Familiarization with the disease and clinical manifestations monitoring	Educate the patient about their disease and physiology, as well as the available diagnostic methods and treatments, in a simple and comprehensible manner. Reliable sources in this area include healthcare providers, the American Heart Association, the National Heart, Lung, and Blood Institute, and educational materials from reputable organizations. Explain the clinical manifestations associated with the disease to the patient. Such as: Shortness of breath Fatigue Sudden weight gain Swelling of the limbs Chest pain Palpitations Dizziness Coughing Constipation Decreased appetite Inform the patient about warning signs and the need for emergency action. Symptoms such as severe shortness of breath, intense chest pain, frothy and blood-tinged sputum, and altered consciousness are critical indicators. In such cases, it is essential to seek emergency medical attention or visit the nearest healthcare facility. Educate the patient to monitor their symptoms according to three zones: green, yellow, and red (see Box 7.2, which illustrates heart failure zones). Instruct the patient to weigh themselves daily in the morning before breakfast and at a specific time (after urination) and to be vigilant for sudden weight increases. Teach the patient and their family caregivers how to measure blood pressure and pulse at home. Educate them about the normal ranges for these measurements. Instruct the patient to undergo regular checkups and routine tests, particularly cardiovascular examinations, as recommended by their healthcare providers. Emphasize the importance of attending all scheduled appointments with their physician and primary care providers to monitor treatment effectiveness and manage potential side effects.

(continued)

Table 7.7 (continued)

Diet modification	Encourage the patient to follow a balanced diet that includes foods from the four main food groups (fruits and vegetables, carbohydrates, dairy products, and proteins). A diet rich in fruits, vegetables, whole grains, lean proteins (such as fish and poultry), and healthy fats (such as those found in nuts and olive oil) is beneficial. The Mediterranean diet is often recommended for heart health. The daily sodium intake should be reduced to 2 grams (less than one teaspoon). Controlling sodium intake, being aware of hidden sodium sources, and adhering to the DASH diet (see Fig. 7.1) are crucial (see Table 7.5). Instruct the patient to reduce their consumption of red meat, high-fat dairy products, foods high in cholesterol such as egg yolks, and processed foods containing saturated or trans fats. Instead, low-fat dairy options, unsaturated fats like olive oil and sesame oil, and lean cuts of meat are appropriate choices. Encourage the patient to use smaller plates or measure portions to prevent overeating. Small, nutritious, and frequent meals can be beneficial. Teach the patient to avoid heavy and gas-producing foods. Advise patients to limit fluid intake to two liters (equivalent to eight glasses) or less per day. All substances that are liquid at room temperature are considered fluids and should be measured and monitored. Even excess liquid in foods and canned fruits should be drained. The use of sugar-free candies or frozen lemon or grape popsicles can help alleviate thirst. Consuming potassium-rich foods may be beneficial for patients taking potassium-depleting medications like furosemide. To manage obesity, the patient should follow weight loss strategies recommended by healthcare providers or a registered dietitian. Teach the patient to limit consumption of sugary beverages, processed drinks, and those containing caffeine. Consumption of fast food can lead to increased blood pressure and may be associated with cardiovascular complications; therefore, it should be eliminated or minimized. Encourage the older patients to quit smoking and avoid alcohol consumption.
Physical activity improvement	Engaging in at least 150 minutes of moderate-intensity aerobic exercise (such as walking and swimming) per week can be beneficial if there are no contraindications. Heavy exercises such as weightlifting, sit-ups, tennis, and squash are not appropriate. Encourage the patient to start exercising slowly with simple movements and gradually increase intensity if possible. If possible, it is advisable to incorporate light resistance training two to three times a week to help maintain muscle mass and strength. Exercises that improve balance and flexibility and reduce the risk of falls (such as yoga or tai chi) can be beneficial. Advise the patient to avoid exercising in extremely hot, cold, or humid environments. Teach the patient to refrain from heavy activities and those beyond their tolerance. Activities that require lifting heavy objects (such as shoveling snow) or those that induce straining (Valsalva maneuver) can be dangerous for these patients. Educate the older patients to pay attention to how their body responds to physical activity and to adjust the intensity and duration accordingly. They should avoid overexertion and rest if they notice any significant changes in vital signs. Monitoring the pulse before, during, and after exercise is crucial for these patients. If fatigue occurs, or if the pulse exceeds 100 beats per minute or symptoms worsen, exercise should be stopped. Encourage the patient to prioritize daily activities. They should distribute various tasks throughout the day to prevent activity intolerance, take breaks between activities, and practice breathing exercises. They should avoid performing all energy-demanding activities in one day or consecutively and refrain from bending or standing for prolonged periods during activities. Educate the patient on methods to lose and maintain weight within a healthy range. It is essential to consult with a healthcare provider before starting any new exercise program to ensure its safety and appropriateness. Teach the patient about the importance of adequate rest, sleep hygiene practices, and strategies for maintaining energy levels.

(continued)

Table 7.7 (continued)

Medication management	Patients with heart failure are prescribed multiple medications. It is essential to familiarize the patient with their prescribed medications, including their overall function, intended purpose, potential side effects, and proper timing and methods of administration. Monitoring vital signs, particularly blood pressure and pulse, prior to medication administration is crucial. If antithrombotic medications (such as antiplatelet and anticoagulant drugs) are prescribed, educate the patient about the risk of bleeding, its symptoms, and important drug and food interactions. Explain to the patient that weight loss, proper nutrition, and lifestyle modifications are critically important alongside pharmacotherapy. For older patients, it is essential to periodically review all medications with healthcare providers to ensure that they are necessary, effective, and do not cause adverse interactions. Any side effects or concerns regarding medications should be promptly communicated to healthcare providers for adjustment or substitution. Advise older patients to avoid self-medicating with any new drugs or abruptly discontinuing prescribed medications and altering dosages without consulting their physician. Explain to the patient that some medications, such as cough syrups, laxatives, sedatives, and alkalizing agents, contain significant amounts of sodium and should not be taken without medical advice. Recommend that patients utilize pill organizers, reminders, or medication management programs to track their medications and dosages and ensure timely administration.
Other considerations	Teach the patient stress management techniques such as yoga, meditation, and deep breathing exercises (see Chap. 3). Encourage participation in activities they enjoy. Encourage them to join support groups for older individuals facing this illness, allowing them to share their experiences and learn from others who are confronting similar challenges. Early integration of palliative care services is beneficial for effective symptom management and improving quality of life alongside medical treatments. Familiarize the patient with palliative care providers in their local area. It is advisable for older people to become acquainted with advance care planning and take action accordingly. This process facilitates discussions about future medical care priorities with family members and healthcare providers to ensure that their wishes are respected. Prepare older patients to utilize new and appropriate technologies that can enhance their self-care behaviors (see Chap. 6).

Box 7.2 Heart Failure Zones

Green zone (safe zone): The patient is having a good day!	
The patient has no symptoms or mild symptoms: The patient can breathe easily and has energy. The patient does not feel discomfort or pressure in the chest. The patient's ability to maintain a normal level of activity has not been reduced. The patient has no swelling in the feet, ankles, or abdomen, or the swelling has not increased compared to before. The patient has not gained more than 2 kg in weight in two consecutive days or more than 2.5 kg in a week.	*Actions that the patient should take in the green zone:* The patient should keep the symptoms under control. The patient should continue their usual activities. The patient should take their medications every day and on time. The patient should weigh themselves every morning after emptying their bladder and write it down. Follow a low-salt diet. The patient should not forget or neglect their next physician's visits.

(continued)

Box 7.2 (continued)

Yellow zone (warning zone): The patient is not having a good day!	
If any of the following symptoms occur, the patient is in the yellow zone: Extreme shortness of breath that worsens when lying down. Feeling more tired and weak than before and not having enough energy to do daily tasks. The patient has a dry and annoying cough or a cough at night. The patient has gained more than 2 kg in weight in two consecutive days or more than 2.5 kg in a week. The patient's ankles/legs or abdomen are swollen more than usual (so their shoes or pants may be tight). The patient experiences dizziness or lightheadedness when he stands up. The patient feels like their heart is beating fast or irregularly. Patient has vomiting or diarrhea that lasts more than two days. Patient has severe nausea or loss of appetite.	*Actions to be taken in the yellow zone:* The patient's symptoms may indicate that they need to adjust their medications. The patient should not wait for their symptoms to improve on their own. The patient should inform their physician immediately.
Red zone (emergency zone): The patient is having a very bad day!	
The patient is in the red zone if any of the following symptoms occur: The patient has difficulty breathing and is feeling scared. The patient has frothy or bloody sputum. The patient has shortness of breath that does not improve even when sitting. The patient has chest pain that is not relieved with rest or medication. The patient feels very dizzy or faint.	*Actions to be taken in the red zone:* The patient should be examined by a physician immediately! Call the emergency room (ER) or 911. The patient should be transported to the nearest emergency center by a family member.

7.5.6 Stroke

Stroke, also known as cerebrovascular accident (CVA), is a focal clinical syndrome. It manifests as a neurological disorder related to vascular injury (infarction or hemorrhage) in the brain. Based on the American Heart Association and the American Stroke Association, this disorder is considered a stroke if it lasts more than 24 hours. Most strokes (about 85%) occur after ischemia and are primarily caused by small-vessel atherosclerosis, cardiac embolism, and large-vessel atherosclerosis or thromboembolism. Other strokes (about 15%) mostly occur after intracranial hemorrhage due to various causes. Stroke is the second leading cause of death worldwide and can lead to long-term and severe disability in survivors. More than 75 percent of people who experience a stroke face disability, making it difficult for them to work. Additionally, over 80 percent of these people suffer from motor function disorders that require rehabilitation. In addition to neurological problems, strokes also cause numerous clinical complications that can interfere with the initial rehabilitation and recovery of these patients. The physical complications of stroke are directly associated with the area involved and the extent of the damage. They can include pain, paralysis of limbs, speech and swallowing disorders, sensory disorders, and ultimately lead to psychological and cognitive problems. The rate of this disease is increasing worldwide. About 7.5 million people died from stroke in 2021, while about 5 million died in 1990. According to statistics provided by the World Stroke Organization, 1 in 4 people over the age of 25 will experience a stroke during their lifetime, making this condition the leading cause of disability worldwide. Its incidence is increasing with aging. This issue can lead to more complications related to this disease and disruption of daily activities and self-care for older people in addition to the disabilities that occur with aging. It is one of the leading causes of morbidity and mortality in people aged 65 and older. Its occurrence is closely related to age-related risk factors such as hypertension, diabetes, and cardiovascular disease. Its prevalence is significantly higher among older people aged over 65 years and has remained relatively stable in recent years (about 7.7% in the United States from 2011 to 2022). Since self-care interventions can help people make decisions and maintain their health, and individuals who have had a stroke face a wide range of problems, some self-care recommendations and tips are summarized in Table 7.8.

Table 7.8 Self-care tips for older adults with stroke

Familiarization with the disease and clinical manifestations monitoring	Educate the older patients about their disease and physiology, types of stroke, and the available diagnostic methods and treatments in a simple and comprehensible manner. Reliable resources in this area include healthcare providers, the American Stroke Association, and educational materials from reputable organizations. Explain the clinical manifestations associated with the disease to the patient. Such as: Weakness or numbness in the face, arm, or leg, typically on one side of the body Difficulty in speaking or swallowing Impaired understanding Vision problems Severe headache Dizziness or issues with balance or coordination Motor difficulties or trouble walking Fainting Seizures Inform the patient about warning signs and the need for emergency action. Any of the above symptoms that occur suddenly may indicate an impending stroke and require immediate emergency care at the nearest healthcare facility. Familiarize older people with the FAST acronym (Face drooping, Arm weakness, Speech difficulties, Time to call emergency services) for the quick identification of stroke symptoms. Teach the patient and their family caregivers how to measure blood pressure and pulse at home. Educate them about the normal ranges for these measurements. Educate patients on the importance of regular checkups (blood sugar and cholesterol levels), routine tests, and particularly neurological, motor, and cardiovascular examinations, as recommended by their healthcare providers. Instruct patients to monitor any changes in physical or cognitive abilities, mood fluctuations, or other symptoms daily and to report these to their healthcare provider as needed. Emphasize the importance of attending all scheduled appointments with their physician and primary care providers to monitor treatment effectiveness and manage potential side effects.

Diet modification	In these patients, diet plays a crucial role both as a factor in enhancing quality of life and as a secondary prevention measure against recurrent strokes. Encourage the older patients to follow a balanced diet that includes foods from the four main food groups (fruits and vegetables, carbohydrates, dairy products, and proteins). The core dietary recommendations for these patients include increased consumption of fruits, vegetables, and unsaturated fatty acids. When it comes to protein intake, plant-based proteins may be appropriate. A heart-healthy diet consists of fruits, vegetables, whole grains, lean proteins (such as fish and poultry), and healthy fats (such as those found in nuts and olive oil). Additionally, a Mediterranean diet has been associated with a reduced risk of stroke. To manage blood pressure and minimize excess sugars for overall health support and to avoid new strokes, it is essential for older people to reduce salt and glucose intake. For this purpose, refer to the guidelines provided in the diabetes and blood pressure sections (Tables 7.3 and 7.5). Reducing sodium intake and consuming potassium-rich foods (if not contraindicated) is beneficial. Instruct the patient to reduce their consumption of red meat, high-fat dairy products, foods high in cholesterol such as egg yolks, and processed foods containing saturated or trans fats. Instead, low-fat dairy options, unsaturated fats like olive oil and sesame oil, and lean cuts of meat are appropriate choices. If there are swallowing difficulties, appropriate measures must be taken to prevent aspiration. Educate the patient and their family that individuals with swallowing disorders should eat while seated and follow a pureed diet. The initiation of oral feeding is contingent upon the physician's approval. Encourage the patient to use smaller plates or measure portions to prevent overeating. Small, nutritious, and frequent meals can be beneficial. Monitoring portion sizes is important for maintaining a healthy weight, improving stroke outcomes, and preventing subsequent strokes. Teach the patient to avoid heavy and gas-producing foods. Encourage the older individuals to drink adequate fluids to stay hydrated (within the limits set by their physician). Dehydration can adversely affect cognitive function and recovery. Teach the patient to limit consumption of sugary beverages, processed drinks, and those containing caffeine. Consumption of fast food can lead to increased blood pressure and may be associated with cardiovascular complications and stroke; therefore, it should be eliminated or minimized. To manage obesity, the patient should follow weight loss strategies recommended by healthcare providers or a registered dietitian. Encourage the older patients to quit smoking and avoid alcohol consumption.

(continued)

Table 7.8 (continued)

Physical activity improvement	A reduction in sedentary lifestyle among individuals with a history of stroke can play a significant role in secondary prevention. Engaging in at least 150 minutes of moderate-intensity aerobic exercise (such as walking and swimming) per week can be beneficial if there are no contraindications. Low-impact exercises, such as walking or chair exercises, are particularly suitable initially if mobility is limited. Encourage the patient to start exercising slowly with simple movements and gradually increase intensity if possible. If possible, it is advisable to incorporate light resistance training two to three times a week to help maintain muscle mass and strength. It is advisable to focus on major muscle groups. Exercises that improve balance and flexibility and reduce the risk of falls (such as yoga or tai chi) can be beneficial. Advise the patient to avoid exercising in extremely hot, cold, or humid environments. Educate the older patients to pay attention to how their body responds to physical activity and to adjust the intensity and duration accordingly. They should avoid overexertion and rest if they notice any significant changes in vital signs. Monitoring the pulse before, during, and after exercise is crucial for these patients. If fatigue occurs, or if the pulse exceeds 100 beats per minute or symptoms worsen, exercise should be stopped. Encourage the patient to prioritize daily activities. They should distribute various tasks throughout the day to prevent activity intolerance, take breaks between activities, and practice breathing exercises. They should avoid performing all energy-demanding activities in one day or consecutively and refrain from bending or standing for prolonged periods during activities. Some stroke survivors may require physical therapy and rehabilitation sessions to restore motor functions. Educate the patient on methods to lose and maintain weight within a healthy range. It is essential to consult with a healthcare provider before starting any new exercise program to ensure its safety and appropriateness. Teach the patient about the importance of adequate rest, sleep hygiene practices, and strategies for maintaining energy levels.
Medication management	Educate the patient about prescribed medications, their overall function, the purpose of their prescription, potential side effects, and the timing and method of administration. Correct and timely medication adherence can be effective in secondary stroke prevention. Monitoring vital signs, particularly blood pressure and pulse, prior to medication administration is crucial. If antithrombotic medications (such as antiplatelet and anticoagulant drugs) are prescribed, educate the patient about the risk of bleeding, its symptoms, and important drug and food interactions. Explain to the patient that weight loss, proper nutrition, and lifestyle modifications are critically important alongside pharmacotherapy. For older patients, it is essential to periodically review all medications with healthcare providers to ensure that they are necessary, effective, and do not cause adverse interactions. Any side effects or concerns regarding medications should be promptly communicated to healthcare providers for adjustment or substitution. Advise older patients to avoid self-medicating with any new drugs or abruptly discontinuing prescribed medications and altering dosages without consulting their physician. Recommend that patients utilize pill organizers, reminders, or medication management programs to track their medications and dosages and ensure timely administration.

Other considerations	Teach the patient stress management techniques such as yoga, meditation, and deep breathing exercises (see Chap. 3). Encourage participation in activities they enjoy. Mindfulness-based stress reduction (MBSR) is another effective intervention for stress management in these patients. Encourage them to join support groups for older individuals facing this illness, allowing them to share their experiences and learn from others who are confronting similar challenges. To support brain health and improve cognitive function poststroke, encourage the patient to engage in cognitive exercises (such as puzzles or memory games). To prevent falls, necessary modifications should be made in the home environment (for example, reducing clutter, using clear signage, ensuring adequate lighting, installing grab bars in bathrooms, and eliminating tripping hazards). These measures are essential to ensure the safety of older people (further strategies are provided in Table 7.13). Prepare older patients to utilize new and appropriate technologies that can enhance their self-care behaviors (refer to Chap. 6 for further details).

7.5.7 Dementia

Changes in mental status are one of the most common symptoms in older patients. They are mostly related to delirium, dementia, and depression (the 3Ds). Among them, dementia is a common, severe, chronic, progressive, and irreversible neurodegenerative disorder in older people. It is characterized by impairments in cognitive function, including impairments in memory, cognition, and executive function; impairments in communication; and changes in mood, personality, and judgment. The prevalence of dementia is increasing exponentially as the population ages worldwide. In a systematic review and meta-analysis of 47 studies, Cao et al. (2019) estimated the prevalence of dementia among people aged 50 years and older at 697 (95% CI: 546–864) per 10,000. It is estimated that 5.2% of people aged 60 years and older have dementia. According to World Health Organization, the number of people with dementia will increase to 115.4 million by 2050. Generally, the clinical manifestations of dementia can be classified into three categories: (1) a significant decline in cognitive function based on normative data; (2) the appearance of peripheral symptoms of dementia, the so-called behavioral and psychological symptoms of dementia; and (3) loss of independence in activities of daily living. Furthermore, the prevalence of behavioral and psychological changes, including apathy, depression, anxiety, irritability, agitation, aggression, sleep disorders, and eating disorders, is high in these patients. Like all older people, those with this disease experience increased disability and poor quality of life. Moreover, the manifestations of this disease make caregiving stressful and increase the burden of caregiving, worsening the mental health of caregivers. Dementia can also be caused by various diseases. Alzheimer's disease (AD) and vascular dementia (VD) are the most common in this regard. AD is currently the most common cause of dementia (60% to 70%). It is characterized by the accumulation of amyloid plaques and tangles of nerve fibers in the brain, leading to changes in cognitive capabilities in a person. The onset of AD, with neurodegeneration, can gradually progress to memory impairment, aphasia, and disability in people's lives to the extent that sometimes they are not even able to perceive and recognize familiar objects through their special senses. A systematic review and meta-analysis study by Cao et al. (2019) revealed that the prevalence of AD was 324 in people over 50 years of age (95% CI: 228–460). Additionally, in people aged 60 to 69 years, its prevalence was estimated to be 1.9 times higher in females than in males (108 cases vs. 56 cases per 10,000 people). Dementia is mostly an irreversible condition, but early diagnosis and treatment can reduce or slow down its progression. Older people with dementia often have comorbidities. The most common comorbidities are diabetes, heart disease, hypertension, stroke, thyroid disorders, osteoporosis, and respiratory problems such as asthma and chronic obstructive pulmonary disease (COPD). Thus, they are highly exposed to polypharmacy and are at higher risk of adverse effects or drug–drug interactions. A cross-sectional study by Muñoz-Contreras et al. (2024) on 100 patients with Alzheimer's or other dementias revealed that 87% of patients experienced drug–drug interactions, and quetiapine (24.5%) and acetylsalicylic acid (10%) were the most frequently involved in these interactions. In such conditions, self-care, especially in the early stages of the disease, is a vital factor for their well-being. Dementia symptoms (including forgetfulness, reduced comprehension, impaired ability to communicate, and behavioral and psychological symptoms) may gradually prevent adherence to a treatment regimen in these individuals, complicating the self-care process. Thus, family caregivers should take over more of the care process due to concerns about the safety of older people. However, these patients can be supported for as long as possible by simplifying routines and reminding them of self-care behaviors. An individualized strategy may be appropriate and promising for patients with dementia or those at risk of AD. Table 7.9 presents some of the most important self-care tips for patients with dementia.

Table 7.9 Self-care tips for older adults with dementia

Familiarization with the disease and clinical manifestations monitoring	Introduce the older individuals and family caregivers to the disease and its physiology, types of dementia (such as AD), diagnostic methods, and available treatments in a simple and comprehensible manner. Reliable resources in this area include healthcare providers, the Alzheimer's Association, and educational materials from reputable organizations. Explain the clinical manifestations associated with the disease. Such as: Memory impairment Cognitive dysfunction Executive function deficits Communication difficulties Changes in mood, orientation, personality, and judgment Inform the patient and his caregiver about warning signs and the need for emergency action. Symptoms such as reduced alertness, respiratory distress, fainting, seizures, and inability to communicate are warning signs that require attention. Additionally, incidents such as falls or any of the aforementioned symptoms that jeopardize the health of the older individuals must be taken seriously. In these situations, it is essential to seek emergency care or visit the nearest healthcare facility. Educate the patient and their family about the importance of regular checkups and routine tests, particularly neurological, motor, and cognitive assessments, as recommended by healthcare providers. Instruct the family to monitor any changes in physical or cognitive abilities, mood fluctuations, or other symptoms on a daily basis and to report these observations to the healthcare provider as needed. Emphasize the importance of attending all scheduled appointments with their physician and primary care providers to monitor treatment effectiveness and manage potential side effects.
Diet modification	Encourage the older patients to follow a balanced diet that includes foods from the four main food groups (fruits and vegetables, carbohydrates, dairy products, and proteins). Family members may need to provide care in these matters. A diet rich in fruits, vegetables, whole grains, lean proteins (such as fish and poultry), and healthy fats (such as those found in nuts and olive oil) is beneficial. Additionally, a Mediterranean diet has been associated with maintaining brain health. Research indicated that a ketogenic diet may be effective in managing many neurodegenerative diseases, particularly Alzheimer's, potentially improving cognitive abilities. Increased consumption of antioxidants, carotenoids, fruits, and vegetables can enhance the functioning of these patients. Higher intake of soy products, vegetables, and dairy while reducing rice consumption may lower the risk of developing dementia. Teach them to reduce the intake of processed foods containing sugars and unhealthy fats, as these can negatively impact overall health. Encourage the older individuals to drink adequate fluids to stay hydrated (within the limits set by their physician). Dehydration can adversely affect cognitive function. If there are swallowing difficulties, appropriate measures must be taken to prevent aspiration. Encourage the patient to have regular meals at consistent times and create a calm dining environment. This approach minimizes distractions and enhances focus on eating. If a patient with dementia refuses to eat, it is necessary to employ appropriate strategies and prepare their favorite foods to stimulate their appetite. Encourage the older patients to quit smoking and avoid alcohol consumption.

(continued)

Table 7.9 (continued)

Physical activity improvement	Increased physical activity has an inverse relationship with the incidence of dementia in patients with Alzheimer's. Regular exercise can generally slow the onset of cognitive problems. Engaging in at least 150 minutes of moderate-intensity aerobic exercise (such as walking or swimming) per week can be beneficial if there are no contraindications. If possible, incorporate light resistance training two to three times a week to maintain muscle mass and strength, focusing on major muscle groups. Exercises that improve balance and flexibility and reduce the risk of falls (such as yoga or tai chi) can be helpful. Patients should avoid exercising in extremely hot, cold, or humid environments. Some patients may require physical therapy and rehabilitation sessions to restore motor functions. For those with mobility impairments, assistive devices can help enhance their movements. Participating in group exercise classes designed for seniors not only promotes physical health but also increases social interaction, which is beneficial for mental well-being. It is essential to consult with a healthcare provider before starting any new exercise program to ensure its safety and appropriateness. Teach the patient about the importance of adequate rest, sleep hygiene practices, and strategies for maintaining energy levels.
Medication management	Educate the patient and their family about prescribed medications, including their overall function, purpose for prescription, potential side effects, and instructions for timing and administration. For older patients, it is essential to periodically review all medications with healthcare providers to ensure that they are necessary, effective, and do not cause adverse interactions. Any side effects or concerns regarding medications should be promptly communicated to healthcare providers for adjustment or substitution. Self-medicating with new drugs or abruptly stopping or changing dosages without consulting the physician can be dangerous. Recommend that patients utilize pill organizers, reminders, or medication management programs to track their medications and dosages and ensure timely administration.
Other considerations	Teach the patient stress management techniques such as yoga, meditation, and deep breathing exercises (see Chap. 3). Encourage participation in activities they enjoy. Encourage them to join support groups for older individuals facing this illness, allowing them to share their experiences and learn from others who are confronting similar challenges. Establishing a daily routine can create stability and predictability, which may help reduce anxiety and confusion. The use of psychotherapeutic methods in neurodegenerative diseases such as Parkinson's and AD can play a significant role in reducing stress for patients and alleviating the caregiving burden on their companions. Encourage the expression of emotions through creative ways such as art or music therapy. Emotional well-being is crucial for the overall health of individuals affected by dementia. To support brain health and improve cognitive function, encourage the patient to engage in cognitive exercises (such as puzzles or memory games). To prevent falls, necessary modifications should be made in the home environment (for example, reducing clutter, using clear signage, ensuring adequate lighting, installing grab bars in bathrooms, and eliminating tripping hazards). These measures are essential to ensure the safety of older people (further strategies are provided in Table 7.13). Propose strategies to alleviate the substantial caregiving burden that family caregivers of these patients experience. Prepare older patients to utilize new and appropriate technologies that can enhance their self-care behaviors (see Chap. 6).

7.5.8 Parkinson

As explained, neurodegenerative diseases are age-related diseases manifesting as the death or degeneration of nerve cells in the central or peripheral nervous system. Parkinson's disease (PD) is another of the most common neurodegenerative disorders in older people after dementia. It manifests as the loss of dopaminergic neurons, especially in the substantia nigra. This disease can be associated with motor symptoms including tremors, postural instability, bradykinesia, and rigidity, and non-motor deficits including anosmia, constipation, autonomic instability, sleep disorders, and problems such as apathy, anhedonia, impulse control disorders, depression, and anxiety. Some patients may even experience feelings of frustration and social stigma. Thus, this disease is significantly associated with a severe reduction in quality of life. The global prevalence of PD has increased more than demographic changes, and one of the reasons for this increase may be the decline in other competing causes of death. The increasing prevalence of PD has more than doubled the global burden of the disease in recent years. Its incidence increases significantly with aging, especially in people aged 65 years and older. It is estimated to be 108 to 212 cases per 100,000 in this age group, with higher rates in males. In addition to age, various environmental factors, genetic predispositions, and lifestyle choices are involved in the onset of the disease. Moreover, there is currently no effective treatment for this disease. Thus, the need for long-term care, which becomes more complex as the disease progresses and the resulting disabilities increase, highlights the importance of promoting self-care behaviors in this population. Behavioral changes and limitations caused by the disease are also widespread in older people with PD, making it necessary to plan an individualized self-care plan. However, the ability to maintain independence decreases, and the need for significant support from caregivers often increases as symptoms progress, including both motor and non-motor symptoms. Considering the frequency of complications and disabilities resulting from this disease, Table 7.10 presents the most important self-care behaviors for these patients.

Table 7.10 Self-care tips for older adults with Parkinson

Familiarization with the disease and clinical manifestations monitoring	Introduce the older patients to their disease and physiology, as well as the available diagnostic methods and treatments, in a simple and comprehensible manner. Reliable resources in this area include healthcare providers, the Parkinson's Foundation, the Michael J. Fox Foundation, and educational materials from reputable organizations. Explain the clinical manifestations associated with the disease. Such as: Tremors in the hands, arms, legs, jaw, or head Postural instability Bradykinesia Rigidity Impairments in balance and coordination Sleep disturbances Mood changes Inform the patient and his caregiver about warning signs and the need for emergency action. Symptoms such as cognitive impairment, reduced alertness, respiratory distress, fainting, seizures, and inability to communicate are warning signs that require attention. Additionally, incidents such as falls or any of the aforementioned symptoms that jeopardize the health of the older individuals must be taken seriously. In these situations, it is essential to seek emergency care or visit the nearest healthcare facility. Educate the patient and their family about the importance of regular checkups and routine tests, particularly neurological, motor, and cognitive assessments, as recommended by healthcare providers. Instruct the family to monitor any changes in physical or cognitive abilities, mood fluctuations, or other symptoms on a daily basis and to report these observations to the healthcare provider as needed. Emphasize the importance of attending all scheduled appointments with their physician and primary care providers to monitor treatment effectiveness and manage potential side effects.
Diet modification	Encourage the older patients to follow a balanced diet that includes foods from the four main food groups (fruits and vegetables, carbohydrates, dairy products, and proteins). Family members may need to provide care in these matters. A diet rich in fruits, vegetables, whole grains, lean proteins (such as fish and poultry), and healthy fats (such as those found in nuts and olive oil) is beneficial. Additionally, a Mediterranean diet has been associated with maintaining brain health. Some individuals may find that protein can interfere with the absorption of certain Parkinson's medications (such as levodopa). In such cases, it is advisable to recommend that they consume protein-rich foods at different times from their medication. Research studies indicated that a ketogenic diet may be effective in managing many neurodegenerative diseases, potentially improving cognitive abilities. Increased consumption of antioxidants, carotenoids, fruits, and vegetables can enhance the functioning of these patients. Higher intake of soy products, vegetables, and dairy while reducing rice consumption may lower the risk of developing dementia. Teach them to reduce the intake of processed foods containing sugars and unhealthy fats, as these can negatively impact overall health. Encourage the older individuals to drink adequate fluids to stay hydrated (within the limits set by their physician). Dehydration can adversely affect cognitive function. If there are swallowing difficulties, appropriate measures must be taken to prevent aspiration. To combat constipation, which is a common issue among Parkinson's patients, it is recommended that patients incorporate high-fiber foods (such as fruits, vegetables, and whole grains) into their diet. Encourage the patient to have regular meals at consistent times and create a calm dining environment. This approach minimizes distractions and enhances focus on eating. If a patient with dementia refuses to eat, it is necessary to employ appropriate strategies and prepare their favorite foods to stimulate their appetite. Encourage the older patients to quit smoking and avoid alcohol consumption.

(continued)

Table 7.10 (continued)

Physical activity improvement	Engaging in at least 150 minutes of moderate-intensity aerobic exercise (such as walking or swimming) per week can be beneficial if there are no contraindications. If possible, incorporate light resistance training two to three times a week to maintain muscle mass and strength, focusing on major muscle groups. Exercises that improve balance and flexibility and reduce the risk of falls (such as yoga or tai chi) can be helpful. Patients should avoid exercising in extremely hot, cold, or humid environments. Some patients may require physical therapy and rehabilitation sessions to restore motor functions. For those with mobility impairments, assistive devices can help enhance their movements. Participating in group exercise classes designed for seniors not only promotes physical health but also increases social interaction, which is beneficial for mental well-being. It is essential to consult with a healthcare provider before starting any new exercise program to ensure its safety and appropriateness. Teach the patient about the importance of adequate rest, sleep hygiene practices, and strategies for maintaining energy levels.
Medication management	Educate the patient and their family about prescribed medications, including their overall function, purpose for prescription, potential side effects, and instructions for timing and administration. For older patients, it is essential to periodically review all medications with healthcare providers to ensure that they are necessary, effective, and do not cause adverse interactions. Any side effects or concerns regarding medications should be promptly communicated to healthcare providers for adjustment or substitution. Self-medicating with new drugs or abruptly stopping or changing dosages without consulting the physician can be dangerous. Recommend that patients utilize pill organizers, reminders, or medication management programs to track their medications and dosages and ensure timely administration.
Other considerations	Teach the patient stress management techniques such as yoga, meditation, and deep breathing exercises (see Chap. 3). Encourage participation in activities they enjoy. Encourage them to join support groups for older individuals facing this illness, allowing them to share their experiences and learn from others who are confronting similar challenges. Establishing a daily routine can create stability and predictability, which may help reduce anxiety and confusion. The use of psychotherapeutic methods in neurodegenerative diseases such as Parkinson's and AD can play a significant role in reducing stress for patients and alleviating the caregiving burden on their companions. Encourage the expression of emotions through creative ways such as art or music therapy. Emotional well-being is crucial for the overall health of individuals affected by dementia. To support brain health and improve cognitive function, encourage the patient to engage in cognitive exercises (such as puzzles or memory games). To prevent falls, necessary modifications should be made in the home environment (for example, reducing clutter, using clear signage, ensuring adequate lighting, installing grab bars in bathrooms, and eliminating tripping hazards). These measures are essential to ensure the safety of older people (further strategies are provided in Table 7.13). Propose strategies to alleviate the substantial caregiving burden that family caregivers of these patients experience. Prepare older patients to utilize new and appropriate technologies that can enhance their self-care behaviors (refer to Chap. 6 for further details).

7.5.9 Respiratory Disorders (Such as Asthma and COPD)

Respiratory diseases in older people are associated with many negative consequences for their health and quality of life. Studies have indicated that these diseases are the third leading cause of death in older people. The diagnosis and management of respiratory diseases in older people are challenging, attributed to age-related changes and the simultaneous occurrence of other diseases. Symptoms of respiratory diseases in older people may differ from those in younger people. For example, dyspnea is a more common symptom in this population than cough and sputum. Additionally, decreased lung function, muscle wasting, and reduced capability to effectively clear the airways exacerbate symptoms and make older people more susceptible to respiratory infections and exacerbations of lung diseases. Age-related changes in the response to medications also put older people at a higher risk for drug interactions and adverse reactions. Among respiratory disorders, asthma and chronic obstructive pulmonary disease (COPD) are the most common chronic airway diseases in this age group. Asthma is a chronic inflammatory disease of the airways characterized by reversible airflow obstruction and airway hyperresponsiveness. It causes bronchospasm and can be triggered by endogenous and exogenous factors, allergens, or irritants. It is characterized by wheezing, shortness of breath, chest tightness, and a persistent cough. It has affected more than 300 million people worldwide. Active asthma is relatively common in people over 65 years of age, although the disease has been considered a childhood disease for a long time. Immunosenescence, characterized by changes in the immune system that may occur during the aging process, may be involved in the development of asthma in older people. The estimated prevalence of asthma in adults over 65 years of age varies from 4% to 13%, and it may be underestimated due to the underdiagnosis of the disease in this population. Asthma in older people can be more severe and associated with higher morbidity and mortality than in younger patients. Undiagnosed or misdiagnosed asthma in older people, along with factors related to geriatric medicine such as cognitive decline, medication misuse, comorbidities, and polypharmacy, could contribute to poorer outcomes in this age group. Generally, asthma is more dangerous for older adults than for younger adults since it causes unique challenges, and its burden regarding costs, quality of life, hospitalizations, and mortality is higher in this age group than in younger adults who suffer from this disease (Braman 2017). COPD is another common respiratory disease in older people. This disease is a progressive lung disorder caused by airflow obstruction due to damage and inflammation of the airways, lung parenchyma, or both. The global prevalence of this disease was estimated at 10.6%, equivalent to 480 million cases, in 2020, and it is projected to increase to 592 million cases in 2050. Furthermore, statistics indicate that the prevalence of this disease has increased significantly among older people over 75 years of age from 2011 to 2021. It is estimated that 20–25% of people over 70 years of age suffer from this disease. This disease often remains undiagnosed, especially in older people. Thus, the real prevalence of this disease is higher than the reported figures. COPD is characterized by symptoms such as shortness of breath, chronic cough, phlegm, wheezing, frequent respiratory infections, and fatigue and weakness. These symptoms usually develop slowly but worsen over time and can eventually limit the person's daily activities. The most important risk factor for this disease is smoking, while other risk factors include advanced age, long-term exposure to chemicals, and genetic factors. The two main types of COPD are emphysema and chronic bronchitis, with emphysema caused by damage to the walls of the alveoli and chronic bronchitis caused by persistent irritation and inflammation in the lining of the airways. Treatment for these diseases involves a combination of lifestyle modifications, medications, oxygen therapy, surgery, and pulmonary rehabilitation. Due to the importance of patient participation in self-care plans for these diseases, Table 7.11 presents the most important tips regarding self-care in these conditions.

Table 7.11 Self-care tips for older adults with asthma and COPD

Familiarization with the disease and clinical manifestations monitoring	Educate the older patients about their disease and physiology, as well as the available diagnostic methods and treatments, in a simple and comprehensible manner. Reliable sources in this area include healthcare providers, the American Lung Association, the National Heart, Lung, and Blood Institute, and educational materials from reputable organizations. Explain the clinical manifestations associated with the disease. Such as: Difficulty breathing Wheezing Low blood oxygen levels (O_2 Saturation) Frequent coughing Tightness in the chest Feelings of fatigue and weakness Low physical endurance for exercise Shortness of breath during routine activities Inform the patient and his caregiver about warning signs and the need for emergency action. Symptoms such as severe shortness of breath, intense chest pain, palpitations, respiratory distress, frothy or bloody sputum, dyspnea or apnea during sleep, feelings of suffocation, significant drops in O_2 saturation, fever, or other signs of respiratory infection and altered consciousness necessitate immediate medical attention. In these situations, it is essential to seek emergency care or visit the nearest healthcare facility. Teach the patient to measure their oxygen saturation levels daily using a pulse oximeter and to be vigilant about any changes. For patients with asthma, the use of a peak flow meter can assist in monitoring lung function at home. Educate the patient on its usage, as it can help detect worsening asthma before it becomes severe. Instruct patients on breathing exercises, such as diaphragmatic breathing (which helps clear airway obstructions) and pursed-lip breathing (which aids in breath control and relaxation). Teach techniques such as effective coughing and huff coughing to help increase mucus clearance. Advise the patient to avoid exposure to extreme temperatures and environments polluted with chemicals, dust, or cigarette smoke. Emphasize the importance of staying indoors on days when air quality alerts are issued. Educate the patient about hygiene practices and personal protective measures to prevent respiratory infections and illnesses. Instruct the patient to follow up on routine checkups and tests, especially respiratory and cardiovascular examinations, as recommended by healthcare providers. Emphasize the importance of attending all scheduled appointments with their physician and primary care providers to monitor treatment effectiveness and manage potential side effects.
Diet modification	Encourage the older patients to follow a balanced diet that includes foods from the four main food groups (fruits and vegetables, carbohydrates, dairy products, and proteins). A diet rich in fruits, vegetables, whole grains, lean proteins (such as fish and poultry), and healthy fats (such as those found in nuts and olive oil) is beneficial. Nutrient-rich foods can support overall health and immune system function. Encourage the patient to use smaller plates or portion sizes to prevent overeating. Small but nutritious and frequent meals can be beneficial. Advise the patient to avoid heavy and gas-producing foods. Educate the patient to refrain from consuming irritating and spicy foods, as certain items may trigger asthma symptoms in some individuals (such as sulfites found in wine or dried fruits). Encourage the older individuals to drink adequate fluids to stay hydrated (within the limits set by their physician). Drinking water not only keeps the patient hydrated but also helps thin mucus for easier clearance. Recommend that the patient sit in a comfortable position while eating to facilitate easier breathing. They should eat slowly, take small bites, rest between bites, and practice deep breathing exercises. It is best to eat when they have more energy to consume an adequate amount of food. If possible, they should drink liquids after meals to avoid early satiety. Teach the patient to limit consumption of sugary beverages, processed drinks, and those containing caffeine. Encourage the older patients to quit smoking and avoid alcohol consumption.

(continued)

Table 7.11 (continued)

Physical activity improvement	Engaging in at least 150 minutes of moderate-intensity aerobic exercise (such as walking and swimming) per week can be beneficial if there are no contraindications. Encourage the patient to start exercising slowly with simple movements and gradually increase intensity if possible. If approved by a physician, attention should be paid to the following guidelines when engaging in exercises or physical activities: Any form of physical activity should be initiated gradually, slowly, and in a relaxed manner. Set achievable goals, such as a daily 20-minute walk or 10 minutes of light stretching exercises. If medications are being taken prior to exercising, it is advisable to wait at least thirty minutes to allow the medications to take effect. Should symptoms such as severe shortness of breath, dizziness, fatigue, weakness, or palpitations occur, the individual should cease physical activity immediately. If oxygen has been prescribed, the patient should exercise while using the oxygen. If possible, it is advisable to incorporate light resistance training two to three times a week to help maintain muscle mass and strength. Exercises that improve balance and flexibility and reduce the risk of falls (such as yoga or tai chi) can be beneficial. Advise the patient to avoid exercising in extremely hot, cold, or humid environments. Educate the older patients to pay attention to how their body responds to physical activity and to adjust the intensity and duration accordingly. They should avoid overexertion and rest if they notice any significant changes in vital signs. Monitoring the pulse before, during, and after exercise is crucial for these patients. If fatigue occurs, or if the pulse exceeds 100 beats per minute or symptoms worsen, exercise should be stopped. Encourage the patient to prioritize daily activities. They should distribute various tasks throughout the day to prevent activity intolerance, take breaks between activities, and practice breathing exercises. They should avoid performing all energy-demanding activities in one day or consecutively and refrain from bending or standing for prolonged periods during activities. Educate the patient on methods to lose and maintain weight within a healthy range. It is essential to consult with a healthcare provider before starting any new exercise program to ensure its safety and appropriateness. Teach the patient about the importance of adequate rest, sleep hygiene practices, and strategies for maintaining energy levels.
Medication management	Educate the patient about the prescribed medications, including their overall function, purpose for prescription, potential side effects, and the appropriate timing and method of administration. Instruct on the proper use of respiratory medications, such as nebulizers, inhalers, turbohalers, and spacers. If oxygen has been prescribed for the patient, provide training on how to use the devices, including appropriate flow rates and duration of use. Additionally, caution the patient against using flammable materials while utilizing oxygen. For some patients, it may be advisable to receive the influenza vaccine at the onset of the cold season, in consultation with their physician. Monitoring vital signs, particularly blood pressure and pulse, is crucial before administering certain medications. Educate the patient to always keep quick-relief (rescue) inhalers readily available. Explain to the patient that weight loss, proper nutrition, and lifestyle modifications are critically important alongside pharmacotherapy. For older patients, it is essential to periodically review all medications with healthcare providers to ensure that they are necessary, effective, and do not cause adverse interactions. Any side effects or concerns regarding medications should be promptly communicated to healthcare providers for adjustment or substitution. Advise older patients to avoid self-medicating with any new drugs or abruptly discontinuing prescribed medications and altering dosages without consulting their physician. Recommend that patients utilize pill organizers, reminders, or medication management programs to track their medications and dosages and ensure timely administration.

(continued)

Table 7.11 (continued)

Physical activity improvement	Engaging in at least 150 minutes of moderate-intensity aerobic exercise (such as walking and swimming) per week can be beneficial if there are no contraindications. Encourage the patient to start exercising slowly with simple movements and gradually increase intensity if possible. If approved by a physician, attention should be paid to the following guidelines when engaging in exercises or physical activities: Any form of physical activity should be initiated gradually, slowly, and in a relaxed manner. Set achievable goals, such as a daily 20-minute walk or 10 minutes of light stretching exercises. If medications are being taken prior to exercising, it is advisable to wait at least thirty minutes to allow the medications to take effect. Should symptoms such as severe shortness of breath, dizziness, fatigue, weakness, or palpitations occur, the individual should cease physical activity immediately. If oxygen has been prescribed, the patient should exercise while using the oxygen. If possible, it is advisable to incorporate light resistance training two to three times a week to help maintain muscle mass and strength. Exercises that improve balance and flexibility and reduce the risk of falls (such as yoga or tai chi) can be beneficial. Advise the patient to avoid exercising in extremely hot, cold, or humid environments. Educate the older patients to pay attention to how their body responds to physical activity and to adjust the intensity and duration accordingly. They should avoid overexertion and rest if they notice any significant changes in vital signs. Monitoring the pulse before, during, and after exercise is crucial for these patients. If fatigue occurs, or if the pulse exceeds 100 beats per minute or symptoms worsen, exercise should be stopped. Encourage the patient to prioritize daily activities. They should distribute various tasks throughout the day to prevent activity intolerance, take breaks between activities, and practice breathing exercises. They should avoid performing all energy-demanding activities in one day or consecutively and refrain from bending or standing for prolonged periods during activities. Educate the patient on methods to lose and maintain weight within a healthy range. It is essential to consult with a healthcare provider before starting any new exercise program to ensure its safety and appropriateness. Teach the patient about the importance of adequate rest, sleep hygiene practices, and strategies for maintaining energy levels.
Medication management	Educate the patient about the prescribed medications, including their overall function, purpose for prescription, potential side effects, and the appropriate timing and method of administration. Instruct on the proper use of respiratory medications, such as nebulizers, inhalers, turbohalers, and spacers. If oxygen has been prescribed for the patient, provide training on how to use the devices, including appropriate flow rates and duration of use. Additionally, caution the patient against using flammable materials while utilizing oxygen. For some patients, it may be advisable to receive the influenza vaccine at the onset of the cold season, in consultation with their physician. Monitoring vital signs, particularly blood pressure and pulse, is crucial before administering certain medications. Educate the patient to always keep quick-relief (rescue) inhalers readily available. Explain to the patient that weight loss, proper nutrition, and lifestyle modifications are critically important alongside pharmacotherapy. For older patients, it is essential to periodically review all medications with healthcare providers to ensure that they are necessary, effective, and do not cause adverse interactions. Any side effects or concerns regarding medications should be promptly communicated to healthcare providers for adjustment or substitution. Advise older patients to avoid self-medicating with any new drugs or abruptly discontinuing prescribed medications and altering dosages without consulting their physician. Recommend that patients utilize pill organizers, reminders, or medication management programs to track their medications and dosages and ensure timely administration.

(continued)

Table 7.11 (continued)

Other considerations	Teach the patient stress management techniques such as yoga, meditation, and deep breathing exercises (see Chap. 3). Encourage them to join support groups for older individuals facing this illness, allowing them to share their experiences and learn from others who are confronting similar challenges. Some patients may require incentive spirometry and respiratory physiotherapy. Teach both the patient and their family how to perform these techniques. Exposure to household allergens and irritants (such as dust, pet dander, and smoke) should be minimized. Patients can utilize air purifiers, regularly clean surfaces, and avoid strong cleaning agents that may trigger symptoms. In addition to quitting smoking, it is essential for these patients to avoid exposure to secondhand smoke. Prepare older patients to utilize new and appropriate technologies that can enhance their self-care behaviors (refer to Chap. 6 for further details).

7.5.10 Kidney Disorders (Such as Chronic Kidney Disease)

Chronic kidney disease (CKD) is a condition in which the kidneys' nephrons are damaged for 3 months or more, and the glomerular filtration rate (GFR) is less than 60 mL/min/1.73 m^2. In this case, the body fails to excrete waste products and excess fluid through the urine, which can have devastating effects on other organs. Many people who suffer from chronic kidney disease do not have any symptoms until the disease is in its advanced stages. As the disease progresses, symptoms that may appear include protein in the urine, increased creatinine in the urine, foamy urine, urinating more or less than usual, itchy and dry skin, feeling tired, nausea, loss of appetite, and unwanted weight loss. It is crucial to understand this disease and identify its early symptoms since failure to diagnose and treat CKD leads to end-stage renal disease (ESRD), which may cause symptoms such as impaired concentration, numbness or swelling in the hands and feet, muscle pain and cramps, shortness of breath, vomiting, sleep disturbances, and ammonia-like breath in the affected person. Risk factors for this disease include obesity, diabetes, hypertension, heart disease, a family history of kidney failure, a history of kidney damage, smoking, kidney stones, recurrent urinary tract infections (UTIs), kidney cancer, autoimmune diseases such as lupus, sepsis, and age over 60.

Studies suggest that the CKD rate is high in older people, with one in two individuals over the age of 75 suffering from this disease, and 20% of older people over 75 in the United States struggle with chronic kidney failure. For this reason, cell destruction increases, and cell repair is impaired with aging. Thus, kidney functions such as glomerular filtration, urine concentration and dilution, and sodium, potassium, and calcium balance are affected. Additionally, chronic diseases such as diabetes and hypertension, which are common in older people, can lead to impaired kidney function. Frailty, reduced protein intake due to age-related anorexia, cognitive impairment, oxidative stress, weight gain, and the use of multiple medications are other risk factors for kidney failure in older people. CKD is also associated with many complications in older people, such as increased incidence of hypertension and cardiovascular disorders, heart failure, atherosclerosis, dyslipidemia, anemia, cognitive disorders, reduced physical activity, impaired vitamin D metabolism, and the development of musculoskeletal diseases such as sarcopenia and bone mineral disorders, especially calcium deficiency. These complications can cause irreparable injuries such as falls, various fractures, and stroke; increase frailty in older people; and reduce their quality of life. Its treatment also varies from medication to dialysis and kidney transplantation in the advanced stages of the disease. The important point in this disease is that patients learn and apply self-care behaviors such as symptom monitoring, diet modification, improved physical activity, and adherence to treatment to control and slow down the progression. Table 7.12 lists some essential self-care techniques for this population.

Table 7.12 Self-care tips for older adults with kidney disorder

Familiarization with the disease and clinical manifestations monitoring	Educate the old patient about their disease and physiology, as well as the available diagnostic methods and treatments, in a simple and comprehensible manner. Reliable sources in this area include healthcare providers and educational materials from reputable organizations. Explain the clinical manifestations associated with the disease. Such as: High blood pressure Edema Sudden weight changes Changes in urine (volume, creatinine, protein) Fatigue Itching and dry skin, feelings of tiredness Nausea and loss of appetite Inform the patient and his caregiver about warning signs and the need for emergency action. Symptoms such as severe shortness of breath, pain, fever, significant edema, difficulty concentrating, numbness, burning during urination, urinary dysfunction, and altered consciousness are critical. In these situations, it is essential to seek emergency care or visit the nearest healthcare facility. Educate the patient on how to measure their blood pressure at home and to monitor their weight daily. Instruct the patient to undergo regular checkups (creatinine, GFR, etc.) and routine tests, especially kidney and cardiovascular examinations, as recommended by healthcare providers. Emphasize the importance of attending all scheduled appointments with their physician and primary care providers to monitor treatment effectiveness and manage potential side effects.
Diet modification	Encourage the older patients to follow a balanced diet that includes foods from the four main food groups (fruits and vegetables, carbohydrates, dairy products, and proteins). Depending on the stage of chronic kidney disease, it may be necessary to limit protein intake to reduce the workload on the kidneys. It is advisable to obtain protein primarily from white meat sources (such as chicken, fish, and poultry). A nutritionist can assist in determining the appropriate amount. Teach the patient to monitor foods high in potassium (such as bananas and oranges) and phosphorus (such as dairy products and nuts), as elevated levels can lead to complications. Instruct the patient to consume less than 2300 mg of sodium per day to help manage blood pressure and reduce fluid retention. They should read food labels and choose low-sodium options while being aware of hidden sodium sources. (Refer to the education provided in the hypertension section and Table 7.5). The intake of sugar in food should be controlled and limited, as high sugar levels can damage the kidneys. Fluid intake should align with the recommendations provided by the physician. Proper hydration is important but may need to be restricted in advanced stages of CKD. Encourage the patient to use smaller plates or portion sizes to prevent overeating. Small but nutritious and frequent meals can be beneficial. Advise the patient to avoid heavy and gas-producing foods. Teach the patient to limit consumption of sugary beverages, processed drinks, and those containing caffeine. Consumption of fast food should be avoided due to its high fat and salt content. Encourage the older patients to quit smoking and avoid alcohol consumption.

(continued)

Table 7.12 (continued)

Physical activity improvement	Engaging in at least 150 minutes of moderate-intensity aerobic exercise (such as walking and swimming) per week can be beneficial if there are no contraindications. Encourage the patient to start exercising slowly with simple movements and gradually increase intensity if possible. If possible, it is advisable to incorporate light resistance training two to three times a week to help maintain muscle mass and strength. Exercises that improve balance and flexibility and reduce the risk of falls (such as yoga or tai chi) can be beneficial. Advise the patient to avoid exercising in extremely hot, cold, or humid environments. Educate the older patients to pay attention to how their body responds to physical activity and to adjust the intensity and duration accordingly. They should avoid overexertion and rest if they notice any significant changes in vital signs. For patients who have undergone kidney transplantation or are on dialysis, moderate exercise can significantly improve quality of life (consult with a physician). Patients who have received a kidney transplant should avoid rough or intense activities, such as martial arts, that may harm the kidneys. Encourage the patient to prioritize daily activities. They should distribute various tasks throughout the day to prevent activity intolerance. Rest between activities and perform breathing exercises. Avoid scheduling all energy-intensive activities for one day or consecutively. During activities, they should refrain from bending or standing for prolonged periods. It is essential to consult with a healthcare provider before starting any new exercise program to ensure its safety and appropriateness. Teach the patient about the importance of adequate rest, sleep hygiene practices, and strategies for maintaining energy levels.
Medication management	Familiarize the patient with prescribed medications, including their overall function, purpose for prescription, potential side effects, and the correct timing and method of administration. Explain to the patient that weight loss, proper nutrition, and lifestyle modifications are critically important alongside pharmacotherapy. For older patients, it is essential to periodically review all medications with healthcare providers to ensure that they are necessary, effective, and do not cause adverse interactions. Any side effects or concerns regarding medications should be promptly communicated to healthcare providers for adjustment or substitution. Advise older patients to avoid self-medicating with any new drugs or abruptly discontinuing prescribed medications and altering dosages without consulting their physician. Explain to the patient that some medications, such as cough syrups, laxatives, sedatives, and alkalizers, contain significant amounts of sodium. Some medications can also increase potassium levels in the blood and should not be taken without medical advice. Be aware that common pain relievers, such as non-steroidal anti-inflammatory drugs (NSAIDs) like ibuprofen, indomethacin, naproxen, diclofenac, aspirin, and meloxicam, can cause kidney damage and should not be taken arbitrarily. Attention to prescribed supplements (such as vitamin D) by the physician is essential to reduce the risk of osteoporosis and anemia. Recommend that patients utilize pill organizers, reminders, or medication management programs to track their medications and dosages and ensure timely administration.

(continued)

Table 7.12 (continued)

Other considerations	*Education related to dialysis:* Care for vascular access points such as fistulas, shunts, and permcaths is crucial. Each vascular access site should be inspected daily for signs of infection, damage, wounds, or bleeding. Teach the patient to check the fistula site for blood flow and to inform their physician if any abnormal conditions are observed. Blood draws and blood pressure measurements should not be performed from the arm with the fistula; this must be communicated to healthcare staff by the patient. Dialysis may have side effects, with low blood pressure being the most common. Symptoms may include lightheadedness, shortness of breath, abdominal cramps, muscle cramps, nausea, or vomiting. Reporting these conditions to a physician is helpful. Between dialysis sessions, it is vital to adhere to dietary and fluid intake guidelines as directed by the physician to prevent waste accumulation in the body and associated complications. For dialysis patients, dietary salt intake must be very low to minimize thirst and reduce fluid consumption between dialysis sessions. Teach the patient stress management techniques such as yoga, meditation, and deep breathing exercises (see Chap. 3). Encourage them to join support groups for older individuals facing this illness, allowing them to share their experiences and learn from others who are confronting similar challenges. Prepare older patients to utilize new and appropriate technologies that can enhance their self-care behaviors (refer to Chap. 6 for further details).

7.5.11 Osteoporosis

Bone density and quality (changes in bone geometry and microarchitecture) decrease with aging. Accordingly, it significantly affects bone strength. This condition causes a chronic, progressive, and common disease called osteoporosis in older people. Osteoporosis is known as the silent epidemic of the twenty-first century. Based on the definition provided by the World Health Organization (WHO) in 1993, it is a systemic skeletal disease in which bone mass decreases and bone tissue microarchitecture deteriorates, followed by increased bone fragility and fractures. Bone is a living and dynamic tissue in constant formation and resorption, so losing the balance in osteoclastic-osteoblastic function, during which resorption (osteoclast activity) increases versus bone formation (osteoblast activity), leads to osteoporosis and bone fragility. Osteoporosis is a major public health concern in this population due to its high prevalence and serious complications. It was estimated in 2010 that 5.5 million males and 22 million females in the European Union had osteoporosis based on the diagnostic criteria used by the WHO. Other statistics in the United States from 2017 to 2018 reported the prevalence of osteoporosis in adults over 50 years of age at about 20% in females and 4% in males. The disease affects females more than males due to hormonal changes caused by menopause. Most females under 50 years of age have normal bone mineral density (BMD), while 27% suffer from osteopenia and 70% from osteoporosis in the hip, lumbar spine, or forearm by the age of 80. It is a multifactorial disease, and a combination of major and minor factors can be involved in its development.

Major risk factors that increase the risk by two times or more include age (over 50 years), gender (female), family history, low weight (body mass index (BMI) of less than 20 kg/m^2), history of some diseases (rheumatoid arthritis, hyperthyroidism, and Crohn's disease), and treatment with corticosteroids. Minor risk factors that increase the risk by less than two times are lifestyle factors including smoking and excessive alcohol consumption (more than three units per day in males and more than two units per day in females). Among these factors, the most important risk factor for osteoporosis and fragility fractures is increasing age. In old age, estrogen deficiency and secondary hyperparathyroidism, along with reduced dietary intake and vitamin D deficiency, are widely considered key determinants of postmenopausal osteoporosis. The two major factors that influence the risk of low-trauma fractures in old age are skeletal fragility (e.g., low bone density and poor bone quality) and trauma (usually a fall). It is estimated that about 30% of people over 60 years of age and 50% of people over 85 years of age fall at least once a year, and half of those who fall experience it more than once. Additionally, sarcopenia is also common in older people, which increases the risk of injury. Common sites of osteoporotic fractures are the spine, hip, distal forearm, and proximal humerus. However, fractures in other bones are also possible. Osteoporosis is usually not painful until a bone breaks, but it can cause severe and acute pain and loss of function when a fracture occurs.

These fractures can even result in hospitalization in healthcare centers and impose heavy costs on patients and societies. In adults with hip fractures, it is estimated that more than 20% will die within 6 to 12 months of the fracture, about 50% will require long-term nursing care, and up to 80% of those who survive will never regain their pre-fracture level of function. In this regard, it is predicted that the number of hip fractures and their associated costs will double or triple by 2040 in many countries worldwide. The disease is diagnosed through various methods, such as bone densitometry and dual-phase X-rays. Treatment of the disease focuses on different aspects and ranges from lifestyle modifications (weight control, smoking cessation, and intake of foods rich in calcium and vitamin D) to pharmacological treatments. However, managing osteoporosis in older people can be challenging.

Clinically, a large number of patients are not adequately treated with pharmacological therapy. A prospective cross-sectional study of nursing home residents with known osteoporosis or recent hip fracture reported that 69% of them used calcium, 63% used vitamin D, and only 19% used bisphosphonates. Thus, prevention may be the best strategy for treating osteoporosis. In this regard, self-care is of particular importance before the onset of osteoporosis and even after its definite diagnosis. According to the results of studies conducted on the self-care of these patients, receiving limited information from healthcare providers is one of the major causes of a reduction in self-care behaviors in older adults. Table 7.13 provides self-care education about this disease.

Table 7.13 Self-care tips about osteoporosis for older adults

Familiarization with the disease and clinical manifestations monitoring	Educate the old patient about their disease and physiology, as well as the available diagnostic methods and treatments, in a simple and comprehensible manner. Reliable sources in this area include healthcare providers and educational materials from reputable organizations. Explain the clinical manifestations associated with the disease. Such as: Shortening of height Changes in skeletal posture, such as stooping Severe pain in the bone areas Inform the patient and his caregiver about warning signs and the need for emergency action. In the event of a fall or any form of trauma, as well as experiencing severe pain, it is essential to consult healthcare professionals. Instruct the patient to undergo regular checkups and routine tests, as recommended by healthcare providers. It is also recommended to undergo routine bone density assessments as directed by a physician. Emphasize the importance of attending all scheduled appointments with their physician and primary care providers to monitor treatment effectiveness and manage potential side effects.

(continued)

Table 7.13 (continued)

Diet modification	Encourage the older patients to follow a balanced diet that includes foods from the four main food groups (fruits and vegetables, carbohydrates, dairy products, and proteins). Consuming calcium-rich foods is the best way to ensure adequate calcium intake. For adults aged 19 to 50 years and for men aged 51 to 70 years, the recommended dietary allowance (RDA) is 1,000 mg of calcium per day. This recommendation increases to 1,200 mg per day for women aged 51 and older and for men aged 71 and above. It is advisable to distribute calcium intake throughout the day in two to three servings. The following foods are rich in calcium: Milk, cheese, yogurt, calcium-fortified soy products, leafy green vegetables, and dried fruits Eggshell powder is high in calcium content and can be consumed daily by incorporating it into food products. Although the primary source of vitamin D is exposure of the skin to sunlight, consuming certain foods and supplements can also be beneficial. For adults aged 19 to 70 years, the RDA for vitamin D is 600 international units (IU) per day, which increases to 800 IU per day for adults aged 71 and older. Good sources of vitamin D include: Fatty fish such as salmon, trout, whitefish, and tuna; mushrooms; eggs; and fortified foods like milk and cereals If there is insufficient intake of these nutrients, calcium and vitamin D supplements can be helpful for older people. It is important to inform seniors about potential side effects of calcium supplements (such as constipation) and vitamin D (adverse effects from excessive intake) as well as methods to manage these issues. Vitamin K is essential for activating bone proteins that contribute to bone health. In bone metabolism, vitamin K has a synergistic effect with vitamin D. Food sources rich in vitamin K include: Green vegetables such as broccoli, Brussels sprouts, and spinach; vegetable oils; and grains, with lesser amounts found in dairy products, meat, and fish. Additionally, natto, a fermented soy product and Japanese food, is the richest dietary source of vitamin K. Prebiotics, probiotics, and synbiotics can aid in enhancing calcium absorption. Protein intake in the diet is recommended at 0.8 grams of protein per kilogram of body weight per day for the general population with moderate activity. However, due to increased protein needs among healthy older adults, the recommended amount for this population is 1.0 to 1.2 grams per kilogram of body weight per day (provided there are no restrictions). Phytoestrogens found in certain plant foods, particularly isoflavones in cherries, oranges, grapes, and soybeans, have a strong affinity for estrogen beta receptors, mimicking estrogenic activity and serving as a therapeutic alternative. Adequate potassium intake in the diet appears to improve calcium balance and reduce bone resorption in the short term (3 to 6 months). In the absence of contraindications, encourage seniors to take advantage of mineral waters rich in bicarbonate and calcium with low sulfate content for bone health. Excessive sodium (salt), caffeine, and high doses of vitamin A (over 2.26–2.40 mmol/L) can have negative effects on bone health. Given that oxidative stress is a contributing factor in accelerating osteoporosis, various antioxidants, including vitamins C and E with antioxidant properties, may help reduce the risk of osteoporosis. Yogurt consumption among seniors can be an excellent source of nutrition. A serving of yogurt contains 270 to 450 mg of calcium (depending on the type), which accounts for nearly half of the daily requirement. Yogurt is better digested and helps achieve optimal balance in gut flora while facilitating proper absorption of nutrients and vitamins. Encourage the older patients to quit smoking and avoid alcohol consumption.

(continued)

Table 7.13 (continued)

Physical activity improvement	Advise older people that physical activities should be within their tolerance levels and should be noninvasive and gradual. Regular exercise, tailored to individuals' fitness levels, is an excellent way to keep bones as strong as possible. Educate seniors to pay attention to how their bodies respond to physical activity and to adjust the intensity and duration accordingly. They should avoid overexertion and rest if they experience significant changes in vital signs. Exercise regimens should be customized to each individual's abilities and tailored specifically for the patient. Frequent walking alone can increase bone density in the pelvis and spine, especially in postmenopausal women. Aerobic, weight-bearing, and resistance exercises are highly beneficial and contribute to increased bone density in the spine. Bodyweight or resistance training effectively enhances bone density, while aerobic exercises improve balance and muscle activity, thereby reducing the risk of falls. Engaging in moderate-intensity aerobic activity for 30 minutes on five days a week is appropriate if tolerated well. Exercises aimed at maintaining or improving balance (such as the Otago Exercise Program (OEP) or Tai Chi) are helpful for seniors at significant risk of falling. Water-based exercises performed in aquatic environments present lower risks of impact-related fractures compared to land-based exercises, and they subject joints to less stress and impact. Additionally, they offer greater benefits for neuromuscular health, functional capacity, and cardiovascular metabolic health. Therefore, such exercises can be recommended for older people. Patients should be instructed to avoid twisting their spines, stretching their toes, or performing sit-ups. Maintaining body weight within a normal and healthy range is recommended. Individuals with low body weight (with a body mass index of 19 or less) typically have more fragile bones, and in the event of a fall, there may not be sufficient fat and muscle to provide protection. It is essential to consult with a healthcare provider before starting any new exercise program to ensure its safety and appropriateness. Teach the patient about the importance of adequate rest, sleep hygiene practices, and strategies for maintaining energy levels.
Medication management	Educate the patient about osteoporosis medications, including the function of each drug, potential side effects, and the appropriate timing and method of administration. Bisphosphonates, which are among the most important medications for osteoporosis, require specific instructions on their use. Teach patients that bisphosphonates should always be taken on an empty stomach with a full glass of water. After taking these medications, individuals must remain upright—either standing or sitting—for at least 30 minutes and should avoid lying down. Additionally, they should wait between 30 minutes and 2 hours before consuming food or other liquids. For older patients, it is essential to periodically review all medications with healthcare providers to ensure that they are necessary, effective, and do not cause adverse interactions. Any side effects or concerns regarding medications should be promptly communicated to healthcare providers for adjustment or substitution. Advise older patients to avoid self-medicating with any new drugs or abruptly discontinuing prescribed medications and altering dosages without consulting their physician. Recommend that patients utilize pill organizers, reminders, or medication management programs to track their medications and dosages and ensure timely administration.

(continued)

Table 7.13 (continued)

Other considerations	Advise older people to spend a short period (10 to 30 minutes) daily in sunlight while adhering to protective measures and without sunscreen. This practice can significantly contribute to meeting the body's vitamin D requirements. However, it is essential to remind them not to remain in the sun for extended periods without sunscreen and to avoid allowing their skin to become red or sunburned. *Fall prevention education* Encourage patients to undergo regular vision and hearing tests (at least once a year) to assess their fall risk. Evaluate cardiovascular causes of falls (such as orthostatic hypotension and arrhythmia) and review medications that may increase the risk of falling (including antipsychotics, antihypertensives, and diuretics). Adjustments or modifications should be made by a physician if necessary. Advise the patient and their family to assess their home for fall hazards and implement corrective measures: Remove or secure slippery rugs or small mats with double-sided tape. Ensure flooring is optimal and free of hazards. Eliminate wires and other obstacles. Install automatic lights in various areas of the home. Add grab bars in the bathroom and near the bathtub. Use nonslip mats in bathrooms. Install handrails and lights on all staircases. Advise against climbing ladders or stools. Ensure that shoes and even slippers worn by seniors are appropriately selected, with nonslip soles. Seniors who feel unstable on their feet should be encouraged to use mobility aids such as canes or walkers. Some older adults may need to wear specialized hip protectors or external pelvic protectors to prevent serious injury from falls. External hip protectors are designed to cover the hip area and reduce impact forces from side falls, although evidence regarding their effectiveness is mixed. Teach seniors that if they experience a fall, instability, or fear of falling, they should immediately inform a family member or healthcare provider. Educate seniors on pain management strategies in case of injury or fracture, including: Pain medications approved by a physician Warm and cold compresses Simple relaxation techniques Therapeutic massage by a qualified professional Teach the patient stress management techniques such as yoga, meditation, and deep breathing exercises (refer to Chap. 3). Encourage them to join support groups for older individuals facing this illness, allowing them to share their experiences and learn from others who are confronting similar challenges. Prepare older patients to utilize new and appropriate technologies that can enhance their self-care behaviors (refer to Chap. 6 for further details).

7.5.12 Chronic Pain (Focusing on Arthritis)

Pain is an unpleasant emotional or physical experience that may be associated with potential or actual tissue damage. It can be nociceptive or neuropathic and can be affected by experiences, cognitive function, and psychological factors. Pain can be chronic or acute. Based on the definition presented in the 11th edition of the International Classification of Diseases (ICD-11), pain is chronic if it lasts for at least three months. Based on the ICD-11, chronic pain is considered a disease and can lead to a high burden of disease and significant social costs, but it is often overlooked and not well perceived.

Almost 20% of the world's population struggles with chronic pain. In addition to causing pain, it has many physical, psychological, and social consequences that can disrupt a person's life. Depression and anxiety are among the most important problems that patients with chronic pain face, and these can worsen the complications of the disease in these patients. Chronic pain is considered an age-related condition, with its occurrence peaking in the seventh decade of life. The incidence of chronic pain in some areas of the body, such as the lower limbs, increases over time, while decreasing in some other parts of the body, such as the waist and back. This issue is mostly related to the way pain is perceived in older people. Generally, the global prevalence of chronic pain among older people has been reported to be about 25% to 85%. Studies have also revealed that its prevalence in individuals aged 80 and older varies from 50.4% to 63%. The number of people with chronic pain is likely higher than reported by the health system since many people with chronic pain do not seek medical attention, and even if they do, they often refer to primary care centers where documentation is inadequate. The important point in this regard is that pain is not a physiological and normal feature of aging and should not be underestimated. Chronic pain leads to functional decline, increases the risk of falls, exacerbates mood disorders, and can ultimately accelerate dependence on organizational care. Pain in older individuals can be due to several causes. Musculoskeletal pain is common and debilitating in older people, and arthritis, which is inflammation of the joints, is one of the most common. Arthritis can arise from various reasons, including gout, autoimmune conditions, and osteoarthritis (which occurs more frequently in older people).

The number of people living with arthritis worldwide was 528 million in 2019, an increase of 113% compared to the figure in 1990. Among them, 73% are over 55 years of age. The knee is the most commonly affected joint. Due to the significant impact of chronic pain on patients and the significant reduction in their ability to perform daily activities, attention to treatment, self-care, and the improvement of its various dimensions is essential. Pain management should be multifaceted and tailored to each patient. A combination of non-pharmacological and pharmacological interventions should be used in this regard. Table 7.14 presents some self-care recommendations for patients with chronic pain, focusing on those with arthritis.

This section discusses common chronic diseases in older people and their self-care tips based on the latest sources. Older people often do not have just one chronic disease, and sometimes having multiple diseases complicates the conditions for a self-care plan. In such conditions, healthcare providers must guide older people and their families with knowledge and expertise in developing a self-care plan appropriate for their specific needs and conditions. In addition to what was stated in this section regarding the physical needs of older people, other aspects of health affected by diseases and their related needs should be considered in developing a holistic self-care plan. Guidance and advice from experts in the same fields may be required in this regard. Box 7.1 provides a template for organizing a holistic self-care plan.

Table 7.14 Self-care tips for older adults with chronic pain (like arthritis)

Familiarization with the disease and clinical manifestations monitoring	Educate older people about the causes of pain (such as arthritis, fibromyalgia, or neuropathy), the related diseases and physiology, diagnostic methods, and available treatments in a simple and understandable manner. Resources like the American Chronic Pain Association can provide valuable information. Explain the clinical manifestations associated with their condition. Pain may sometimes be accompanied by symptoms such as shortness of breath, nausea, vomiting, restlessness, aggression, fatigue, and changes in vital signs. If the pain is severe enough to interfere with daily activities or is accompanied by changes in vital signs, vomiting, or shortness of breath, it is crucial to inform a physician. Suggest that patients keep a diary to record their pain levels, triggers, and patterns. They should use a scale from 0 to 10 to assess pain intensity and pay attention to factors that exacerbate or alleviate their discomfort. This information can be helpful during discussions with healthcare providers. Teach older people pain management techniques, such as: Pain medications approved by a physician Warm and cold compresses Simple relaxation techniques Therapeutic massage by a qualified professional Instruct the patient to undergo regular checkups and routine tests, as recommended by healthcare providers. Emphasize the importance of attending all scheduled appointments with their physician and primary care providers to monitor treatment effectiveness and manage potential side effects.
Diet modification	Encourage the older patients to follow a balanced diet that includes foods from the four main food groups (fruits and vegetables, carbohydrates, dairy products, and proteins). Recommend that patients incorporate anti-inflammatory foods into their diets, such as fatty fish (rich in omega-3 fatty acids), fruits (berries, cherries), vegetables (leafy greens, broccoli), whole grains, nuts, and seeds. The Mediterranean diet is often recommended. Instruct patients to reduce their intake of processed foods, refined sugars, trans fats, and excessive alcohol, as these substances can contribute to inflammation and worsen pain. Encourage the older people to drink sufficient fluids to stay hydrated (within the limits advised by their physician). Dehydration can exacerbate fatigue and discomfort. Consuming foods high in branched-chain amino acids (BCAAs), such as poultry, salmon, eggs, and tuna, may reduce the risk of developing rheumatoid arthritis. The use of magnesium supplements may improve the prognosis for patients with arthritis, particularly female patients. Zinc supplements may help reduce the risk of osteoporosis in patients with rheumatoid arthritis. Encourage the older patients to quit smoking and avoid alcohol consumption.
Physical activity improvement	Advise older people that physical activity should be conducted within their tolerance levels and should be noninvasive and non-sudden. Engaging in at least 150 minutes of moderate-intensity aerobic exercise (such as walking and swimming) per week can be beneficial if there are no contraindications. Encourage the patient to start exercising slowly with simple movements and gradually increase intensity if possible. If possible, it is advisable to incorporate light resistance training two to three times a week to help maintain muscle mass and strength. Exercises that improve balance and flexibility and reduce the risk of falls (such as yoga or tai chi) can be beneficial. Educate the older patients to pay attention to how their body responds to physical activity and to adjust the intensity and duration accordingly. They should avoid overexertion and rest if they notice any significant changes in vital signs. Encourage the patient to prioritize daily activities. They should distribute various tasks throughout the day to prevent activity intolerance, take breaks between activities, and practice breathing exercises. They should avoid performing all energy-demanding activities in one day or consecutively and refrain from bending or standing for prolonged periods during activities. Educate the patient on methods to lose and maintain weight within a healthy range. It is essential to consult with a healthcare provider before starting any new exercise program to ensure its safety and appropriateness. Teach the patient about the importance of adequate rest, sleep hygiene practices, and strategies for maintaining energy levels.

(continued)

Table 7.14 (continued)

Medication management	Familiarize patients with painkillers, including their range and allowable dosages, the function of each drug, potential side effects, and the appropriate timing and method of administration. There are various analgesics available, including simple analgesics (such as paracetamol or acetaminophen), NSAIDs, stronger analgesics (i.e., opioids), and adjuvant medications. Each has unique concerns regarding its side effect profile. Continuous use of any medication should be regularly assessed to ensure its ongoing effectiveness. If corticosteroid medications are prescribed to arthritis patients, it is essential to educate them about potential side effects, such as increased blood sugar levels and an elevated risk of infection. For older patients, it is essential to periodically review all medications with healthcare providers to ensure that they are necessary, effective, and do not cause adverse interactions. Any side effects or concerns regarding medications should be promptly communicated to healthcare providers for adjustment or substitution. Advise older patients to avoid self-medicating with any new drugs or abruptly discontinuing prescribed medications and altering dosages without consulting their physician. Recommend that patients utilize pill organizers, reminders, or medication management programs to track their medications and dosages and ensure timely administration. Patients can discuss non-pharmacological treatments such as physical therapy, occupational therapy, acupuncture, or cognitive-behavioral therapy (CBT) with their healthcare provider as effective options for managing chronic pain.
Other considerations	Educate patients and their families about fall prevention strategies (as outlined in Table 7.13). Arthritis can lead to nocturia in patients over 60 years old; therefore, ensuring adequate nighttime lighting in the home is essential to prevent falls. Teach the patient stress management techniques such as yoga, meditation, and deep breathing exercises (see Chap. 3). Encourage them to join support groups for older individuals facing this illness, allowing them to share their experiences and learn from others who are confronting similar challenges. Prepare older patients to utilize new and appropriate technologies that can enhance their self-care behaviors (refer to Chap. 6 for further details).

7.6 Developing a Self-Care Plan in Older Adults with Chronic Disorders

Different theories, models, and strategies have been developed and evaluated for the design and implementation of self-care plans, as self-care is an essential aspect of health management. Evidence suggests that self-management interventions, especially those guided by established nursing theories, target specific behaviors such as health literacy, effective communication, and psychosocial support, and help improve health outcomes. The process of developing self-care plans in this population is inherently complex due to the complexities of chronic disease and the need for long-term care in older people. Thus, it is necessary to use them in developing a self-care plan and apply the best method according to the patient and his family's conditions. This section presents some appropriate models and strategies that are effective in improving self-care in older people with chronic diseases:

7.6.1 Theoretical Models

1. *Orem's Self-Care Deficit Theory*

Orem's model emphasizes one's ability to perform self-care and identifies factors that may lead to self-care deficits. Based on this theory, self-care is a learned behavior that can be improved through education and support. The core assumption of this theory is that the nurse is responsible for identifying and addressing self-care deficits among patients and promoting agency to promote a return to independence and health. Studies have indicated that interventions based on this model, such as individualized education programs for chronic disease management, can significantly promote self-care behaviors in older adults.

2. *The Health Promotion Model*

The health promotion model was first developed by Nola Pender in 1982. She developed several versions and revisions to address health behavior by focusing on factors such as spiritual growth, interpersonal relations, nutrition, physical activity, health responsibility, and stress management necessary in promoting health.

The three components of the health promotion model include individual characteristics and experiences, specific behavioral cognitions, and health-promoting behavior. Based on this theory, several intentions must be present for patients to seek and achieve health promotion. In this model, older adults must see the value of the benefits, feel competent to achieve the results, and receive positive attitudes and support from others.

3. *Roy Adaptation Model (RAM)*

RAM, presented by Roy in 1970, considers the person as a bio-psycho-social being interacting constantly with a changing environment. This model believes that humans are a complete adaptive system and that life is a process of continuous adaptation to various stimuli from the internal and external environment. Many self-care behaviors can be institutionalized by creating adaptation in older people. In this regard, some studies have been conducted to design a self-care plan for chronic patients using the RAM model and have shown several benefits.

4. *Theory of Interpersonal Relations*

This model was presented by Hildegard Peplau in the mid-twentieth century and has four stages, including orientation, identification, exploitation, and resolution. It depicts the evolving relationship between a nurse and a patient and highlights the nurse's role in each stage. Peplau's theory is grounded in the belief that interpersonal interactions are central to the therapeutic process and that these relationships can facilitate personal growth and healing. By applying this model, healthcare providers can foster strong therapeutic relationships that enhance patient engagement in their own care, ultimately leading to better health outcomes.

5. *The Health Belief Model (HBM)*

The HBM believes that a person's beliefs about health risks and benefits affect their engagement in health-promoting behaviors. This model is a theoretical framework that explains that engagement in health behaviors occurs based on perceived susceptibility to receiving health status, severity of health status, benefits of recommended action, barriers to taking recommended action, signs of engagement in health behavior, and self-efficacy to engage in it. The HBM is one of the most extensively applied theoretical frameworks for explaining health behavior change. Studies indicate that older adults who perceive a higher risk of health problems are more likely to adopt self-care practices.

6. *Social Cognitive Theory (SCT)*

SCT highlights the role of observational learning, social influences, and self-efficacy in behavior change. This well-established theoretical model, explaining the dynamic relationship between behavior and individual and environmental factors, has been extensively applied in the study of various behaviors of older adults, including their physical activity. For example, interventions that include peer support or coaching have indicated that they increase self-efficacy and promote self-care behaviors among older adults. Programs that enhance social relations can lead to better adherence to self-care regimens.

7. *Chronic Care Model (CCM)*

CCM, developed by Wagner, provides a framework for improving chronic disease management by emphasizing the need for informed and active patients and a prepared and proactive healthcare team. CCM is an approach applied extensively in various healthcare settings to guide system improvement for chronic care. The model encourages cooperation between healthcare providers and patients and creates an environment for effective self-care. It has been shown that the implementation of CCM in primary care improves self-management and health outcomes among older adults with multiple chronic conditions.

8. *Illness Representation Theory*

Illness representation theory states that a person's beliefs about their chronic illness include multiple dimensions. In other words, people have unique perceptions of their condition, including dimensions such as perceptions of symptoms, outcomes and complications, chronicity, and level of control over the illness. These different dimensions of illness representation can affect health-related outcomes and self-care behaviors.

9. *COM-B Model*

Applying behavior change theories, such as the COM-B model, which identifies capability, opportunity, and motivation-behavior as critical components of behavior change, can be beneficial in improving self-care in older adults. This model, first proposed by Michie, states that to facilitate behavior change, interventions should improve three domains, including capabilities (psychological or physiological capacities, such as self-efficacy and hope), opportunities (physical and social environments, such as family influences), and motivations (reflective and autonomous mechanisms, such as goals and motivation), and finally, remove the barriers that older adults face in managing their chronic conditions.

Models and theories related to behavior change and self-care in older adults are not limited to those mentioned above. See Chap. 1 to gain more information on theories related to self-care in older adults.

7.6.2 Strategies

1. *Education and Training Programs*

Educational interventions have been beneficial in increasing self-management skills. Many review studies on patients with various chronic diseases have indicated that structured educational programs significantly improve self-care knowledge and behaviors in older adults with chronic diseases. These programs often include information about medication management, dietary changes, and physical activity.

2. *Technology-Enhanced Interventions*

Utilizing technology, such as mobile health applications and telehealth services, has emerged as a promising strategy for improving self-care. Many studies have recently designed innovative interventions based on new technologies and digital interventions. They have indicated that these methods are beneficial in improving health outcomes in older patients with chronic diseases despite numerous limitations. They can also be used in the design and development of self-care plans.

3. *Behavioral Interventions*

It has been shown that behavioral strategies, including motivational interviewing and cognitive-behavioral techniques, are effective in promoting self-care behaviors. These approaches can lead to significant improvements in physical activity levels and dietary habits among older adults. Many self-care programs target behavioral changes.

4. *Community-Based Programs*

Community resources play a vital role in supporting self-care. Programs that integrate social support, such as group exercise classes or nutrition workshops, are associated with improved self-care outcomes. These initiatives not only provide education but can also foster a sense of belonging and responsibility.

5. *Peer Support Programs*

Peer support is a valuable resource for promoting self-care among older adults. Programs that connect people with similar health challenges can increase motivation and responsibility. It has been shown that self-management programs, along with peer support, lead to improved health outcomes and higher confidence in managing chronic conditions.

6. *Family Involvement*

Involving family members in the self-care process can increase adherence to health regimens. Many self-care programs have been designed and implemented to involve family members. Family support positively affects older adults' capability to effectively manage chronic conditions. It has been proven that interventions that include education and family involvement lead to better health outcomes.

This section presented some of the most popular and commonly used models and related strategies to improve self-care behaviors in older adults suffering from a disease. Since each of the mentioned cases is linked to a vast body of information and studies, it is essential to thoroughly study each of them before implementing them.

7.7 Barriers and Challenges to Self-Care in Older Individuals with Chronic Diseases

Despite the importance of self-care in old people with chronic diseases and its many benefits, the aging process and life in old age inherently cause barriers and challenges for old adults in their self-care. It sometimes makes older adults fail despite their efforts to implement, maintain, and continue self-care behaviors. This section presents some of the most important barriers and challenges that older individuals with chronic diseases face based on the results of studies conducted, especially qualitative studies on this population, and solutions to deal with them:

1. *Physical Limitations:* Many seniors face physical limitations and movement disorders for various reasons, such as frailty due to aging, chronic pain, or diseases such as arthritis, osteoporosis, or other musculoskeletal conditions. These problems can even limit seniors in performing daily tasks, exercising, preparing food, or even observing basic health.
   - *Solution:* Avoiding fatigue and managing pain based on the methods discussed before are vital in this population. Implementing tailored exercise programs within the tolerance range can increase physical activity levels. Programs such as tai chi or yoga have shown benefits in improving balance and strength in older adults. Additionally, home modifications (e.g., grab bars, ramps, etc.) can facilitate easier access to daily activities in this population. Telehealth services can also significantly compensate for delays in in-person medical visits due to physical limitations.
2. *Cognitive Deficits:* Cognitive deficits in older adults are often associated with deficits in attention, memory, executive function, language, and response speed. They can impair older people's ability to understand health-related information, remember medication schedules, adhere to dietary restrictions, or recognize symptoms that require medical attention. Older adults may also have difficulty making informed decisions about their healthcare due to cognitive deficits, leading to poor self-care practices.
   - *Solution:* Providing health information in words that are as understandable and simple as possible can help reduce this problem. Using blister packs is also beneficial. Moreover, using memory aids, such as phone reminders or alarms, can help support adherence to self-care routines. Many new technologies are nowadays available to help seniors with cognitive impairments improve self-care and maintain safety.
3. *Psychosocial Factors:* Mental health issues such as anxiety, depression, and isolation are common among older adults and can significantly affect the motivation and energy levels needed for self-care. Social isolation can lead to a lack of support systems to encourage and assist with self-care activities.
   - *Solution:* It is crucial to pay attention to mental health issues and symptoms of anxiety, sadness, hopelessness, or depression in older people and take action immediately. In some cases, counseling, psychotherapy, or referral to a psychiatrist may be essential. Programs that promote social interaction, such as older people's houses or community groups, can help combat isolation and depression.

4. *Health Literacy Deficiencies:* Lack of knowledge about conditions, medications, and effective self-care practices complicates older people's ability to engage in this process. Inadequate awareness and low health literacy among older adults make it difficult to understand medical advice, treatment plans, or self-management guidelines. This issue can even lead older adults to trust unreliable sources and engage in behaviors that put their health at greater risk.
   - *Solution:* Educational interventions using various approaches, in-person or virtual, can increase the level of health awareness and literacy among older people. Easy access to reliable information about health and disease through appropriate media and software can be very beneficial.
5. *Uncertainty in the Disease Trajectory:* Many chronic diseases have an uncertain trajectory and prognosis, making older people lose hope of recovery or maintaining their abilities. Thus, they consider self-care futile. Additionally, many diseases, such as heart failure and cancer, are accompanied by instabilities, making the course of the disease unpredictable. As the disease worsens, the patient loses previous abilities in self-care behaviors. Suddenly entering the final stages of the disease without having the necessary preparation makes the patient fail to adapt to his new condition and causes confusion among older adults.
   - *Solution:* Providing comprehensive education through personal care programs can help clarify the course of the disease and its management strategies. Healthcare providers should engage in shared decision-making and ensure that patients understand their condition and feel comfortable raising their questions and concerns. Specifying advance directives and healthcare proxies when old people have the power to make decisions reduces confusion for family members in the event of an acute disease.
6. *Complexity of Comorbid Conditions:* Older people often experience comorbid conditions that can complicate disease management due to the interaction between different health issues. The complexity of managing multiple medications, adhering to multiple diets, and physical activities that may sometimes conflict with each other in some situations makes the process of self-care difficult and overwhelming.
   - *Solution:* In such conditions, a self-care program should be planned in an integrated and coordinated manner with the help of healthcare professionals. Coordinated care approaches, such as those offered in patient-centered medical homes (PCMHs), allow for better communication between healthcare providers and ensure that treatment plans are coordinated across specialties. Fragmented self-care programs can have inadequate or even inappropriate effects in some situations. The skills of health-related decision-making, problem-solving, and prioritizing self-care behaviors in a way that does not worsen the disease are among the most important capabilities that older people and their families must acquire in these situations.
7. *Frustration and Fatigue in Medical Adherence:* A chronic disease requires long-term self-care. This complex, uncertain, difficult, and ongoing process often causes fatigue and frustration in older people. In some cases, this makes older people consider self-care behaviors futile.
   - *Solution:* Emotional and social support, incorporating regular recreational programs into their daily routine, and communicating with peers can prevent fatigue and frustration. The use of assistive technologies for older people, such as medication management programs or automated drug dispensing systems, can help with adherence by providing reminders and tracking consumption. Educational programs that focus on the importance of adherence and involve family members or caregivers can also increase motivation. Moreover, simplifying medication regi-

mens and aligning them with personal daily routines can reduce the burden of self-care in patients.

8. *Lack of Social and Emotional Support:* Social isolation and inadequate informal social and emotional support systems are among the barriers that weaken self-care in older people with chronic diseases. Many older people report feelings of loneliness and a lack of reliable support from family and friends. Geographic distance from family and friends often complicates maintaining social relationships and contributes to isolation.
   - *Solution:* Family plays a vital role in providing emotional support to older adults and should be addressed by healthcare providers. Maintaining relationships with family, friends, and acquaintances allows older adults to have access to a good social network and meet their emotional needs. Additionally, developing community support programs that strengthen social relations, such as older people's houses or peer support groups, can provide emotional support and encouragement for self-care practices. Telehealth services can also offer opportunities for virtual social interaction for those who are at home and help reduce feelings of isolation.
9. *Financial Constraints:* The financial burden of medications, treatments, and healthcare services can be a major barrier for older people with fixed incomes. In other words, economic costs significantly affect access to care and the ability to engage in self-care. Financial constraints can deprive older people of access to many technologies that facilitate the process of self-care. Financial pressure can lead to nonadherence to medication and inadequate self-care practices.
   - *Solution:* Introducing counseling and financial assistance centers can help reduce some of the financial burden. Introducing donors to them can be beneficial for some patients. Furthermore, identifying and introducing alternative solutions that are less expensive or centers that provide free or low-cost services by healthcare providers help older people in this regard.
10. *Cultural and Environmental Factors:* Cultural attitudes toward aging and healthcare can affect older people's perception of their ability to participate in self-care. In some cultures, family care may be preferred over self-care. Self-care education may not be taken seriously in some cultures. Additionally, unfavorable environmental conditions, such as unsafe housing and lack of adequate access, can impair an older person's self-care ability. Limited access to transportation can cause older people in some areas to avoid attending medical appointments or accessing community resources that support self-care.
    - *Solution:* Cultural barriers must be identified in older people. It is often difficult to change issues that are specific to the culture of a particular population or group. However, culturally sensitive health education programs must be carefully delivered in a way that respects the values of different populations. Implementing home environment modifications tailored to the needs and limitations of older people can reduce environmental barriers. Technologies like smart homes or monitoring tools can be very instrumental in some situations.
11. *Healthcare System Barriers:* The structure of healthcare systems can create additional barriers to effective self-care. Many current care models focus on individual diseases rather than a holistic approach to managing multiple chronic conditions, which can ignore the complexities faced by older patients. Additionally, complex healthcare systems and processes can overwhelm older people and make it challenging for them to access the resources or services needed for self-care. Furthermore, fragmented services, long wait times, and inadequate communication between providers can create significant barriers to effective self-care.

- *Solution:* Implementing coordinated care models that emphasize communication between healthcare providers can ensure that older patients receive consistent information and support. The use of care coordinators or case managers can also facilitate better management of chronic conditions across specialties. Moreover, telehealth options can reduce barriers related to transportation and access to professionals.

These barriers should be considered in the development of a self-care plan and proactively addressed to eliminate them, ensuring that self-care behaviors are established and sustained. Eliminating these barriers requires a multifaceted approach that involves considering the patient's limitations and the complexities of disease management, strengthening support systems, improving health literacy, providing mental health resources, and ensuring access to cost-effective healthcare options.

Recommendations for Family Caregivers and Older Individuals

This section offers some recommendations for the implementation of self-care strategies for older people with minor ailments or chronic diseases.

- *Patient–Caregiver Dyads:* A dyadic approach involves both the patient and their caregivers in the self-care process. Caregivers assist and facilitate the patient's self-care in chronic conditions by providing support, supervision, and management. Older patients and family caregivers are better able to make joint health-related decisions.
- *Continual Learning:* Health issues in aging and self-care strategies during disease are extensive. Much of the information and self-care methods may be constantly changing. Thus, older people and their family caregivers need to be educated about their diseases, symptoms, treatment options, and management strategies. For this purpose, follow reputable and up-to-date scientific sources and seek help from your healthcare providers.
- *Routine Health Monitoring*: Older people and their caregivers should be sensitive to the development of new symptoms or changes in existing symptoms. Encouraging them to establish a routine for monitoring vital signs (such as blood pressure, body temperature, and blood sugar) and manifestations of disease will help them identify complications early and allow for timely interventions if needed.
- *Regular Health Checkups*: Regular checkups with healthcare providers are essential for diagnosing and managing health conditions. Older people should prioritize routine tests (blood sugar and cholesterol levels, kidney, thyroid, and liver function tests, etc.), screenings (such as blood pressure, cancer screenings, and eye and dental exams), and vaccinations (flu vaccine, COVID-19, etc.) to detect potential problems early and prevent rapid and severe disease progression.
- *Keeping Patience:* The process of accepting and adapting to diseases, especially chronic ones, varies among individuals. This process requires lifestyle modifications and self-care strategies, which may take more practice and time for older people. Allow older individuals to progress at their own pace and be patient.
- *Ongoing Support:* Family is the primary source of support for older people in

coping with a chronic disease, even if older people perform self-care activities well. Emotional support makes older people not feel lonely and less tired. Active listening, empathy, compassion, and encouraging older people to express their feelings and concerns about health and the future are examples of this emotional support. In addition, providing social and community support for the older people based on the training provided can improve their well-being.

- *Utilizing Technology:* Many new technologies, such as e-health services, monitoring devices and applications, robotic developments, and smart home technology, are designed to improve the self-care and safety of older people and to assist their family caregivers. Introducing new and appropriate technologies for older people and encouraging them to utilize them can facilitate the self-care process for older people.
- *Flexibility of Self-Care Plan*: The self-care plan should be updated based on new conditions and the slightest change in the patient's health. Health status is not stable and constantly changes in old age, making it impossible to implement a fixed self-care plan. Thus, the self-care plan should be modified based on new conditions. However, flexibility does not mean that people can stop adhering to the self-care plan and abandon self-care whenever they want.
- *Considering Family Caregivers' Health*: Family caregivers who care for older people with chronic diseases often experience a high level of physical, psychological, and financial stress. These people should not neglect their health and need to be educated on self-care behaviors. Obtaining proper counseling, maintaining necessary recreation during the week, and considering respite programs can be beneficial.

7.8 Summary of the Chapter

This chapter emphasizes the importance of self-care in the management of minor ailments and chronic diseases among older adults. It discusses and introduces the most important and common minor ailments and chronic diseases in this age group. Additionally, practical recommendations will be provided to promote self-care behaviors for older people and their caregivers by emphasizing the significance of self-care in increasing the quality of life. It highlights the importance of developing a holistic self-care program and implementing self-care in all aspects of human life and important points in developing a comprehensive care plan. Models related to self-care in chronic conditions and evidence-based strategies for integrating self-care into the lives of older people are discussed. Then, barriers to implementing self-care in older people with chronic conditions are investigated. After providing recommendations for family caregivers and older people and referring to studies conducted in this field, scenarios are presented to actively engage the reader's mind in applying what they have learned from this chapter.

7.9 Summary of Research Studies

Self-care in various diseases, especially chronic diseases, has always been an interesting research topic for researchers worldwide. Various methodologies, including qualitative and quantitative studies (ranging from cross-sectional to clinical trials and systematic reviews), have been used to gain a complete perspective on this concept. Some of these have theoretical applications, while others have practical applications.

The application and effectiveness of nursing-based theories and models is one of the aspects that have been investigated by various researchers in this field to improve patients' self-care behaviors. Theory-guided action helps people know what they are doing and why they are doing it. In this regard, an integrated review study by Younas and Quennell (2019) reviewed 35 studies on the application of nursing theories in guiding care practices. They showed that most studies in this field were from Iran, the United States, and Turkey. In addition, Orem's self-care model, Roy's adaptation model, and Peplau's interpersonal relations theory were the most frequently used. The effect of theory-guided interventions was more pronounced on outcomes such as quality of life, self-efficacy, self-care, and stress in patients, especially those with chronic illnesses and cardiac conditions. Three included studies had high quality, and all found that the nursing theory-guided interventions were beneficial. In addition, nursing theory-guided interventions mostly improved all the outcomes studied. A systematic review by Nasiri et al. (2023) outlines the application of Orem's self-care deficit theory and shows that interventions rooted in this framework significantly increase self-efficacy and improve psychosocial outcomes such as anxiety and depression in adults with chronic diseases. Such studies suggest that theory, as a framework for practice, paves the way for the development of coherent self-care programs, particularly relevant to older people facing multiple health challenges.

One of the important issues is that the conducted studies are often on chronic diseases, and researchers have paid less attention to minor ailments. Thus, a significant limitation is felt in studies in this field. Several reasons can be involved in this regard. One of the important reasons is that self-care is done periodically for minor ailments, so researchers do not pay much attention to them. Moreover, sampling and interventions in these conditions will be more limited than in chronic diseases. All of these factors lead researchers to pay less attention to minor ailments.

Although several studies have been conducted on self-care in chronic diseases, a review of the studies indicates that there are gaps and limitations in this field. Self-care is a fundamental aspect of recovery for patients with chronic diseases and serves as the focus of many interventions. However, numerous studies describing various self-care interventions lack comparative analysis under different conditions. A thorough examination and comparison of these interventions can provide valuable insights into effective approaches tailored for different groups of patients with chronic diseases. One of the most important issues in evaluating interventions for older adults is that many studies that assess different self-care promotion methods have focused on patients with a mean age of less than 70 years. Many studies evaluating interventions have excluded older people due to the challenges and barriers associated with teaching and implementing self-care behaviors.

However, several studies have also targeted only the older population. A meta-analysis by Chodosh et al. (2005) reviewed 53 studies and revealed that self-management programs for chronic diseases, especially diabetes and hypertension, have crucial clinical benefits. Many studies in recent years have examined the applications of new technologies and telehealth in the self-care of older patients with chronic conditions. For example, a systematic review and meta-analysis by Wong et al. (2022) reviewed 13 clinical trials to investigate nurse-led remote self-care promotion programs in community-dwelling older people. The results showed that the overall quality of life of intervention groups and their self-efficacy improved significantly, and their depression levels decreased compared to control groups. In addition, a systematic review by Alhussein and Hadjileontiadis (2022) reported the potential of mobile health (m-Health) applications to empower self-management among osteoporosis patients. This study revealed that these programs significantly relieve pain and improve disability, although there are still criticisms regarding the inadequacy of clinically valid tools.

Regarding factors related to self-efficacy, Sadeghi et al. (2024) conducted a qualitative study of content analysis on 26 participants, including older people with multiple chronic conditions, family caregivers, and professionals. In this study, the obtained categories included individual factors (with sub-categorization of biological factors, cognitive factors, comorbidities, mental health, economic status, and health-centered behaviors), interpersonal factors (with sub-categorization of interaction with the medical care team and family relationships), factors related to the health system (facilities of health centers, staff empowerment, and health policy), and external factors (cultural and social factors). One of the significant issues in the studies is that lifestyle modification and control of physical symptoms are often addressed, while other dimensions related to self-care, such as social, psychological, and spiritual dimensions, are less considered.

Investigating the role of family caregivers in improving the self-care behaviors of older adults and the self-care and health of caregivers affected by caring for chronically ill older adults has been a hot topic in studies. For example, Lusardi et al. (2017) investigated the multifactorial risk of falls among community-dwelling older adults. Although this study primarily focused on assessing fall risk, it emphasized the need for caregivers to participate in active management strategies to minimize risks. A systematic review study by Huang et al. (2023) highlighted the importance of home education not only for patients with chronic wounds but also for their caregivers. This study revealed that patient and caregiver involvement in chronic wound management improved self-care behaviors and, thus, patient outcomes. The study by Morkisch et al. (2020) discussed the transitional care model and showed that the transition from hospital to home care requires the active involvement of caregivers, especially in maintaining continuity of care and preventing readmission. High-intensity interventions that include caregiver education in the area of transitional care can further enhance patient independence and encourage self-management. Moreover, the caregiving burden and its consequences have been extensively reported as an important issue that affects both caregiver and care recipient health outcomes. A systematic review by Tu et al. (2022) reported that caregivers of older adults with dementia experience significant stress, which is associated with higher rates of depression and adverse health outcomes. This burden often leads to a reduced capacity for effective self-care among caregivers, highlighting a cyclical pattern of stress in which caregivers' poor health negatively affects their ability to meet the needs of older adults.

This section discussed the strengths and weaknesses of the studies conducted on self-care in older adults with chronic diseases and minor ailments. Reviewing these studies and benefiting from their results will provide opportunities for designing innovative interventions and improving the quality of future self-care-related studies.

7.10 Critical Thinking (Scenario-Based)

- *Scenario case 1*

Mr. John is a 70-year-old businessman diagnosed with moderate heart failure due to left ventricular systolic dysfunction last year. His long-term condition has been well controlled with prescribed medication. He has recently been under much stress at work and has experienced heartburn attacks, for which he has started taking an OTC antacid (magnesium hydroxide). The antacid is very soothing, and he has been taking it regularly since he thought it was a relatively harmless substance. He has currently visited his general practitioner since he noticed that he has shortness of breath and swollen ankles. He is also suffering from diarrhea and frequent burping.

Discussion Points:

1. What do you think is the problem?
2. What part of self-care is impaired that caused this problem? What do you suggest to solve it?
3. Using the training in this chapter and Orem's theory, how would you develop a self-care program for him to manage his heart failure?
4. What training would you suggest for controlling his diarrhea?

- *Scenario Case 2*

Mr. Robert is an 89-year-old man with a history of hypertension and is struggling to keep his blood pressure within the desired range. He lives alone in a rural area and is unable to visit a healthcare provider regularly. Although he is taking his prescribed medications and following a recommended diet, he has recently been experiencing mild headaches and fatigue. Believing that his hypertension is the cause, he decides to start a strict diet without consulting his healthcare provider to improve his condition. He eliminates salt from his meals and significantly reduces his fluid intake, believing that this will help him better control his blood pressure. After one week, he begins to feel dizzy and faint and informs his family.

Discussion Points:

1. What do you think is wrong with his self-care, and where does the problem stem from?
2. How can his family help him?
3. How do you train him to develop and follow a self-care plan?

- *Scenario Case 3*

Ms. Mary is a 68-year-old woman experiencing abdominal pain, fatigue, nocturnal epigastric pain, and postprandial pain over the last week. She reports no hematemesis and has no significant underlying medical history. There is mild tenderness on abdominal examination. During history taking, she reports that she has been taking naproxen 500 mg twice daily for the past month due to an ankle sprain and minor pain. She has been taking it for the past two days.

Discussion Points:

1. What is the most likely diagnosis?
2. What is the best diagnostic method?
3. What is the cause of this problem in the patient?
4. What is the most important training to prevent its recurrence?
5. What recommendations do you have for improving self-care behaviors to control the current problem?

- *Scenario Case 4*

Ms. Brenda is a 78-year-old woman with early-stage Parkinson's disease. She also suffers from chronic obstructive pulmonary disease (COPD). She lives with her 90-year-old husband, and their only source of income is his limited pension. She has become anxious and confused as her functional abilities declined. She feels that managing both conditions is beyond her control, which makes her very frustrated. She avoids many foods and adheres to her COPD medication regimen because she is afraid of worsening her Parkinson's disease. She avoids performing activities to prevent shortness of breath, believing that this decision will prevent the progression of her Parkinson's disease.

Discussion Points

1. Review the problem from different angles.
2. How will you help Ms. Brenda with the training provided in this chapter?

Bibliography

Abdi S, Spann A, Borilovic J, de Witte L, Hawley M. Understanding the care and support needs of older people: a scoping review and categorisation using the WHO international classification of functioning, disability and health framework (ICF). BMC Geriatr. 2019;19:1–5.

ADA, American Diabetes Association. Patient Education Library [Internet]. 2024. Available from: https://professional.diabetes.org/clinical-support/patient-education-library

Addae S, Kim J, Smith A, Kang M, Rajana P. Smart solutions for detecting, predicting, monitoring, and managing dementia in the older people: a survey IEEE Access. 2024.

Aghajanloo A, Negarandeh R, Janani L, Tanha K, Hoseini-Esfidarjani SS. Self-care status in patients with heart failure: systematic review and meta-analysis. Nurs Open. 2021;8(5):2235–48.

Aibar-Almazán A, Voltes-Martínez A, Castellote-Caballero Y, Afanador-Restrepo DF, Carcelén-Fraile MD, López-Ruiz E. Current status of the diagnosis and management of osteoporosis. Int J Mol Sci. 2022;23(16):9465.

Al-kuraishy HM, Jabir MS, Albuhadily AK, Al-Gareeb AI, Jawad SF, Swelum AA, et al. Role of ketogenic diet in neurodegenerative diseases focusing on Alzheimer diseases: the guardian angle. Ageing Res Rev. 2024;95:102233.

Alhussein G, Hadjileontiadis L. Digital health technologies for long-term self-management of osteoporosis: systematic review and meta-analysis. JMIR mHealth and uHealth. 2022;10(4):e32557

Alonso Salinas GL, Cepas-Guillén P, León AM, Jiménez-Méndez C, Lozano-Vicario L, Martínez-Avial M, Díez-Villanueva P. The impact of geriatric conditions in older patients with coronary heart disease: a state-of-the-art review. J Clin Med. 2024;13(7):1891.

Alqahtani J, Alqahtani I. Self-care in the older adult population with chronic disease: concept analysis. Heliyon. 2022;8(7).

Ambrose KR, Golightly YM. Physical exercise as non-pharmacological treatment of chronic pain: why and when. Best Pract Res Clin Rheumatol. 2015;29(1):120–30.

American Diabetes Association. 12. Older adults: standards of medical care in diabetes—2021. Diabetes Care. 2021;44(Supplement_1):S168–79.

American Lung Assocation [Internet]. COPD; [Last updated July 11, 2024]. Available from: https://www.lung.org/lung-health-diseases/lung-disease-lookup/copd/living-with-copd

Amin MB, Greene FL, Edge SB, Compton CC, Gershenwald JE, Brookland RK, et al. The Eighth Edition AJCC Cancer Staging Manual: Continuing to build a bridge from a population-based to a more "personalized" approach to cancer staging. CA Cancer J Clin. 2017;67(2):93–9.

Ansari A, Fahimfar N, Noruzi A, Fahimifar S, Hajivalizadeh F, Ostovar A, Larijani B, Sanjari M. Health information–seeking behavior and self-care in women with osteoporosis: a qualitative study. Arch Osteoporos. 2021;16(1):78.

Armitage AE, Fonkem E. Supportive care of neurodegenerative patients. Front Oncol. 2023;13:1029938.

Arnold M, Rajagukguk YV, Gramza-Michałowska A. Functional food for older people high in antioxidant and chicken eggshell calcium to reduce the risk of osteoporosis—a narrative review. Foods. 2021;10(3):656.

Aroesty JM. Patient education: angina treatment — medical versus interventional therapy (Beyond the basics) [Internet]. Uptodate.com. 2024 [cited 2024 Dec 11]. Available from: https://www.uptodate.com/contents/angina-treatment-medical-versus-interventional-therapy-beyond-the-basics

Asante S, Bang EJ. Chronic illnesses and fatigue in older individuals: a literature review. Innov Aging. 2019;3(S1):319.

Asthma and Allergy Foundation of America. Asthma in older adults [internet]. Asthma & Allergy Foundation of America. 2022. Available from: https://aafa.org/asthma/living-with-asthma/asthma-in-older-adults/

Ayele AA, Mekuria AB, Tegegn HG, Gebresillassie BM, Mekonnen AB, Erku DA. Management of minor ailments in a community pharmacy setting: findings from simulated visits and qualitative study in Gondar town, Ethiopia. PLoS One. 2018;13(1):e0190583.

Baker LA, March DS, Wilkinson TJ, Billany RE, Bishop NC, Castle EM, et al. Clinical practice guideline exercise and lifestyle in chronic kidney disease. BMC Nephrol. 2022;23(1):75.

Bakhshi F, Safavi SR, Sadeghi R. Social cognitive theory and healthy lifestyle among older people. Health Educ Health Promot. 2024;12(2):315–22.

Battaglia S, Benfante A, Spatafora M, Scichilone N. Asthma in the older people: a different disease? Breathe. 2016;12(1):18–28.

Bayliss EA, Ellis JL, Steiner JF. Barriers to self-management and quality-of-life outcomes in seniors with multimorbidities. Ann Fam Med. 2007;5(5):395–402.

Bednarski BK. Patient education: Colon and rectal cancer (Beyond the basics) [Internet] Uptodatecom. 2019. Available from: https://www.uptodate.com/contents/colon-and-rectal-cancer-beyond-the-basics

Benetos A, Petrovic M, Strandberg T. Hypertension management in older and frail older patients. Circ Res. 2019;124(7):1045–60.

Ben-Shlomo Y, Darweesh S, Llibre-Guerra J, Marras C, San Luciano M, Tanner C. The epidemiology of Parkinson's disease. Lancet. 2024;403(10423):283–92.

Berk T, Ashina S, Martin V, Newman L, Vij B. Diagnosis and treatment of primary headache disorders in older adults. J Am Geriatr Soc. 2018;66(12):2408–16.

Berns JS. Patient education: hemodialysis (beyond the basics) [Internet]. Uptodate.com. 2019. Available from: https://www.uptodate.com/contents/hemodialysis-beyond-the-basics

Berns J. Patient education: chronic kidney disease (beyond the basics). UpToDate, Waltham. Accessed. 2021;4.

Bhat S, Acharya UR, Hagiwara Y, Dadmehr N, Adeli H. Parkinson's disease: cause factors, measurable indicators, and early diagnosis. Comput Biol Med. 2018;102:234–41.

Bianchi VE, Herrera PF, Laura R. Effect of nutrition on neurodegenerative diseases. A systematic review. Nutr Neurosci. 2021;24(10):810–34.

Bianchi VE, Rizzi L, Somaa F. The role of nutrition on Parkinson's disease: a systematic review. Nutr Neurosci. 2023;26(7):605–28.

Bico I, Afonso A, Sousa L, Bule MJ, Lopes MJ. Empowering Cancer patients with self-care and Pain management skills: a quasi-experimental study. Pain Manag Nurs. 2024;25(4):369–76.

Boers E, Barrett M, Su JG, Benjafield AV, Sinha S, Kaye L, et al. Global burden of chronic obstructive pulmonary disease through 2050. JAMA Netw Open. 2023;6(12):e2346598.

Bokermann J, König HH, Hajek A. Pain: its prevalence and correlates among the oldest old. Aging Clin Exp Res. 2024;36(1):2.

Bordin D, Luíza Pinto A, Leme Trupel LL, Borgo P, Luiza da Silva C, Messias Floriano LS. Symptoms of mood change in hospitalized older people people: prevalence and associated factors. Saúde e Pesquisa. 2024;17(2).

Bouya S, Balouchi A, Rafiemanesh H, Hesaraki M. Prevalence of chronic kidney disease in Iranian general population: a meta-analysis and systematic review. Ther Apher Dial. 2018;22(6):594–9.

Bożek A. Clinical outcomes of AIT in the older people population. Curr Opin Allergy Clin Immunol. 2023;23(4):341–5.

Braman SS. Asthma in the older people. Clin Geriatr Med. 2017;33(4):523–37.

Brewster GS, Riegel B, Gehrman PR. Insomnia in the older adult. Sleep Med Clin. 2018;13(1):13–9.

Brown JS, Amend SR, Austin RH, Gatenby RA, Hammarlund EU, Pienta KJ. Updating the definition of Cancer. Mol Cancer Res. 2023;21(11):1142–7.

Bruera E, Yennurajalingam S. Overview of fatigue in palliative care [Internet]. www.uptodate.com 2024. Available from: https://www.uptodate.com/contents/overview-of-fatigue-in-palliative-care

Cacciatore S, Spadafora L, Bernardi M, Galli M, Betti M, Perone F, Nicolaio G, Marzetti E, Martone AM, Landi F, Asher E. Management of coronary artery disease in older adults: recent advances and gaps in evidence. J Clin Med. 2023;12(16):5233.

Cahan JG, Abbott SM. Use of light therapy for insomnia in the older people: role of circadian rhythm disorders. Curr Sleep Med Rep. 2020;6:176–83.

Cancer Pain. Current clinical medicine. 2nd ed. Philadelphia: W.B. Saunders; 2010. p. 666–71.e1.

Cao Q, Tan CC, Xu W, Hu H, Cao XP, Dong Q, Tan L, Yu JT. The prevalence of dementia: a systematic review and meta-analysis. J Alzheimer's Dis. 2019;73(3):1157–66.

Cardol M, Schellevis FG, Spreeuwenberg P, van de Lisdonk EH. Changes in patients' attitudes towards the management of minor ailments. Br J Gen Pract. 2005;55(516):516–21.

Cardona V, Guilarte M, Luengo O, Labrador-Horrillo M, Sala-Cunill A, Garriga T. Allergic diseases in the older people. Clin Transl Allergy. 2011;1:1.

Carney EF. The impact of chronic kidney disease on global health. Nat Rev Nephrol. 2020;16(5):251–2.

Carter E. Most common cancers in the older people | Caring Senior Service [Internet]. Caring Senior Service. 2023 [cited 2024 Dec 9]. Available from: https://caringseniorservice.com/blog/common-cancers-in-olderpeople/

CDC [Internet]. About High Blood Pressure; [Last updated May 15, 2024]. Available from: https://www.cdc.gov/high-blood-pressure/about/index.html

Chahine L. Insomnia, daytime sleepiness, and other sleep disorders in Parkinson disease [Internet]. Uptodate.com. 2024 [cited 2024 Nov 29]. Available from: https://www.uptodate.com/contents/insomnia-daytime-sleepiness-and-other-sleep-disorders-in-parkinson-disease

Chait MM. Gastroesophageal reflux disease: important considerations for the older patients. World J Gastroint Endosc. 2010;2(12):388.

Chambe J, Reynaud E, Maruani J, Fraih E, Geoffroy PA, Bourgin P. Light therapy in insomnia disorder: a systematic review and meta-analysis. J Sleep Res. 2023;32(6):e13895.

Chapman EJ, Edwards Z, Boland JW, Maddocks M, Fettes L, Malia C, et al. Practice review: evidence-based and effective management of pain in patients with advanced cancer. Palliat Med. 2020;34(4):444–53.

Chen W, Huang Y, Chong CM, Zheng H. Editorial: post-stroke complications: mechanisms, diagnosis, and therapies. Front Neurol. 2023;14:1292562.

Cho SJ, Stout-Delgado HW. Aging and lung disease. Annu Rev Physiol. 2020;82:433–59.

Chodosh J, Morton SC, Mojica W, Maglione M, Suttorp MJ, Hilton L, Rhodes S, Shekelle P. Meta-analysis: chronic disease self-management programs for older adults. Ann Intern Med. 2005;143(6):427–38.

Cleveland Clinic. Low Fodmap Diet: what it is, uses & how to follow [Internet]. Cleveland Clinic. 2022. Available from: https://my.clevelandclinic.org/health/treatments/22466-low-fodmap-diet

Clinic C. Blood Sugar Monitoring [Internet]. 2023. Available from: https://my.clevelandclinic.org/health/treatments/17956-blood-sugar-monitoring

Cohen M, Quintner J. Is "Chronic Pain" a Meaningful Diagnosis? In: van Rysewyk S, editor. Meanings of pain: volume 2: common types of pain and language. Cham: Springer International Publishing; 2019. p. 249–60.

Colucci W. Patient education: heart failure (Beyond the basics) [Internet]. Uptodate.com. 2024. Available from: https://www.uptodate.com/contents/heart-failure-beyond-the-basics

Cong Z, Huo M, Jiang X, Yu H. Factors associated with the level of self-management in older patients with chronic diseases: a pathway analysis. BMC Geriatr. 2024;24(1):377.

Creighton SD, Palmer D, Mitchnick KA, Winters BD. Chapter 6 - Exploiting novelty and oddity exploratory preferences in rodents to study multisensory object memory and perception. In: Ennaceur A, de Souza Silva MA, editors. Handbook of behavioral neuroscience. 27: Elsevier; 2018. p. 103–23.

Curto E, Crespo-Lessmann A, González-Gutiérrez MV, Bardagí S, Cañete C, Pellicer C, Bazús T, Vennera MD, Martínez C, Plaza V. Is asthma in the older people different? Functional and clinical characteristics of asthma in individuals aged 65 years and older. Asthma Res Pract. 2019;5:1–6.

Dalgleish L, Campbell J. Xerosis in Older Adults. Adv Skin Wound Care. 2022;35(1):62–3.

Danby SG, AlEnezi T, Sultan A, Lavender T, Chittock J, Brown K, Cork MJ. Effect of olive and sunflower seed oil on the adult skin barrier: implications for neonatal skin care. Pediatr Dermatol. 2013;30(1):42–50.

Danielsen R, Thorgeirsson G, Einarsson H, Ólafsson Ö, Aspelund T, Harris TB, Launer L, Gudnason V. Prevalence of heart failure in the older people and future projections: the AGES-Reykjavík study. Scand Cardiovasc J. 2017;51(4):183–9.

Dawod E, Crawford CV. Common diarrheal illnesses in the older people. Clin Geriatr Med. 2021;37(1):103–17.

De Maria M. Self-care in chronic diseases The patient-caregiver dyad in the Albanian reality. Medicus 7(7).

Dharmarajan K, Rich MW. Epidemiology, pathophysiology, and prognosis of heart failure in older adults. Heart Fail Clin. 2017;13(3):417–26.

Díez-Villanueva P, Jiménez-Méndez C, Alfonso F. Heart failure in the older people. J Geriatr Cardiol. 2021;18(3):219.

Dineen-Griffin SM. Minor ailment services from community pharmacy. University of Technology Sydney (Australia); 2020.

Dobarrio-Sanz I, Hernández-Padilla JM, López-Rodríguez MM, Fernandez-Sola C, Granero-Molina J, Ruiz-Fernández MD. Non-pharmacological interventions to improve constipation amongst older adults in long-term care settings: a systematic review of randomised controlled trials. Geriatr Nurs. 2020;41(6):992–9.

Dorak MT, Karpuzoglu E. Gender differences in cancer susceptibility: an inadequately addressed issue. Front Genet. 2012;3:268.

Doris SF, Lee DT, Man NW. Fatigue among older people: a review of the research literature. Int J Nurs Stud. 2010;47(2):216–28.

Dorner TE. Pain and chronic pain epidemiology. Wien Klin Wochenschr. 2018;130(1):1–3.

Dragan S, Şerban MC, Damian G, Buleu F, Valcovici M, Christodorescu R. Dietary patterns and interventions to alleviate chronic Pain. Nutrients. 2020;12(9).

Dumic I, Nordin T, Jecmenica M, Stojkovic Lalosevic M, Milosavljevic T, Milovanovic T. Gastrointestinal tract disorders in older age. Can J Gastroenterol Hepatol. 2019;2019(1):6757524.

Dunn RM, Busse PJ, Wechsler ME. Asthma in the older people and late-onset adult asthma. Allergy. 2018;73(2):284–94.

ElSayed NA, Aleppo G, Aroda VR, Bannuru RR, Brown FM, Bruemmer D, et al. 13. Older adults: standards of care in diabetes-2023. Diabetes Care. 2023;46(Suppl 1):S216–29.

Endomba FT, Tchebegna PY, Chiabi E, Angong Wouna DL, Guillet C, Chauvet-Gelinier JC. Epidemiology of insomnia disorder in older persons according to the Diagnostic and Statistical Manual of Mental Disorders: a systematic review and meta-analysis. Eur Geriatr Med. 2023;14(6):1261–72.

Estape T. Cancer in the older people: challenges and barriers. Asia Pac J Oncol Nurs. 2018;5(1):40–2.

Fadah K, Hechanova A, Mukherjee D. Epidemiology, pathophysiology, and management of coronary artery disease in the older people. Int J Angiol. 2022;31(04):244–50.

Falaschi P, Marsh D. Orthogeriatrics: the management of older patients with fragility fractures. Cham: Springer; 2021.

Fang D, Jiang D, Shi G, Song Y. The association between dietary zinc intake and osteopenia, osteoporosis in patients with rheumatoid arthritis. BMC Musculoskelet Disord. 2024;25(1):710.

Faniyi AA, Hughes MJ, Scott A, Belchamber KBR, Sapey E. Inflammation, ageing and diseases of the lung: potential therapeutic strategies from shared biological pathways. Br J Pharmacol. 2022;179(9):1790–807.

Fathidokht H, Mansour-Ghanaei R, Darvishpour A, Maroufizadeh S. The effect of communication using Peplau's theory on satisfaction with nursing care in hospitalized older adults in cardiac intensive care unit: a quasi-experimental study. J Educ Health Promot. 2023;12(1):426.

Fitzcharles MA, Lussier D, Shir Y. Management of chronic arthritis pain in the older people. Drugs Aging. 2010;27:471–90.

Forman DE, Maurer MS, Boyd C, Brindis R, Salive ME, Horne FM, Bell SP, Fulmer T, Reuben DB, Zieman S, Rich MW. Multimorbidity in older adults with cardiovascular disease. J Am Coll Cardiol. 2018;71(19):2149–61.

Foster M, Xiong W, Quintiliani L, Hartmann CW, Gaehde S. Preferences of older adult veterans with heart failure for engaging with mobile health technology to support self-care: qualitative interview study among patients with heart failure and content analysis. JMIR Format Res. 2022;6(12):e41317.

Fotouhi F, Rezvan F, Hashemi H, Javaherforoushzadeh A, Mahbod M, Yekta A, et al. High prevalence of diabetes in older people of Iran: an urgent public health issue. J Diabetes Metab Disord. 2022;21(1):777–84.

Fowler H, Belot A, Ellis L, Maringe C, Luque-Fernandez MA, Njagi EN, et al. Comorbidity prevalence among cancer patients: a population-based cohort study of four cancers. BMC Cancer. 2020;20(1):2.

Franceschi M, Di Mario F, Leandro G, Maggi S, Pilotto A. Acid-related disorders in the older people. Best Pract Res Clin Gastroenterol. 2009;23(6):839–48.

Gervais-Hupé J, Filleul A, Perreault K, Gaboury I, Wideman TH, Charbonneau C, et al. "How can we help you?": results of a scoping review on the perceived needs of people living with chronic pain regarding physiotherapy. BMC Health Serv Res. 2024;24(1):1401.

Glickman L, Friedman SA. Changes in behavior, mood, or thinking in the older people: diagnosis and management. Med Clin North Am. 1976;60(6):1297–313.

Goede V. Frailty and Cancer: current perspectives on assessment and monitoring. Clin Interv Aging. 2023;18:505–21.

Gogia B, Fang X. Differentiating delirium versus dementia in the older people. In: StatPearls [Internet]. 2023. StatPearls Publishing.

Goldberg JI, Schulman-Green D, Hernandez M, Nelson JE, Capezuti E. Self-management interventions for psychological distress in adult Cancer patients: a systematic review. West J Nurs Res. 2019;41(10):1407–22.

Greater Austin Allergy. Understanding allergies in seniors: a comprehensive guide for 55+ – part 1 [Internet]. Greater Austin Allergy. 2023. Available from: https://www.austinallergist.com/understanding-allergies-in-seniors-a-comprehensive-guide-for-55-part-1/

Griñán-Ferré C, Bellver-Sanchis A, Guerrero A, Pallàs M. Advancing personalized medicine in neurodegenerative diseases: the role of epigenetics and pharmacoepigenomics in pharmacotherapy. Pharmacol Res. 2024;205:107247.

Guasti L, Gaudio G. Hypertension in older adults [internet]. www.escardio.org. 2023. Available from: https://www.escardio.org/Councils/Council-for-Cardiology-Practice-(CCP)/Cardiopractice/hypertension-in-older-adults

Gulia KK, Kumar VM. Sleep disorders in the older people: a growing challenge. Psychogeriatrics. 2018;18(3):155–65.

Harte N, Aaron RV, Bhattiprolu K, Bisby MA, Gandy M, Hathway T, et al. The association between anxiety and depression symptoms and pain and function in adolescents and young adults with chronic pain: a meta-analysis. J Psychosom Res. 2024;187:111945.

Heart Failure Patient Guide [Internet]. www.ottawaheart.ca. 2022. Available from: https://www.ottawaheart.ca/sites/default/files/uploads/heart-failure-patient-guide.pdf

Heart Failure Zones [Internet]. Heart and Stroke Foundation of Canada. 2019 [cited 2024]. Available from: https://www.heartandstroke.ca

Heidenreich PA, Bozkurt B, Aguilar D, Allen LA, Byun JJ, Colvin MM, Deswal A, Drazner MH, Dunlay SM, Evers LR, Fang JC. 2022 ACC/AHA/HFSA guideline for the management of heart failure. J Card Fail. 2022;28(5):e1–67.

Hershey LA, Bednarczyk EM. Treatment of headache in the older people. Curr Treat Options Neurol. 2013;15:56–62.

Hinkle JL, Cheever KH, Overbaugh KJ. Brunner & Suddarth's textbook of medical-surgical nursing. 15th ed. S.L.: Wolters Kluwer Medical; 2022.

Ho A, Nair S. Chapter Nine - Global chronic Pain: public and population health responses. In: Buchman DZ, Davis KD, editors. Developments in neuroethics and bioethics. 1. Academic Press; 2018. p. 171–89.

Ho LY, Ng SS. Non-pharmacological interventions for fatigue in older adults: a systematic review and meta-analysis. Age Ageing. 2020;49(3):341–51.

Hosseini M, Soltanian M. Application of Roy's adaptation model in clinical nursing: a systematic review. J Iran Med Council. 2022;

Hsu YY, Chen CJ, Wu SH, Chen KH. Cold intervention for relieving migraine symptoms: a systematic review and meta-analysis. J Clin Nurs. 2023;32(11–12):2455–65.

Huang JK, Jarjour AA, Nait Oumesmar B, Kerninon C, Williams A, Krezel W, Kagechika H, Bauer J, Zhao C, Evercooren AB, Chambon P. Prevalence and attributable health burden of chronic respiratory diseases, 1990-2017: a systematic analysis for the Global Burden of Disease Study 2017. Lancet Respir Med. 2020;8(6):585–96.

Huang Y, Hu J, Xie T, Jiang Z, Ding W, Mao B, Hou L. Effects of home-based chronic wound care training for patients and caregivers: a systematic review. Int Wound J. 2023;20(9):3802–20.

Imoisili OE, Chung A, Tong X, Hayes DK, Loustalot F. Prevalence of stroke—behavioral risk factor surveillance system, United States, 2011–2022. Morb Mortal Wkly Rep. 2024;73(20):449.

Jaarsma T, Hill L, Bayes-Genis A, La Rocca HP, Castiello T, Čelutkienė J, Marques-Sule E, Plymen CM, Piper SE, Riegel B, Rutten FH. Self-care of heart failure patients: practical management recommendations from the Heart Failure Association of the European Society of Cardiology. Eur J Heart Fail. 2021;23(1):157–74.

Jadoul M, Aoun M, Imani MM. The major global burden of chronic kidney disease. Lancet Glob Health. 2024;12(3):e342–3.

Jafarnejad S, Shab-Bidar S, Speakman JR, Parastui K, Daneshi-Maskooni M, Djafarian K. Probiotics reduce the risk of antibiotic-associated diarrhea in adults (18–64 years) but not the older people (> 65 years) a meta-analysis. Nutr Clin Pract. 2016;31(4):502–13.

Jaqua EE, Hanna M, Labib W, Moore C, Matossian V. Common sleep disorders affecting older adults. Perm J. 2023;27(1):122.

Jenerette CM, Brewer C, Leak AN. Self-care recommendations of middle-aged and older adults with sickle cell disease. Nurs Res Pract. 2011;2011(1):270594.

Jin Y, Bratzke L, Baumann LC. Helping persons with multiple chronic conditions overcome barriers to self-management. Nurse Pract. 2021;46(3):20–8.

Jojan L, Carroll K. Peplau's theory of interpersonal relations: scholarly practice. Nurs Sci Q. 2025;38(1):27–30.

Kang SJ, Cho YS, Lee TH, Kim SE, Ryu HS, Kim JW, Park SY, Lee YJ, Shin JE, of the Korean CR. Medical management of constipation in older patients : systematic review. J Neurogastroenterol Motil. 2021;27(4):495.

Kaniecki RG, Levin AD. Headache in the older people. Handb Clin Neurol. 2019;167:511–28.

Kannam JP, Aroesty JM, Gersh, BJ. Chronic coronary syndrome: overview of care [Internet]. www.uptodate.com. 2024. Available from: https://www.uptodate.com/contents/chronic-coronary-syndrome-overview-of-care

Katsimbri P, Grivas A, Papadavid E, Tzannis K, Flouda S, Moysidou G-S, et al. Mediterranean diet and exercise are associated with better disease control in psoriatic arthritis. Clin Rheumatol. 2024;43(9):2877–87.

Kennedy A, Rogers A, Bower P. Support for self care for patients with chronic disease. BMJ. 2007;335(7627):968–70.

Khan MAB, Hashim MJ, King JK, Govender RD, Mustafa H, Al KJ. Epidemiology of type 2 diabetes - global burden of disease and forecasted trends. J Epidemiol Glob Health. 2020;10(1):107–11.

Khorsandi M, Fekrizadeh Z, Roozbahani N. Investigation of the effect of education based on the health belief model on the adoption of hypertension-controlling behaviors in the older people. Clin Interv Aging. 2017;27:233–40.

Kim BR, Lee J, Sohn MK, Kim DY, Lee SG, Shin YI, et al. Risk factors and functional impact of medical complications in stroke. Ann Rehabil Med. 2017;41(5):753–60.

Kim M, Seol J, Sato T, Fukamizu Y, Sakurai T, Okura T. Effect of 12-week intake of nicotinamide mononucleotide on sleep quality, fatigue, and physical performance in older Japanese adults: a randomized, double-blind placebo-controlled study. Nutrients. 2022;14(4):755.

Knoop V, Cloots B, Costenoble A, Debain A, Azzopardi RV, Vermeiren S, Jansen B, Scafoglieri A, Bautmans I, Bautmans I, Verté D. Fatigue and the prediction of negative health outcomes: a systematic review with meta-analysis. Ageing Res Rev. 2021;67:101261.

Kuijsters A, Redi J, De Ruyter B, Heynderickx I. Lighting to make you feel better: improving the mood of older people people with affective ambiences. PLoS One. 2015;10(7):e0132732.

Kunsmann-Leutiger E, Straßner C, Schalhorn F, Stolz R, Stotz-Ingenlath G, Buhlinger-Göpfarth N, Bentner M, Joos S, Valentini J, Frick E. Training general practitioners and medical assistants within the framework of HoPES3, a holistic care program for older patients to integrate spiritual needs, social activity, and self-care into disease management in primary care. J Multidiscip Healthc. 2021;13:1853–61.

Kwon CY, Lee B. Prevalence of behavioral and psychological symptoms of dementia in community-dwelling dementia patients: a systematic review. Front Psych. 2021;12:741059.

Laevski AM, Doucet MR, Doucet MS, LeBlanc AA, Pineau PE, Hébert MPA, et al. Dietary omega-3 fatty acids modulate the production of platelet-derived microvesicles in an in vivo inflammatory arthritis model. Eur J Nutr. 2024;63(6):2221–34.

Lamptey RNL, Chaulagain B, Trivedi R, Gothwal A, Layek B, Singh J. A review of the common neurodegenerative disorders: current therapeutic approaches and the potential role of nanotherapeutics. Int J Mol Sci. 2022;23(3).

LaRocque R, Harris JB. Patient education: acute diarrhea in adults [Internet]. www.uptodate.com. 2024. Available from: https://www.uptodate.com/contents/acute-diarrhea-in-adults-beyond-the-basics/print

LeBlanc RG, Jacelon CS. Self-care among older people living with chronic conditions. Int J Older People Nursing. 2018;13:e12191. https://doi.org/10.1111/opn.12191.

Lee E, Park E. Self-care behavior and related factors in older patients with uncontrolled hypertension. Contemp Nurse. 2017;53(6):607–21.

Lee J, Yeom I, Chung ML, Kim Y, Yoo S, Kim E. Use of mobile apps for self-care in people with parkinson disease: systematic review. JMIR Mhealth Uhealth. 2022;10(1):e33944.

Liddy C, Blazkho V, Mill K. Challenges of self-management when living with multiple chronic conditions: systematic review of the qualitative literature. Can Fam Physician. 2014;60(12):1123–33.

Ligibel JA, Bohlke K, May AM, Clinton SK, Demark-Wahnefried W, Gilchrist SC, et al. Exercise, diet, and weight management during cancer treatment: ASCO guideline. J Clin Oncol. 2022;40(22):2491–507.

Lintel H, Corpuz T, Paracha SU, Grossberg GT. Mood disorders and anxiety in Parkinson's disease: current concepts. J Geriatr Psychiatry Neurol. 2021;34(4):280–8.

Lipska KJ. Patient education: hypoglycemia (low blood glucose) in people with diabetes (Beyond the basics) [Internet]. 2024. Available from: https://www.uptodate.com/contents/hypoglycemia-low-blood-glucose-in-people-with-diabetes-beyond-the-basics

Liu Y, Carlson SA, Watson KB, Xu F, Greenlund KJ. Trends in the prevalence of chronic obstructive pulmonary disease among adults aged ≥18 years — United States, 2011–2021. MMWR Morb Mortal Wkly Rep. 2023;72:1250–6. https://doi.org/10.15585/mmwr.mm7246a1.

Liu B, Zhou H, Tan L, Siu KTH, Guan X-Y. Exploring treatment options in cancer: tumor treatment strategies. Signal Transduct Target Ther. 2024a;9(1):175.

Liu H, Zhang K, Xiong L. Dietary magnesium intake and rheumatoid arthritis patients' all-cause mortality: evidence from the NHANES database. J Health Popul Nutr. 2024b;43(1):112.

Lusardi MM, Fritz S, Middleton A, Allison L, Wingood M, Phillips E, Criss M, Verma S, Osborne J, Chui KK. Determining risk of falls in community dwelling older adults: a systematic review and meta-analysis using posttest probability. J Geriatr Phys Ther. 2017;40(1):1–36.

Macfarlane GJ. The epidemiology of chronic pain. Pain. 2016;157(10):2158–9.

Madhavan MV, Gersh BJ, Alexander KP, Granger CB, Stone GW. Coronary artery disease in patients≥ 80 years of age. J Am Coll Cardiol. 2018;71(18):2015–40.

Makhlouf AM, Ibrahim MI, Awaisu A, Vyas SK, Yusuff KB. Management of common minor ailments in Qatar: community pharmacists' self-perceived competency and its predictors. PLoS One. 2021;16(8):e0256156.

Mann JF. Patient education: high blood pressure in adults (beyond the basics) [Internet] wwwuptodatecom 2023. Available from: https://www.uptodate.com/contents/high-blood-pressure-in-adults-beyond-the-basics

Mann EG, LeFort S, VanDenKerkhof EG. Self-management interventions for chronic pain. Pain Manage. 2013;3(3):211–22.

Maresova P, Javanmardi E, Barakovic S, Barakovic Husic J, Tomsone S, Krejcar O, Kuca K. Consequences of chronic diseases and other limitations associated with old age–a scoping review. BMC Public Health. 2019;19:1–7.

Marosi C, Köller M. Challenge of cancer in the older people. ESMO Open. 2016;1(3):e000020.

Martin SS, Aday AW, Almarzooq ZI, Anderson CAM, Arora P, Avery CL, et al. 2024 heart disease and stroke statistics: a report of US and global data from the American Heart Association. Circulation. 2024;149(8):e347–913.

Martinelli E, Di Stefano A, Gareri P, Sapone P, Carlucci R, Brandino M, Maina E, Piscioneri S, Cagnoli G, Cotroneo AM. Heart failure in older people: from pathophysiology to diagnosis and management. OBM Geriatr. 2023;7(3):1–26.

Mayo Clinic. Cold remedies: what works, what doesn't [Internet]. Mayo Clinic. 2018. Available from: https://www.mayoclinic.org/diseases-conditions/common-cold/in-depth/cold-remedies/art-The National Council on Aging (NCOA). 20046403

Mayo Clinic. Diarrhea - diagnosis and treatment - Mayo Clinic [internet]. Mayoclinic.org 2019. Available from:

https://www.mayoclinic.org/diseases-conditions/diarrhea/diagnosis-treatment/drc-20352246

Mayo Clinic. How to keep your bones healthy [internet]. Mayo Clinic. 2022. Available from: https://www.mayoclinic.org/healthy-lifestyle/adult-health/in-depth/bone-health/art-20045060

Mayo Clinic. DASH diet: healthy eating to lower your blood pressure [internet]. Mayo Clinic. 2023. Available from: https://www.mayoclinic.org/healthy-lifestyle/nutrition-and-healthy-eating/in-depth/dash-diet/art-20048456

Mayo Clinic. Tension-type headaches: Self-care measures for relief [Internet]. mayoclinic.org. [cited 2024a Oct 4]. Available from: https://www.mayoclinic.org/diseases-conditions/tension-headache/in-depth/headaches/art-20047631

Mayo Clinic. mayoclinic.org. Indigestion - Diagnosis and treatment - Mayo Clinic [Internet]. www.mayoclinic.org. [cited 2024b Nov 8]. Available from: https://www.mayoclinic.org/diseases-conditions/indigestion/diagnosis-treatment/drc-20352215

Mayo Clinic. Osteoporosis - diagnosis and treatment - Mayo Clinic [internet]. Mayoclinic.org. 2024c. Available from: https://www.mayoclinic.org/diseases-conditions/osteoporosis/diagnosis-treatment/drc-20351974

Mayo Clinic [Internet]. High blood pressure (hypertension); [Last updated Feb 29, 2024]. Available from: https://www.mayoclinic.org/diseases-conditions/high-blood-pressure/symptoms-causes/syc-20373410

McCrea GL, Miaskowski C, Stotts NA, Macera L, Varma MG. Pathophysiology of constipation in the older adult. World J Gastroenterol: WJG. 2008;14(17):2631.

MedlinePlus [Internet]. Bethesda: National Library of Medicine (US). COPD; [Last updated October 5, 2021]. Available from: https://medlineplus.gov/copd.html [Internet].

Merchant RA, Vathsala A. Healthy aging and chronic kidney disease. Kidney Res Clin Pract. 2022;41(6):644.

Moadab Kazerouni S, Hatami M, Seifaddini R. Comparison of the effectiveness of self-care education and process emotion regulation in the mitigation of depression symptoms among the caregivers of older adults with dementia. Razavi Int J Med. 2024;12(3):18–25.

Mordarska K, Godziejewska-Zawada M. Diabetes in the older people. Menopause Rev/Przegląd Menopauzalny. 2017;16(2):38–43.

Morkisch N, Upegui-Arango LD, Cardona MI, van den Heuvel D, Rimmele M, Sieber CC, Freiberger E. Components of the transitional care model (TCM) to reduce readmission in geriatric patients: a systematic review. BMC Geriatr. 2020;20:1–8.

Muñoz-Contreras MC, Cerdá B, López-Román FJ, Segarra I. Patients with dementia: prevalence and type of drug–drug interactions. Front Pharmacol. 2024;15:1472932.

Murat B, Stewart G, Rea J. Do I need to see the doctor? John Wiley & Sons; 2013.

Murphy SJ, Werring DJ. Stroke: causes and clinical features. Medicine (Abingdon). 2020;48(9):561–6.

N Rosen H, Lewiecki M. Overview of the management of low bone mass and osteoporosis in postmenopausal women [Internet]. www.uptodate.com. 2024. Available from: https://www.uptodate.com/contents/overview-of-the-management-of-low-bone-mass-and-osteoporosis-in-postmenopausal-women

Nakano Y, Mandai S, Naito S, Fujiki T, Mori Y, Ando F, et al. Effect of osteosarcopenia on longitudinal mortality risk and chronic kidney disease progression in older adults. Bone. 2024;179:116975.

Nakhjiri LZ, Darvishpour A, Pourghane P, Chaboki BG. The relationship between frailty syndrome and self-care ability in the older people with heart failure. J Educ Health Promot. 2021;10:475.

Nakhla N, Taylor J. Self-care and minor ailments: the view from Canada. Explor Res Clin Soc Pharm. 2024;13:100412.

Nasiri M, Jafari Z, Rakhshan M, Yarahmadi F, Zonoori S, Akbari F, Sadeghi Moghimi E, Amirmohseni L, Abbasi M, Keyvanloo Sharstanaki S, Rezaei M. Application of Orem's theory-based caring programs among chronically ill adults: A systematic review and dose–response meta-analysis. Int Nurs Rev. 2023;70(1):59–77.

National Health Service (NHS). Osteoporosis [Internet]. NHS. 2022. Available from: https://www.nhs.uk/conditions/osteoporosis/

National Health Service (NHS). Living with Chronic obstructive pulmonary disease (COPD) [Internet] [Last reviewed: 11 April, 2023]. Available from: https://www.nhs.uk/conditions/chronic-obstructive-pulmonary-disease-copd/living-with/

National Heart, Lung, and Blood Institute. COPD; [Last updated October 6, 2024]. Available from: https://www.nhlbi.nih.gov/health/copd [Internet].

National Institute on Aging. Skin care and aging [Internet]. National Institute on Aging. 2017. Available from: https://www.nia.nih.gov/health/skin-care/skin-care-and-aging

National Institute on Aging. Fatigue in Older Adults [Internet]. 2023. Available from: https://www.nia.nih.gov/health/fatigue/fatigue-older-adults

Naughton MJ, Weaver KE. Physical and mental health among cancer survivors: considerations for long-term care and quality of life. N C Med J. 2014;75(4):283–6.

Neeraj G, Meenakshi C. The quality of life in Cancer patients. In: Bassam Abdul Rasool H, editor. Supportive and palliative care and quality of life in oncology. Rijeka: IntechOpen; 2023.

Negarandeh R, Aghajanloo A, Seylani K. Barriers to self-care among patients with heart failure: a qualitative study. J Caring Sci. 2021;10(4):196.

Nguyen TN, Whitehead L, Saunders R, Dermody G. Systematic review of perception of barriers and facilitators to chronic disease self-management among older adults: implications for evidence-based practice. Worldviews Evid-Based Nurs. 2022;19(3):191–200.

Niams. NIAMS health information on arthritis. National Institute of Arthritis and Musculoskeletal and Skin Diseases; 2019.

NIDDK. Eating Right for Chronic Kidney Disease [Internet]. NIH. Available from: https://www.niddk.nih.gov/health-information/kidney-disease/chronic-kidney-disease-ckd/eating-nutrition

NKF, National Kidney Disease. Chronic Kidney Disease (CKD) [Internet] 2023. Available from: https://www.kidney.org/kidney-topics/chronic-kidney-disease-ckd

NKF, National Kidney Disease. Chronic kidney disease [Internet]. Available from: https://www.kidney.org.uk/chronic-kidney-disease?gad_source=1&gclid=CjwKCAiArva5BhBiEiwA-oTnXV4dGiThRhN6WjAX-FL9xHk6MCvkWO%2D%2D9F5RSZl1MAR-oq7v-LjmgajxoC-00QAvD_BwE

Nomali M, Mohammadrezaei R, Keshtkar AA, Roshandel G, Ghiyasvandian S, Alipasandi K, Zakerimoghadam M. Self-monitoring by traffic light color coding versus usual care on outcomes of patients with heart failure reduced ejection fraction: protocol for a randomized controlled trial. JMIR Res Protoc. 2018;7(11):e9209.

O'Brien L, Wall C, Wilkinson TJ, Gearry RB. Chronic diarrhoea in older adults and the role of dietary interventions. Nutr Health Aging. 2022;7(1–2):39–50.

Ogurtsova K, da Rocha Fernandes JD, Huang Y, Linnenkamp U, Guariguata L, Cho NH et al IDF diabetes atlas: global estimates for the prevalence of diabetes for 2015 and 2040. Diabetes Res Clin Pract [Internet]. 2017;128:40–50. Available from: https://www.sciencedirect.com/science/article/pii/S0168822717303753

Oliveros E, Patel H, Kyung S, Fugar S, Goldberg A, Madan N, et al. Hypertension in older adults: assessment, management, and challenges. Clin Cardiol. 2020;43(2):99–107.

Orkaby AR, Onuma O, Qazi S, Gaziano JM, Driver JA. Preventing cardiovascular disease in older adults: one size does not fit all. Cleve Clin J Med. 2018;85(1):55–64.

Öteleş S, Ayan G, Ekici M, Ünal E, Bilgiç P, Kalyoncu U. The dietary acid load is associated with disease severity in psoriatic arthritis. Mod Rheumatol. 2024;34(5):1019–26.

Pandya N, Hames E, Sandhu S. Challenges and strategies for managing diabetes in the older people in long-term care settings. Diabetes Spectrum. 2020;33(3):236–45.

patient.info. Indigestion (Dyspepsia) [Internet]. patient.info. [cited 2024 Nov 8]. Available from: https://patient.info/digestive-health/dyspepsia-indigestion

Pavasini R, Biscaglia S, Kunadian V, Hakeem A, Campo G. Coronary artery disease management in older adults: revascularization and exercise training. Eur Heart J. 2024;45(31):2811–23.

Pender N. Health promotion model. 1982. http://deepblue.lib.umich.edu/bitstream/handle/2027.42/85350/HEALTH_PRO MOTIONMANUAL_Rev_5-2011.pdf?sequence=1. Accessed 1 Nov 2024.

Peplow PV, Martinez B, Gennarelli TA. Prevalence, needs, strategies, and risk factors for neurodegenerative diseases. In: Peplow PV, Martinez B, Gennarelli TA, editors. Neurodegenerative diseases biomarkers: towards translating research to clinical practice. New York: Springer US; 2022. p. 3–8.

Pilleron S, Soto-Perez-de-Celis E, Vignat J, Ferlay J, Soerjomataram I, Bray F, Sarfati D. Estimated global cancer incidence in the oldest adults in 2018 and projections to 2050. Int J Cancer. 2021;148(3):601–8.

Pinto C, Geraghty AWA, McLoughlin C, Pagnini F, Yardley L, Dennison L. Experiences of psychological interventions in neurodegenerative diseases: a systematic review and thematic synthesis. Health Psychol Rev. 2023;17(3):416–38.

Pirmohamed A, Kitzman DW, Maurer MS. Heart failure in older adults: embracing complexity. J Geriatr Cardiol. 2016;13(1):8.

Popa-Wagner A, Dumitrascu DI, Capitanescu B, Petcu EB, Surugiu R, Fang WH, et al. Dietary habits, lifestyle factors and neurodegenerative diseases. Neural Regen Res. 2020;15(3):394–400.

Pound SE, Heading RC. Diagnosis and treatment of dyspepsia in the older people. Drugs Aging. 1995;7:347–54.

Prevention. C for DC and, Report NDS. National Diabetes Statistics Report. 2020.

Punthakee Z, Goldenberg R, Katz P. Definition, classification and diagnosis of diabetes, prediabetes and metabolic syndrome. Can J Diabetes [Internet]. 2018;42:S10–5. Available from: https://doi.org/10.1016/j.jcjd.2017.10.003

Rajati F, Rajati M, Rasulehvandi R, Kazeminia M. Prevalence of stroke in the older people: a systematic review and meta-analysis. Interdisc Neurosurg. 2023;32:101746.

Rao SS. Constipation in the older adult [Internet]. Uptodate.com. 2022. Available from: https://www.uptodate.com/contents/constipation-in-the-older-adult

Ravasco P. Nutrition in cancer patients. J Clin Med [Internet]. 2019; 8(8).

Rees J, Tuijt R, Burton A, Walters K, Cooper C. Supporting self-care of long-term conditions in people with dementia: a systematic review. Int J Nurs Stud. 2021;116:103432.

Ricci C. Study on genotypes and phenotypes of neurodegenerative diseases. Genes [Internet]. 2024; 15(6).

Richardson M, Khouja C, Sutcliffe K, Hinds K, Brunton V, Stansfield C, Thomas J. Self-care for minor ailments: systematic reviews of qualitative and quantitative research.

Rico TM, dos Santos Machado K, Fernandes VP, Madruga SW, Santin MM, Petrarca CR, et al. Use of text messaging (SMS) for the Management of Side Effects in Cancer patients undergoing chemotherapy treatment: a randomized controlled trial. J Med Syst. 2020;44(11):193.

Riegel B, Westland H, Iovino P, Barelds I, Slot JB, Stawnychy MA, Osokpo O, Tarbi E, Trappenburg JC, Vellone E, Strömberg A. Characteristics of self-care

interventions for patients with a chronic condition: a scoping review. Int J Nurs Stud. 2021;116:103713.
Rinninella E, Mele MC, Cintoni M, Raoul P, Ianiro G, Salerno L, et al. The facts about food after Cancer diagnosis: a systematic review of prospective cohort studies. Nutrients [Internet]. 2020;12(8).
Rivera E, Corte C, Steffen A, DeVon HA, Collins EG, McCabe PJ. Illness representation and self-care ability in older adults with chronic disease. Geriatrics. 2018;3(3):45.
Robbins RN, Cortes T, O'Connor JC, Jiwani R, Serra MC. The influence of branched-chain amino acid supplementation on fatigue and tryptophan metabolism after acute and chronic exercise in older adults: protocol for a pilot randomized controlled trial. JMIR Res Protoc. 2023;12(1):e52199.
Robblee J, Singh RH. Headache in the older population: causes, diagnoses, and treatments. Curr Pain Headache Rep. 2020;24:1–9.
Roeland EJ, Bohlke K, Baracos VE, Bruera E, del Fabbro E, Dixon S, et al. Management of Cancer Cachexia: ASCO guideline. J Clin Oncol. 2020;38(21):2438–53.
Rosen H. Calcium and vitamin D supplementation in osteoporosis [internet]. Uptodate.com. 2024. Available from: https://www.uptodate.com/contents/calcium-and-vitamin-d-supplementation-in-osteoporosis
Roshandel M, Rakhshan M, Najafi KM. The effect of using peer on self-care, quality of life, and adherence in older people with coronary artery disease. Sci World J. 2021;2021(1):4770721.
Sacco RL, Kasner SE, Broderick JP, Caplan LR, Connors JJ, Culebras A, et al. An updated definition of stroke for the 21st century: a statement for healthcare professionals from the American Heart Association/American Stroke Association. Stroke. 2013;44(7):2064–89.
Sadeghi H, Shahbolaghi FM, Hosseini M, Fallahi-Khoshknab M, Harouni GG. Self-management in older adults with Multiple Chronic Conditions (MCCs): a qualitative content analysis. IJ Psychiatry Behav Sci. 2024 Sep 1(In Press).
Saini V, Guada L, Yavagal DR. Global epidemiology of stroke and access to acute ischemic stroke interventions. Neurology. 2021;97(20_Supplement_2):S6–S16.
Salari N, Ghasemianrad M, Ammari-Allahyari M, Rasoulpoor S, Shohaimi S, Mohammadi M. Global prevalence of constipation in older adults: a systematic review and meta-analysis. Wien Klin Wochenschr. 2023;135(15):389–98. https://doi.org/10.1007/s00508-023-02156-w.
Salzberg L. Risk factors and lifestyle interventions. Prim Care. 2022;49(2):201–12.
Sandelowsky H, Weinreich UM, Aarli BB, Sundh J, Høines K, Stratelis G, et al. COPD - do the right thing. BMC Fam Pract. 2021;22(1):244.
Santiago JA, Potashkin JA. Physical activity and lifestyle modifications in the treatment of neurodegenerative diseases. Front Aging Neurosci. 2023;15:1185671.
Schulman-Green D, Feder SL, Dionne-Odom JN, Batten J, En Long VJ, Harris Y, Wilpers A, Wong T, Whittemore R. Family caregiver support of patient self-management during chronic, life-limiting illness: a qualitative metasynthesis. J Fam Nurs. 2021;27(1):55–72.
Self-Care Tips for Heart Health [Internet]. National Institutes of Health (NIH). 2024. Available from: https://www.nhlbi.nih.gov/sites/default/files/publications/SelfCareTips-for-HeartHealth-508.pdf
Sell K, Amella E, Mueller M, Andrews J, Wachs J. Use of social cognitive theory to assess salient clinical research in chronic disease self-management for older adults: an integrative review. Open J Nurs. 2016;6(3):213–28.
Sendall M, McCosker L, Crossley K, Bonner A. A structured review of chronic care model components supporting transition between healthcare service delivery types for older people with multiple chronic diseases. Health Inform Manage J. 2017;46(2):58–68.
Sexton DJ, McClain MT. The common cold in adults: treatment and prevention [Internet]. Uptodate.com 2024 [cited 2024 Dec 10]. Available from: https://www.uptodate.com/contents/the-common-cold-in-adults-treatment-and-prevention
Shamekh A, Tahmasbi F, Mousavi SE, Nejadghaderi A, Sullman MJM, Kolahi A-A. Burden of chronic kidney disease for adults 70 years and older in Iran during 1990-2021. Int J Aging. 2024;2(1):e12.
Shetty A, Delanerolle G, Cavalini H, Deng C, Yang X, Boyd A, et al. A systematic review and network meta-analysis of pharmaceutical interventions used to manage chronic pain. Sci Rep. 2024;14(1):1621.
Sinclair A, Saeedi P, Kaundal A, Karuranga S, Malanda B, Williams R. Diabetes and global ageing among 65–99-year-old adults: findings from the International Diabetes Federation Diabetes Atlas. Diabetes Res Clin Pract. 2020;162:108078.
Singh SP, Dwivedi D, Ahsan R, Srivastava A, Shukla AK. A systematic review of neurodegenerative diseases: etiology, clinical symptoms, pathogenesis, and future developments. In: Advances in diagnostics and immunotherapeutics for neurodegenerative diseases; 2024. p. 1–16.
Soleimani Damaneh M, Aryaeian N, Khajoenia S, Azadbakht L, Hosseini-Baharanchi FS. The association between dietary intake of branched-chain amino acids and odds and severity of rheumatoid arthritis. Sci Rep. 2024;14(1):6309.
Sözen T, Özışık L, Başaran NÇ. An overview and management of osteoporosis. Eur J Rheumatol. 2017;4(1):46.
Starling AJ. Diagnosis and management of headache in older adults. In: Mayo Clinic Proceedings, vol. 93(2), pp. 252–262). Elsevier; 2018.
Stompór M, Grodzicki T, Stompór T, Wordliczek J, Dubiel M, Kurowska I. Prevalence of chronic pain, particularly with neuropathic component, and its effect on overall functioning of older patients. Med Sci Monitor. 2019;25:2695.
Straßner C, Frick E, Stotz-Ingenlath G, Buhlinger-Göpfarth N, Szecsenyi J, Krisam J, Schalhorn F,

Valentini J, Stolz R, Joos S. Holistic care program for older patients to integrate spiritual needs, social activity, and self-care into disease management in primary care (HoPES3): study protocol for a cluster-randomized trial. Trials. 2019;20:1–1.

Suzuki K, Miyamoto M, Hirata K. Sleep disorders in the older people: diagnosis and management. J General Fam Med. 2017;18(2):61–71.

Talley NJ, Evans JM, Fleming KC, Harmsen WS, Zinsmeister AR, Joseph Melton III, L. Nonsteroidal antiinflammatory drugs and dyspepsia in the older people. Dig Dis Sci. 1995;40(6):1345–50.

Talley NJ, Napthali K, McQuaid K. Practical gastroenterology and hepatology board review toolkit. Wiley; 2016. p. 70–3.

Tang Y, Jiang J, Zhao Y, Du D. Aging and chronic kidney disease: epidemiology, therapy, management and the role of immunity. Clin Kidney J. 2024a;17(9):sfae235.

Tang S, Zhang C, Feng S. The relationship between arthritis and nocturia among adults under 60: a cross-sectional study based on National Health and Nutrition Examination Survey. Neurourol Urodyn. 2024b;43(8):2229–39.

The National Council on Aging (NCOA). The common cold: No-nonsense tips for older adults [Internet]. The National Council on Aging (NCOA); [cited 2024 Nov 8]. Available from: https://www.ncoa.org/article/a--common-sense-guide-to-the-common-cold-for-older-adults/

The University of Maryland Medical System [Internet]. Breathing exercises for COPD; [November11, 2024]. Available from: https://www.umms.org/bwmc/health-services/pulmonary-disease/copd/treatment/breathing-exercises

Tinkham M. Health promotion in the older people with coronary artery disease. J Vasc Nurs. 2014;32(4):151–5.

Tomisa G, Horváth A, Sánta B, Keglevich A, Tamási L. Epidemiology of comorbidities and their association with asthma control. Allergy, Asthma Clin Immunol. 2021;17:1–4.

Torregrosa C, Chorin F, Beltran EE, Neuzillet C, Cardot-Ruffino V. Physical activity as the best supportive Care in Cancer: the clinician's and the researcher's perspectives. Cancers [Internet]. 2022;14(21)

Trinh C, Prabhakar K. Diarrheal diseases in the older people. Clin Geriatr Med. 2007;23(4):833–56.

Tu JY, Jin G, Chen JH, Chen YC. Caregiver burden and dementia: a systematic review of self-report instruments. J Alzheimer's Dis. 2022;86(4):1527–43.

United Medicare Advisors. Senior Seasonal Allergies | How allergies affect adults over 65 [Internet]. United Medicare Advisors. 2019 [cited 2024 Nov 8]. Available from: https://unitedmedicareadvisors.com/blog/health/senior-seasonal-allergies-overview/

University of Maryland Medical System. Heart disease symptom warning signs [Internet]. UMMS Health. 2022. Available from: https://health.umms.org/2022/01/07/heart-failure-warning-signs/

Vaezi MF, Swoger J. Gastroesophageal reflux disease in the older people. In: Gastroesophageal reflux disease: Principles of disease, diagnosis, and treatment. 2006:23–43.

Vaidya SR, Aeddula NR, Doerr C. Chronic kidney disease (Nursing). 2021.

Valenzuela-Martínez S, Ramírez-Expósito MJ, Carrera-González MP, Martínez-Martos JM. Physiopathology of osteoporosis: nursing involvement and management. Biomedicine. 2023;11(4):1220.

van der Linden R, Bolt T, Veen M. 'If it can't be coded, it doesn't exist'. A historical-philosophical analysis of the new ICD-11 classification of chronic pain. Stud Hist Phil Sci. 2022;94:121–32.

Ventura MT, D'Amato A, Giannini M, Carretta A, Tummolo RA, Buquicchio R. Incidence of allergic diseases in an older people population. Immunopharmacol Immunotoxicol. 2010;32(1):165–70.

Vidán MT, Martín Sánchez FJ, Sánchez E, Ortiz FJ, Serra-Rexach JA, Martínez-Sellés M, Bueno H. Most older patients hospitalized for heart failure lack the abilities needed to perform the tasks required for self-care: impact on outcomes. Eur J Heart Fail. 2019;21(11):1434–42.

Vincenzo JL, Patton SK, Lefler LL, McElfish PA, Wei J, Curran GM. Older adults' perceptions and recommendations regarding a falls prevention self-management plan template based on the health belief model: a mixed-methods study. Int J Environ Res Public Health. 2022;19(4):1938.

Vondracek SF, Linnebur SA. Diagnosis and management of osteoporosis in the older senior. Clin Interv Aging. 2009;14:121–36.

Walker MM, Talley NJ. Functional dyspepsia in the older people. Curr Gastroenterol Rep. 2019;21:1–6.

Wang W, Lin B, Mei Y, Zhang Z, Zhou B. Self-care interventions in stroke survivor–caregiver dyads: a protocol for systematic review and meta-analysis. BMJ Open. 2021;11(12):e051860.

Wang F, Fei M, Hu WZ, Wang XD, Liu S, Zeng Y, Zhang JH, Lv Y, Niu JP, Meng XL, Cai P. Prevalence of constipation in older people and its association with dementia and mild cognitive impairment: a cross-sectional study. Front Neurosci. 2022;15:821654.

Warner V, Nguyen D, Bayles T, Hopper I. Management of heart failure in older people. J Pharm Pract Res. 2022;52(1):72–9.

Watson A, Wilkinson TM. Respiratory viral infections in the older people. Ther Adv Respir Dis. 2021;15:1753466621995050.

White SM, Wójcicki TR, McAuley E. Social cognitive influences on physical activity behavior in middle-aged and older adults. J Gerontol B Psychol Sci Soc Sci. 2012;67(1):18–26.

White MC, Holman DM, Boehm JE, Peipins LA, Grossman M, Henley SJ. Age and cancer risk: a potentially modifiable relationship. Am J Prev Med. 2014;46(3 Suppl 1):S7–15.

White-Chu EF, Reddy M. Dry skin in the older people: complexities of a common problem. Clin Dermatol. 2011;29(1):37–42.

Whitman A, Erdeljac P, Jones C, Pillarella N, Nightingale G. Managing polypharmacy in older adults with Cancer across different healthcare settings. Drug Healthc Patient Saf. 2021;13:101–16.
WHO [Internet]. Hypertension; [Last updated March 16, 2023]. Available from: https://www.who.int/news-room/fact-sheets/detail/hypertension
Willis AW, Roberts E, Beck JC, Fiske B, Ross W, Savica R, Van Den Eeden SK, Tanner CM, Marras C, Parkinson's Foundation P4 Group Alcalay Roy Schwarzschild Michael Racette Brad Chen Honglei Church Tim Wilson Bill Doria James M. Incidence of Parkinson disease in North America. npj Parkinson's Dis. 2022;8(1):170.
Winkelman JW. Overview of the treatment of insomnia in adults [Internet]. www.uptodate.com. 2024. Available from: https://www.uptodate.com/contents/overview-of-the-treatment-of-insomnia-in-adults
Wong AK, Bayuo J, Wong FK, Yuen WS, Lee AY, Chang PK, Lai JT. Effects of a nurse-led telehealth self-care promotion program on the quality of life of community-dwelling older adults: systematic review and meta-analysis. J Med Internet Res. 2022;24(3):e31912.
World Health O. Osteoarthritis. 2023. www.who.int.
World Health Organization. Diabetes. 2020. https://www.who.int/diabetes/country-profiles/irn_en.pdf?ua=1. Accessed 4 Sept 2020.
World Stroke Organization. Available from: https://www.sciencedirect.com/science/article/abs/pii/S0738399124001757.
Wu C, Chang EH. An investigation of minor ailments management by older people in non-urban areas. Value Health. 2018;21:S43.
Yang Y, Li W, Guo Y, Liu Y, Li Q, Yang K, et al. Early COPD risk decision for adults aged from 40 to 79 years based on lung Radiomics features. Front Med. 2022;9:845286.
Yeoh EK, Wong MC, Wong EL, Yam C, Poon CM, Chung RY, Chong M, Fang Y, Wang HH, Liang M, Cheung WW. Benefits and limitations of implementing Chronic Care Model (CCM) in primary care programs: a systematic review. Int J Cardiol. 2018;258:279–88.
Yildirim Duman JG. Self-management of chronic diseases: a descriptive phenomenological study. Soc Work Public Health. 2021;36(2):300–10.
Younas A, Quennell S. Usefulness of nursing theory-guided practice: an integrative review. Scand J Caring Sci. 2019;33(3):540–55.
Zaib S, Javed H, Khan I, Jaber F, Sohail A, Zaib Z, et al. Neurodegenerative diseases: their onset, epidemiology, causes and treatment. ChemistrySelect. 2023;8(20):e202300225.
Zhang J, Guo L, Mao J, Qi X, Chen L, Huang H, Sun Y, Yang X. The effects of nursing of Roy adaptation model on the older people hypertensive: a randomised control study. Ann Palliat Med. 2021;10(12):121492158–12158.

MIX
Papier aus verantwortungsvollen Quellen
Paper from responsible sources
FSC® C105338

If you have any concerns about our products,
you can contact us on
ProductSafety@springernature.com

In case Publisher is established outside the EU,
the EU authorized representative is:
Springer Nature Customer Service Center GmbH
Europaplatz 3, 69115 Heidelberg, Germany

Printed by Libri Plureos GmbH
in Hamburg, Germany